Perspectives in Nursing

THE IMPACTS ON THE NURSE, THE CONSUMER, AND SOCIETY

Clinton E. Lambert, Jr., RN, MSN, CS
Private Practitioner
Psychiatric/Mental Health Nursing
and
Doctoral Student
School of Nursing
University of Maryland
Baltimore, Maryland

Vickie A. Lambert, RN, DNSc, FAAN
Associate Professor and Associate Dean of Nursing
Frances Payne Bolton School of Nursing
Case Western Reserve University
Cleveland, Ohio

Copyright © 1989 by Appleton & Lange
A Publishing Division of Prentice Hall

89 90 91 92 93 / 10 9 8 7 6 5 4 3 2 1

Prentice Hall International (UK) Limited, *London*
Prentice Hall of Australia Pty. Limited, *Sydney*
Prentice Hall Canada, Inc., *Toronto*
Prentice Hall Hispanoamericana, S.A., *Mexico*
Prentice Hall of India Private Limited, *New Delhi*
Prentice Hall of Japan, Inc., *Tokyo*
Simon & Schuster Asia Pte. Ltd., *Singapore*
Editora Prentice Hall do Brasil Ltda., *Rio de Janeiro*
Prentice Hall, *Englewood Cliffs, New Jersey*

Library of Congress Cataloging-in-Publication Data

Perspectives in nursing : the impacts on the nurse, the consumer, and
    society / [edited by] Clinton E. Lambert, Jr., Vickie A. Lambert.
        p.   cm.
    ISBN 0-8385-7826-8
    1. Nursing. 2. Nursing--Research. 3. Nursing--Study and
teaching. 4. Nursing--Social aspects. I. Lambert, Clinton E.
II. Lambert, Vickie A.
    [DNLM: 1. Delivery of Health Care. 2. Education, Nursing.
3. Nursing.   WY 16 P467]
RT42.P42 1989
610.73--dc19
DNLM/DLC
for Library of Congress   88-7501
                                                               CIP

Acquisitions Editor: Marion Kalstein-Welch
Managing Editor: Gale Burnick

Text Designer: Harry Rinehart
Cover Designer: Kathy Ceconi
Production: Falletta Associates

PRINTED IN THE UNITED STATES OF AMERICA

Contents

Preface

The profession of nursing does not and never will exist in a vacuum. Many important societal factors influence nursing's ability to function at an optimal level. Knowledge of the perspectives that influence the practice, educational, research, and sociopolitical arenas of nursing are a must for today's professional nurse. Therefore, the purposes of this book are to present salient perspectives that influence the profession of nursing; to assess the impact that each perspective has upon the nurse, the consumer, and society; and to discuss aspects of the perspective that need to be considered for the future.

The text is divided into three units with specific focuses. **UNIT I: Practice Perspectives in Nursing** addresses aspects and issues that can and do influence the actual "practice" of nursing. **UNIT II: Educational and Research Perspectives in Nursing** discusses educational and research issues that influence the entire profession of nursing. **UNIT III: Sociopolitical Perspectives in Nursing** presents how various societal and political components of our environment affect nursing's ability to adequately meet the demands of today's health care needs.

Within a unit each chapter presents a separate perspective, organized around a framework that includes: 1) background information on the perspective including its historical evolution, if appropriate; 2) the impacts that the perspective creates on the nurse, the consumer, and society; 3) factors that need to be considered in regards to the future development, evolution and/or resolution of the perspective; 4) a vignette demonstrating the perspective in the "real world" with a series of related questions that can be used for further classroom discussion; and 5) a list of additional sources of information on the perspective under discussion. Since many of the chapters use terms that may be unfamiliar to the student, new terms are not only defined but appear in bold print for easy identification.

Each chapter is written by an expert or experts in the field who have indepth knowledge and understanding of the perspective under discussion. The authors come from a variety of experiential backgrounds, are employed by institutions from all over the country, and represent various career options in nursing.

v

UNIT I: Practice Perspectives in Nursing addresses nursing's evolution as a bonafide profession, the features and characteristics of technical and professional nursing practice, the process of credentialing, how nurses can and are engaging in entrepreneurial activities, how and why academicians are engaging in faculty practice, the various types of nursing care assignment systems, the development and future of nursing diagnosis; various patient classification systems; how quality assurance appraises the delivery of health care delivery; the ethical dimensions of health care delivery, and how health care litigation can affect nursing practice.

In **UNIT II: Educational and Research Perspectives in Nursing** the authors present the types and benefits of the various continuing education offerings, the various graduate educational programs and their purposes, the influence of nursing research, the structure and function of the National Center for Nursing Research, and the common goals of nursing education and nursing service.

In the final section of the text, **UNIT III: Sociopolitical Perspectives in Nursing** deals with the existing inequalities in health care delivery, how DRG's are attempting to control health care costs, the diversification and decentralization of the various health care delivery systems, how nursing is obtaining financial equity for services rendered, the evolution and need for home health care, who is responsible for paying for society's health/illness care, what deinstitutionalization of the mentally ill has done to health care delivery, nursing's participation in public policy formation, and the demystification of political involvement.

There are various unique aspects and benefits of *Perspectives in Nursing: The Impacts on the Nurse, the Consumer, and Society.* The text presents a vignette that allows the student the opportunity to discuss the perspective at hand within the context of the "real world." The additional information sources listed at the end of each chapter provide the student and the faculty with possible sources for obtaining additional indepth information on the perspective under discussion. The text provides a diverse scope of perspectives not addressed in any other book. Finally, the authors of each chapter are experts on the perspective presented and have not only theoretical knowledge, but working knowledge of the related content.

An instructor's manual for *Perspectives in Nursing: The Impacts on the Nurse, the Consumer, and Society* is available. The manual's purpose is to assist faculty in reinforcing students' acquisition of knowledge about modern day perspectives in nursing. The manual's content consists of chapter overviews, chapter outlines, key words, learning activities, supplemental publications and audiovisual aids, and over 350 test questions.

The editors hope that you will find the text and its accompanying manual thought provoking and stimulating. It is the intent of the text to stimulate thought and raise further questions about salient perspectives that can and do influence the profession of nursing.

Contributors

Rita M. Carty, RN, DNSc, FAAN
Professor and Dean, School of Nursing
George Mason University
Fairfax, VA

Ann H. Cary, RN, PhD
Chairperson, Graduate Level Community
Health Nursing and
Project Director, Home Health Administration Project
School of Nursing
The Catholic University of America
Washington, DC

Brenda J. Cherry, RN, PhD
Dean, College of Nursing
University of Massachusetts, Boston
Harbor
Boston, MA

Janet Niemi Chubb, RN, MS
Assistant Administrator
Charter Hospital By-The-Sea
St. Simons Island, GA

Jacqueline F. Clinton, RN, PhD, FAAN
Professor and Director
Center for Nursing Research and Evaluation
School of Nursing
University of Wisconsin
Milwaukee, WI

Frances Crosby, RN, EdD
Research Associate, Research Foundation
State University of New York
Buffalo, NY

Constance R. Curran, RN, EdD, FAAN
President, The Curran Group
Chicago, IL

Vivien DeBack, RN, PhD
Project Director, Implementation Project
National Commission on Nursing
Milwaukee, WI

Jane Lynne Echols, RN, PhD
Assistant Professor, College of Nursing
University of Nebraska Medical Center
Omaha, NE

Beverly C. Flynn, RN, PhD, FAAN
Professor and Chairperson
Department of Community Health Nursing
School of Nursing
Indiana University
Indianapolis, IN

Sara T. Fry, RN, PhD
Associate Professor, School of Nursing
University of Maryland
Baltimore, MD

Barbara C. Gaines, RN, EdD
Associate Professor and Chairperson
Department of Community Health Care
Systems
School of Nursing
The Oregon Health Sciences University
Portland, OR

Susan B. Gantz, RN, MSN
Executive Director, Self-Care Institute
School of Nursing
George Mason University
Fairfax, VA

Andrea O. Hollingsworth, RN, PhD
Assistant Professor, Department of Health
Care of Women and the Childbearing
Family
School of Nursing
University of Pennsylvania
Philadelphia, PA

Hazel W. Johnson-Brown, RN, PhD, FAAN
Professor, School of Nursing
George Mason University
Fairfax, VA

Trudy Knicely Henson, PhD
Associate Professor, Department of Soci-
ology
University of South Carolina
Aiken, SC

Arlene Lowenstein, RN, PhD
Associate Professor and Chairperson
Department of Nursing Administration
School of Nursing
Medical College of Georgia
The Health Sciences University of the State
of Georgia
Augusta, GA

Ann Marriner-Tomey, RN, PhD, FAAN
Professor, Department of Nursing Admin-
istration/Teacher Education
School of Nursing
Indiana University
Indianapolis, IN

Joanne B. Martin, RN. DrPH
Associate Professor
Department of Community Health Nursing
School of Nursing
Indiana University
Indianapolis, IN

Virginia Layng Millonig, RN, PhD
Consultant, Potomac, MD
Former Associate Professor and
Director of Nursing Continuing Education
Program
School of Nursing
George Mason University
Fairfax, VA

Sue Popkess-Vawter, RN, PhD
Professor, Department of Medical-Surgical
Nursing
School of Nursing
The University of Kansas Medical Center
Kansas City, KS

Donna Rae Richardson, RN, JD
Congressional and Agency Relations
Division of Government Affairs
American Nurses' Association
Washington, DC

Virginia Peterson Tilden, RN, DNSc, FAAN
Professor, Department of Mental Health
Nursing
School of Nursing
Oregon Health Sciences University
Portland, OR

Mary Graney Trainor, RN, PhD
Associate Professor, School of Nursing
George Mason University
Fairfax, VA

James D. Vail, RN, DNSc
Associate Professor, School of Nursing
George Mason University
Fairfax, VA

Marlene R. Ventura, RN, EdD, FAAN
Associate Chief, Department of Nursing
Service for Research
Veterans Administration Medical Center
Buffalo, NY

Dorothy Jean Walker, RN, PhD, JD
Professor, School of Nursing
George Mason University
Fairfax, VA

Nancy Wiederhorn, RN, DNSc
Assistant Professor, School of Nursing
George Mason University
Fairfax, VA

Reviewers

Fran Hicks, RN, PhD
School of Nursing
University of Portland
Portland, OR

Judith Lewis, RN, PhD
School of Nursing
University of Massachusetts
Boston, MA

Irene Joos, RN, PhD
School of Nursing
University of Pittsburgh
Pittsburgh, PA

Mary Ann Schroeder, RN, DNSc
School of Nursing
Catholic University
Washington, DC

Mary Ann Haw, RN, PhD
Department of Nursing
San Francisco State University
San Francisco, CA

The authors would like to thank the educators who responded to their questionnaire concerning the content taught in their issues course. The results of this questionnaire were instrumental in developing this book.

UNIT I

Practice Perspectives in Nursing

This unit addresses aspects and issues that can and do influence the actual "practice" of nursing. The chapters in this section address how nursing is evolving as a profession; the characteristics of technical and professional nursing practice; the various types and processes of credentialing; how nurses are involved in entrepreneurial endeavors; the evolvement of faculty practice; the pros and cons of the types of nursing care assignment systems that exist in the acute care setting; the development and future evolvement of nursing diagnoses; the development and use of different patient classification systems; how quality assurance assists in the appraisal of health care delivery; the ethical dimensions of technology; and how health care litigation can influence nursing practice. The reader must keep in mind that each chapter is written by a different author(s) and thus the writing styles will vary to some degree. The chapter that addresses health care litigation might be more difficult for some individuals to read than some of the other chapters, due to the nature of the topic presented. Many new terms, which are legal in nature, appear in the chapter and the approach to the content is from a legal perspective. However, all legal terms are defined and identified in bold print. After reading each chapter in this unit, the student should have an eclectic perception as to what salient issues and perspectives influence the nurse's professional practice.

VICKIE A. LAMBERT, RN, DNSc, FAAN

CLINTON E. LAMBERT, JR., RN, MSN, CS

CHAPTER 1

Nursing: An Evolving Profession

Background and Overview

The issue of whether nursing meets the criteria of an established profession has been a matter of discussion and debate for the past eight decades. No doubt the continuation of such discussion and debate is due to an inadequate interpretation of the term *profession*. Although many nurses would contend that nursing is a "full-fledged" profession, in the true sense of the word, nursing is an evolving profession like education, social work, and pharmacy, since it does not meet all the criteria of the established professions of law, the ministry, and medicine. How nursing measures up to the criteria of the established professions; what impact nursing's evolving status has upon nurses, consumers, and society; and what future considerations must be addressed so that nursing can continue to enhance its professional status will be the focus of this chapter.

CHARACTERISTICS OF A PROFESSION

Numerous social scientists have studied and delineated a variety of characteristics that are used to identify and define an established profession.[1-6] Some of these characteristics include: knowledge, altruism, theoretical

3

base, code of ethics, autonomy, service, competence, commitment, professional association, prestige, authority, and trustworthiness. Although most social scientists have similar ideas about what constitutes the distinguishing characteristics of an established profession, there remains some disagreement as to how one should differentiate a profession from an occupation. The occupation-profession continuum model developed by Ronald Pavalko[7] seems to provide not only the most comprehensive list of characteristics that identify and describe a profession, but also one of the most logical frameworks for explaining how nursing's professionalism is evolving.

Pavalko[7] perceives occupations and professions to exist on a continuum with occupations at the low end of the continuum and professions at the high end. By using the context of a continuum, one can ask, "How do the activities one does at the workplace or on the job make the activities a profession as opposed to an occupation?" The idea of the continuum implies that the difference among professions and occupations lies in the existing *degree* of eight specific "work characteristics." A profession manifests the eight work characteristics to a high degree, while an occupation manifests the characteristics to a low degree. The eight work characteristics delineated by Pavalko[7] include: theory or intellectual technique, relevance to basic social values, a training period, motivation, autonomy, sense of commitment, sense of community, and a code of ethics. The established

TABLE 1-1

*The Occupation—Profession Model**

Dimensions	Occupation		Profession
1. Theory, intellectual technique	Absent	——	Present
2. Relevance to social values	Not relevant	——	Relevant
3. Training period A	Short	——	Long
B	Non-specialized	——	Specialized
C	Involves things	——	Involves symbols
D	Subculture unimportant	——	Subculture important
4. Motivation	Self-interest	——	Service
5. Autonomy	Absent	——	Present
6. Commitment	Short term	——	Long term
7. Sense of community	Low	——	High
8. Code of ethics	Undeveloped	——	Highly developed

*Taken from: Pavalko R. (1971). *Sociology of occupations and professions*, Itasca, IL: F.E. Peacock Publishers, Inc., p. 26.

professions exhibit this complex of work characteristics to the highest degree. The degree to which each work characteristic is possessed by a particular work activity determines where the activity lies on the continuum. (See Table 1-1.)

Theory or Intellectual Technique.   This characteristic refers to the degree to which a work activity has a systematic body of theory and esoteric, abstract knowledge upon which the work is based. This knowledge base generally, but not necessarily, represents the results of scientific research. Medicine, for example, is a work activity whose knowledge base is built upon scientific research, whereas legal practice is an example of a work activity whose knowledge base is built upon an elaborate system of changing rules and customs that are normative (or the standard) rather than scientific. The work activity's body of knowledge provides the basis for legitimizing the actions of a "professional." A professional's claim to expertise rests upon a presumed mastery of this body of knowledge.

Relevance to Basic Social Values.   This characteristic refers to the relationship that the work activity has to the basic central values of society. "Professionals" claim that their work activities "maximize the realization of such values"[7] and, therefore, are applied to the most severe crises that people have to face. For example, medicine maximizes the societal value of health, while law maximizes the value of justice.

*Training (Educational) Period.**   This characteristic involves: the amount of education that the individual must undergo in order to be prepared to carry out the specific work activity, the extent to which the education is specialized, the degree to which the work activity is symbolic and involves the formation of ideas and thoughts, and the acquisition of a specific set of values, norms, and role conceptions. It must be kept in mind that all types of work activities involve some type of education; however, the longer the period of education required for a specific work activity, the closer the activity is to the profession end of the continuum.

The degree of knowledge specialization involved in the work activities' educational period is a dimension that sets a profession apart from an occupation. Although specialization tends to be widespread in today's society, the *degree* of specialization in one's education for a work activity varies widely. The greater the degree of specialization, the closer the work activity is to the profession end of the occupation-profession continuum.

In addition to being highly specialized, professional education involves the ability to manipulate ideas, thoughts, and symbols, as well as things or

---

* Although society often tends to place a higher value on training than education and Pavalko uses the term *training* in his occupation-profession conceptual model, the authors have chosen to use the term *education* in place of the word *training*.

physical objects. No one's work activity is completely non-thought oriented, nor is it completely thought oriented. Again, the point to be made is that the *degree* of manipulation of ideas, thoughts, and symbols by the professional is greater. For example, the computer repair person's work involves primarily the manipulation of tools and materials; however, there are principles of thought involved if one is to perform the work activity appropriately. The education of a physician, on the other hand, involves the use of medical tools and equipment; however, greater emphasis is placed upon the learning of scientific principles, concepts, and ideas.

The acquisition of a specific set of values, norms, and role expectations is a dimension of the professional educational period. The greater the *degree* to which the values, norms, and role expectations are either intentionally or unintentionally learned, the more likely the work activity is to be placed on the profession end of the continuum.

Motivation. The characteristic of motivation involves the degree to which the work group emphasizes the fact that their primary goal is to provide service to the client and public. In other words, work activities at the profession end of the continuum are assumed to be motivated by the desire to serve clients, rather than by the desire for monetary gain and self-interest. Such a belief implies that the professional's dedication to the client precludes the possibility of self-serving behavior. For example, if a client goes to the professional because of need for specialized services, the client believes (because society has publicly acknowledged the fact) that the professional has his or her best interests in mind. By comparison, work activities at the occupational end of the continuum, such as activities related to business, are more likely to be geared toward seeking and maintaining customers for the purpose of monetary gain.

Autonomy. The freedom to regulate one's work behavior constitutes autonomy for the professional. **Autonomy** on the part of the professional involves controlling matters related to the activities of the work members. Such control is reflected by guarding access to the work activity through **credentialing** (licensing, certification, registration, and accreditation). Taking part in the work activity without proper credentialing constitutes illegal practice.

In addition to the activity of credentialing, the ability of the individual practitioner to function freely, without supervision by someone from outside of the work activity, constitutes another dimension of autonomy. Such autonomy implies that the existence of the specialized competence, embodied by the individual, allows for *only* others with similar training to judge the quality of the work activity. A high degree of autonomy lays claim to a high degree of monopoly and control of the right to perform the particular work activity. Although some work activities at the occupational end of the continuum may have a degree of monopoly over their work activity through such mechanisms as the "unions," the degree of monopoly is much less than that achieved by the work activities at the profession end of the continuum.

Sense of Commitment. This characteristic involves the sentiment that individuals have toward their work activity. At the profession end of the continuum the work activity may be viewed as a "calling," in that one's engagement in the activity is not a "passing fancy," but a lifelong involvement. For example, one who selects to engage in the profession activities of the ministry, law, or medicine is assumed to remain in the work activity during his or her entire life. By comparison, work activities that are closer to the occupation end of the continuum are seen as a means to an end, such as an activity that simply provides one with money for paying living expenses.

Sense of Community. The sense of a common identity and destiny, the possession of a distinctive culture, and the presence of shared values and norms constitute a sense of community. While the sense of community primarily controls one's work behavior, it may extend into controlling non-work behavior, such as leisure activities and political orientations. According to Goode,[8] the professional's demonstration of community involves: a sense of identity, a lifelong status, shared values, agreed-upon role behaviors, a common language, power over its members, clear social limits, and control over the selection and socialization of trainees. By comparison, work activities that are on the occupation end of the continuum are more rudimentary and less likely to impose standardization over the behavior of members or trainees.

Code of Ethics. The final characteristic of Pavalko's[7] occupation-profession continuum is the code of ethics. Codes of ethics may be written or unwritten and cover such activities as practitioner-public relationships, relationships among practitioners, and relationships between practitioners and members of other work groups. A code of ethics is a normative or standardizing system for the members of the work activity and serves to assure clients and the public that only the highest degree of performance will be provided and/or tolerated by members of the work group. Codes of ethics aid in reinforcing the characteristics of motivation (service orientation) and autonomy. They emphasize the practitioner's primary concern to be that of the welfare of the client and the practitioner's work group to be the only one capable of judging the quality of the service rendered.

In summary, the eight characteristics of Pavalko's[7] occupation-profession continuum provide a means of assessing where a work activity lies in regard to the traditional professions or to occupations. As Pavalko pointed out, assessment of a work activity must be based upon the *degree* to which the activity embodies each of the eight characteristics. No work activity will exhibit all of the characteristics to the highest degree, nor will a work activity exhibit none of the characteristics. Keeping these facts in mind, where does nursing lie on the continuum? Before proceeding, however, the reader should keep in mind that not everyone will agree with the authors' assessment of nursing's evolving professional status and that the author's assessment of where nursing lies on Pavalko's occupation-profession continuum is only one interpretation of this health perspective.

NURSING'S PLACEMENT ON THE OCCUPATION-PROFESSION CONTINUUM

In order for nursing to be considered an established profession, according to Pavalko's[7] occupation-profession continuum, nursing must possess a high degree of the eight dimensions delineated in the model (see Table 1-2). First and foremost of the eight dimensions is the existence of a systematic body of knowledge that is esoteric and abstract and upon which work activities are based. The existence of a comprehensive, esoteric body of knowledge for nursing is in the early to middle stages of development, thereby placing nursing toward the middle of the occupation-profession continuum. One must keep in mind that the development and refinement of nursing theory was not considered an issue of extreme importance until the middle 1960s.[9] Developing a scientific knowledge base upon which to build nursing

TABLE 1-2

Nursing's Evolving Professional Status Based on Pavalko's*
Occupation-Profession Continuum

Dimensions	Occupation		Middle		Profession
1. Theory, intellectual technique			▬		
2. Relevance to social values					▬
3. Training (Education) period*					
a. Length		▬			
b. Specialization				▬	
c. Idea manipulation		▬			
d. Subculture		▬			
4. Motivation					▬
5. Autonomy	▬				
6. Commitment				▬	
7. Sense of community	▬				
8. Code of ethics					▬

* Pavalko's model uses the term *training*. The authors have substituted the term *education*.

practice is considered one of nursing's most important and demanding tasks.[9,16] Development of a scientific knowledge base will provide nursing with a theoretical basis for practice and, subsequently, the ability to exercise greater control over practice (ie, autonomy). Today there are a number of well-developed and increasingly refined theories that nurses can and are using to guide practice, research, and education.[10-15]

Schlotfeldt[17] points out that "nursing is the appraisal and the enhancement of the health status, health assets, and health potentials of human beings." If one accepts this definition, then nursing's work-related activities may be viewed as ranking high on the profession end of the continuum for relevance to basic social values. Such ranking seems appropriate, since nursing's work activities reflect society's long-established value of health.

A long and specialized educational period that involves the manipulation of ideas, thoughts, and symbols and consists of a specific set of values and norms denotes an established profession and constitutes the third dimension of the continuum. Nursing tends to rank more toward the lower middle section of the continuum in regard to a long and specialized educational period, since a variety of programs preparing beginning practitioners of nursing exist (diploma, associate degree, baccalaureate, and ND—nursing doctorate). These programs range in length of study from two (associate degree) to six (ND) years. Although the American Nurses' Association (ANA)[18] in 1965 and the National League for Nursing (NLN)[19] in 1986 stated that the entry level for *professional* nursing should occur at the baccalaureate level, the practice of such a position remains unactualized and continues to create heated debates among many nurses.

Concerning specialization within the work activity, nursing tends to rank toward the upper half of the occupation-profession continuum. Specialization in nursing tends to occur more readily at the master's level, with master's degree prepared specialists working in areas such as neo-natal intensive care, oncology, psychiatry, midwifery, rheumatology, cardiology, community health, home health care, gerontology, anesthesia, and pediatrics—just to name a few. Many nurses, however, with less than a baccalaureate degree proclaim themselves as specialists simply by the nature of the work they perform and not by the nature of their educational preparation, as denoted by the more established professions. With the increasing development of technology and increasing demands placed upon nursing by society's health care needs, nursing specialization is becoming more sophisticated. This especially is noted when one looks at the variety of master's degree programs being offered by NLN accredited schools and by the types of certifications offered by the ANA and other certifying bodies.

Nursing involves the ability to manipulate ideas, thoughts, and symbols, in addition to things or physical objects such as syringes or intravenous infusions. Since nursing continues to work on a well-established theoretical base and, in the not so distant past, focused very heavily upon the task oriented rather than upon the holistic aspects of care, nursing is somewhat new to the art and science of manipulating ideas, thoughts, and symbols. Therefore, nursing tends to rank more toward the middle of the continuum in idea manipulation. Great strides and advancements in this arena are being made, as demonstrated by the increasing number of nurses holding graduate degrees, by the increasing number of well developed and executed nursing research studies, and by the increasing number of curriculums that offer courses requiring the analysis of theory and its application.

Acquiring a specific set of values, norms, and role expectations either intentionally or unintentionally during one's educational experience constitutes the last dimension of the educational period. The educational process in nursing does provide, to some degree, the incorporation of a specific set of values, norms, and role expectations. However, unlike individuals prepared in the established professions, nursing prepares its beginning workers in such a variety of educational programs (diploma, AD, BSN, ND) that it is impossible to instill the same set of values, norms, or role expectations. Therefore, nursing tends to rank toward the lower middle section of the continuum. Nurses prepared at the AD level are likely to hold a similar set of values, norms, or role expectations, whereas nurses prepared at the BSN level will have an entirely different set of values, norms, and role expectations, simply due to the nature of their educational experience.

The degree to which the work group emphasizes the fact that their primary goal is to provide service to the client and public constitutes the fourth dimension, motivation. Nursing tends to rank high on the profession end of the continuum concerning this component of the model. Such a ranking is based on the fact that, since Florence Nightingale's time, nursing has espoused the goal of service to the client and public versus the goal of self-serving behavior. Even today service to the client remains a key aspect in the delivery of quality nursing care.

Autonomy, or the freedom to regulate work behavior, is the fifth dimension of the model. Due to the incompleteness of nursing's freedom to regulate its work behavior, nursing tends to rank closer to the occupation end than to the profession end of the continuum for this dimension. According to Moloney,[20] nurses' lack of autonomy can, in part, be attributed to the fact that most nurses are employed by hospitals or other types of organizations in which the precise definition of client has not been made. Working in large bureaucratic organizations, such as hospitals, weakens the autonomy of the nurse, since the organization tends to tell the nurse what to do and how it is to be done. Along with the lack of a well-delineated body of theoretical knowledge, the lack of autonomy is a major factor in keeping nursing from becoming an established profession. Nursing is redefining its function in order to claim autonomy over its services, as can be noted by the increasing number of nurses who have gone into private practice or who have established their own health care related businesses. However, not until nursing delineates what constitutes its unique work activity will nursing be able to have complete autonomy and monopoly over services rendered, as does medicine and the other established professions.

Nursing tends to rank more toward the middle of the continuum for commitment, the sentiment that individuals have toward their work activity, since in the past nursing was viewed as a nice means of income until the responsibilities of a family occurred. Lack of commitment most likely is related to nursing being a predominately female-dominated work activity. It was not until the women's rights movement in the 1960s and 1970s that women viewed themselves as having long-term involvement in a work activity and as enactors of the multiple roles of wife, mother, homemaker, and professional. Today more individuals are assuming the multiple roles demanded by the work force and the family and, as a result, are entering nursing with the perception that it is a professional endeavor that requires long-term involvement.

In recognizing that nursing has not agreed upon role behaviors, a common language, power over its members, or clear social limits, it tends to rank toward the lower end of the continuum for the seventh dimension of the model, a sense of community, the existence of a distinctive culture, and the presence of shared values and norms. This became apparent to Gorman and Clark[21] when their findings in the "Nursing Knowledge Project" suggested that the collegiality demonstrated among nurses was not strong. Nurses tended to function on the **basis of hierarchy,** that is, receiving most of their information from supervisors with little information or support received from nurses outside the immediate work environment. Again, this was due to the existence of the varied educational programs that prepare nurses for their work activity. It is difficult to create and sustain a sense of community that fosters shared values and norms when practitioners with differing educational preparation fail to share the same values and norms from the onset.

The eighth and final dimension of the model, a code of ethics, is the normative or standardizing system for the members of the work activity. Nursing tends to rank very high on the profession end of the model in this dimension, since its first formal code of ethics, although developed later than the ethical codes of many of the other health-related work activities, was developed in 1950.[22] Since codes of ethics assist in reinforcing the characteristics of motivation and autonomy,[7] the fact that nursing ranks high on the profession end of the continuum, regarding its code of ethics, cannot help but assist nursing in its evolution toward established professionalism.

In summary (see Table 1-2), nursing tends to rank high on the profession end of Pavalko's[7] continuum in regard to relevance to social values, motivation, code of ethics, and specialization. On the other hand, nursing appears to rank more toward the middle of the continuum on theory and intellectual technique, length of the educational period, idea manipulation, subculture, and commitment. For autonomy and sense of community, nursing ranks toward the lower end of the continuum. Thus nursing, although not an established profession, when measured against Pavalko's[7] continuum, certainly is an *evolving* one. In the words of Carr-Saunders[2] and Etzioni,[3] nursing is in the *process* of emerging. Being a part of an evolving profession can be an exciting experience for nurses, consumers, and society. However, it can also impose a variety of impacts upon each of these groups.

Impacts on the Nurse, the Consumer, and Society

THE NURSE

Since nursing does not appear to manifest a high degree of *all* of the characteristics of an established profession, difficulties tend to be created for nurses regarding their abilities to achieve a position of high and powerful status in the health care system. Often nurses tend not to be perceived as having the power that established professionals have to negotiate within the health care organization. Thus, when demands are made by nurses to leaders in the bureaucratic health care system about issues surrounding nursing's work activities, these demands often fall upon deaf ears. The lack of power within the organization often tends to lead to lessened autonomy.

When nurses are perceived as having limited power within the health care organization, collegial relationships between nurses and the established professionals may be compromised. Rather than being perceived to be on "equal footing," nurses often are seen as "workers" who are present to carry out activities under the direction of the established professionals. However, with the increasing number of nurses who hold master's and doctoral degrees, power bases and interdisciplinary collegial relationships are greatly improving and nurses are being viewed more as colleagues rather than as subservient workers.

Although a professional does not work for the primary purpose of monetary gain, the fact that nursing is an emerging profession is likely to influence the monetary status of nurses. Nursing has not been a profession that has provided the reaping of substantial monetary rewards. Such an act has added to the decline of individuals pursuing nursing as a work activity.[23] Economic remuneration tends to be related to the value of one's contribution to the work activity and, unfortunately, the health care industry and society often have been unwilling to acknowledge nursing services by way of salaries.[24]

The fact that nursing has not been perceived as an established profession has created disparity in the courts of law. As Segal[25] points out, most lawsuits brought against nurses have resulted from negligence, "acting in a manner that no reasonable person, guided by considerations that normally regulate human behavior, would act," whereas most lawsuits brought against physicians have resulted from malpractice, the act of negligence committed in the course of carrying out *professional* responsibilities. It may seem beneficial to the nurse to be charged with negligence instead of malpractice; however, being charged with malpractice, according to Segal,[25] has three advantages. These advantages include 1) the **statute of limitations,** which governs the time limit during which a lawsuit may be brought; 2) the court's determination of the proper standard of care against which the defendant's actions will be judged; and 3) the calling of an expert witness to aid the court in determining the proper standard of care.

Statutes of limitations have been established to ensure that lawsuits are brought against the accused within a reasonable time after the alleged act has occurred. Since there have been an increasing number of malpractice cases, the courts have been unduly burdened and, as a result, many state legislatures have enacted shorter statutes of limitations for professional negligence (about an average of one year) than for ordinary negligence (about an average of two years).[25] When a patient brings a lawsuit against both a physician (for malpractice) and a nurse (for ordinary negligence), the statute of limitations may protect the physician, but not the nurse, from having to stand trial.

Standards of care are always used by the courts when evaluating the actions of a professional. In order to apply a professional standard of care, there needs to exist a clear definition of the scope or domain of the practice being evaluated. Unfortunately, the states' nurse practice acts often are unclear, restrictive, inconsistent between states, and generally unrepresentative of the actual scope or domain of nursing practice. Such facts leave the question of nursing's scope or domain of practice open to considerable interpretation and, in turn, may place the nurse experiencing litigation in jeopardy.

Generally an expert witness is called to testify in malpractice cases. In regard to nurses, however, the courts are in a quandary. Sometimes an expert witness will be called and sometimes not. As a rule, the more technical the act, the more likely an expert witness will be called to testify. The dilemma lies in the fact that the courts sometimes accept the statements of physicians, rather than nurses, as experts on nursing care.[26] Such a practice creates a distinct disadvantage for the nurse on trial, since juries tend to have a higher opinion of physicians than nurses and may subconsciously give more credence to the physician's testimony than to the nurse's testimony, even though the nurse is more knowledgeable about nursing standards of practice than is the physician. Thus, from a legal point of view, not being an established profession often places nursing in additional legal jeopardy.

THE CONSUMER AND SOCIETY

Nursing's status as an evolving profession has an impact upon the consumer and society, since the nurse's role in the health care system often remains unclear. Health care consumers and members of society are aware that the physician's role is one of diagnosis and treatment of illness, along with the prescription of medications. Precisely what role the nurse plays in the health care system remains a mystery to many consumers and members of society.

The decreasing number of individuals selecting nursing as a career option possibly is related to nursing's emerging professional status. There has been a considerable decline in the enrollment of students in basic nursing education programs and subsequently a shortage of nurses nation-wide. From 1984 to 1985 enrollments were down an average of 8.1 percent.[24] Preliminary estimates suggest that a steeper decline in enrollments will occur over the next few years. The impact that the present and projected shortage of nurses has and will have upon the delivery of quality health care could be devastating to the consumer and society. Services in various health care agencies will have to be limited or stopped, patients will have to be discharged from acute care facilities earlier than desired, and long-term follow-up care in the community will have to be curtailed due to the lack of qualified nurses to carry out needed care. It will become increasingly difficult to provide the best possible nursing care to the consumer if nursing is not able to recruit and retain the caliber of nurses needed to meet the health care demands of society.

The fact that nursing has not been perceived as an established profession has influenced the development of scientifically based nursing care. In the past federal monies to fund research endeavors carried out by nurses frequently have been limited. Nursing studies often have been viewed with skepticism and seen as less than scientific because they were not designed like studies done in the basic sciences, nor did they address issues similar to those of the basic sciences. However, with the creation of the National Center for Nursing Research on the campus of the National Institutes of Health, more federal recognition is being given to the support of nursing research. Such recognition will enhance the development and, subsequently, the delivery of scientifically based nursing care to the consumer and society.

Future Considerations

Over the past three decades, nursing has made great strides in evolving as a profession. However, it is imperative that nursing continue its development and emergence toward established professionalism. Established professionalism will enhance nursing's autonomy, power within the health care system, collegial equivalency, social status, monetary reward, and scientific credibility. To enhance nursing's continued professional evolution, the following steps need to be considered:

- standardizing the educational entry level for professional practice
- identifying and describing nursing's uniqueness as a provider of health care
- clarifying to the public nursing's role in the health care system
- marketing nursing's unique health care services to consumers and to society
- continuing to develop and refine nursing theory and research
- developing nursing care based upon nursing theory and research
- developing and instituting nursing services that address not only the immediate needs of the health care consumer, but also long-term needs
- encouraging entrepreneurial endeavors that would enhance nursing's autonomy
- instituting mentor relationships that enhance a sense of community
- being actively involved in the formulation of health policy

Each nurse needs to be involved and committed to the charge of carrying out activities that promote and foster nursing's evolving professionalism. Being a part of such a movement can be exciting and a challenge to each nurse who partakes.

Dr. Mary Jones is an associate professor who teaches health related issues and perspectives to second semester senior nursing students. She is in the process of presenting a lecture on nursing's status as an evolving profession. As part of her classroom presentation, she asks the class the following questions. How would you answer each of these questions?

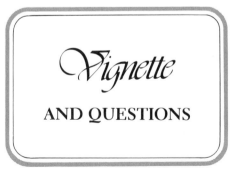

Vignette

AND QUESTIONS

1. How does nursing compare to medicine, law, and the ministry in regard to each of the following?
   a. theory and intellectual technique
   b. specialization
   c. autonomy
   d. code of ethics

2. What impact does nursing's evolving status have upon nurses, the consumer, and society?

3. What actions could be taken by nurses to enhance nursing's movement toward established professionalism?

INFORMATION SOURCES

American Nurses' Association
2420 Pershing Road
Kansas City, MO 64108

National League for Nursing
10 Columbus Circle
New York, NY 10019

Kalish P, Kalish B: *The Advance of American Nursing*, ed 2. Boston, Little, Brown, 1986

Moloney M: *Professionalization of Nursing*. Philadelphia, Lippincott, 1986

REFERENCES

1. Becker H: The nature of a profession. In *Education for the Professions: The Sixty-First Yearbook of the National Society for the Study of Education, Part II*. Chicago, University of Chicago Press, 1962

2. Carr-Saunders A, Wilson P: *The Professions*. Oxford, Clarendon Press, 1933

3. Etzioni A: *The Semi-Professions and Their Organization*. New York, Free Press, 1969

4. Flexner A: Is social work a profession? In *Proceedings of the National Conference of Charities and Corrections*. Chicago, Hildermann Printing Co, 1915

5. Greenwood E: Attributes of a profession. *Soc Work* 2:45, 1957

6. Goode W: The theoretical limits of professionalization. Etzioni A (ed): *The Semi-Professions and Their Organizations: Teacher, Nurses, Social Workers*. New York, Free Press, 1969

7. Pavalko R: *Sociology of Occupations and Professions*. Itasca, IL, FE Peacock Publishers, Inc, 1971

8. Goode W: Community within a community: The professions. *Am Soc Rev* 22:194, 1957

9. Meleis A: *Theoretical Nursing: Development and Progress*. Philadelphia, Lippincott, 1985

10. Johnson D: The behavioral system model for nursing. In Riehl J, Roy C (eds): *Conceptual Models for Nursing Practice*, ed 2. New York, Appleton-Century-Crofts, 1980

11. Neuman B: *The Neuman Systems Model: Application to Nursing Education and Practice*. Norwalk, CT, Appleton-Century-Crofts, 1982

12. Roy C, Roberts S: *Theory Construction in Nursing: An Adaptation Model*. Englewood Cliffs, NJ, Prentice-Hall, 1981

13. Orem D: *Nursing: Concepts of Practice*, ed 2. New York, McGraw-Hill, 1980

14. Rogers M: Science of unitary human being: A paradigm for nursing. In Clements I, Roberts F (eds): *Family Health: A Theoretical Approach to Nursing Care*. New York, Wiley, 1983

15. King I: *A Theory for Nursing: Systems, Concepts, Process*. New York, Wiley, 1981

16. Conway M: Prescription for professionalization. In Chaska N (ed): *The Nursing Profession: A Time to Speak*. New York, McGraw-Hill, 1983

17. Schlotfeldt R: Defining nursing: A historic controversy. *Nurs Res* 36:64, 1987

18. American Nurses' Association: Position on education for nursing. *Am J Nurs* 65:101, 1965

19. Board of Directors, National League for Nursing: Interpretative statement on NLN position in support of two levels of nursing practice. *Nurs Health Care* 7:234, 1986

20. Moloney M: *Professionalization of Nursing: Current Issues and Trends*. Philadelphia, Lippincott, 1986

21. Gorman S, Clark N: Power and effective nursing practice. *Nurs Outlook* 34:124, 1986

22. Wilensky H: The professionalization of everyone? *Am J Soc* 70:143, 1964

23. Clark M, Turque B, Hutchinson S, Gosnell M, Rotenberek L: Nurses: Few and fatigued. *Newsweek* June 29:59, 1987

24. Selby T: RN shortage threatens quality of care. *The Am Nurse* March 1, 1987

25. Segal E: Is nursing a profession? *Nursing '85* 17:41, 1987

26. Murphy E: The professional status of nursing: A view from the courts. *Nurs Outlook* 35:12, 1987

VIVIEN DeBACK, RN, PhD

Technical Versus Professional Practice

CHAPTER 2

Background and Overview

Nursing, from the early 1800s to the mid-1950s, was essentially an apprentice-type educational system, in spite of the fact that the first collegiate programs in nursing in the United States were instituted at the turn of the century. Teachers College in New York opened the first baccalaureate program in 1899, and the University of Minnesota opened a baccalaureate program for nurses in 1909. Generally, however, nursing education throughout the 1950s could be best described as "nursing training" and was found in hospital schools throughout the country.

Studies about nursing and nursing education that began as early as 1912[1-4] consistently recommended that schools of nursing be moved out of hospital control and placed in schools of higher education.

In 1948 Esther Lucille Brown[3] supported the earlier studies that questioned apprenticeship training for nurses. Furthermore, she suggested that there existed both technical and professional functions in nursing and that nurses could be prepared for technical functions in less time than it took to prepare them for professional functions. Brown also recommended that programs to prepare technical nurses be located in institutions of higher education. Brown's study began almost 40 years of discussion about professional and technical nursing.

Following the Brown study, Mildred Montag[5] in 1951 developed a program to prepare nurses predominately for technical functions with an associate degree in nursing as an outcome of the course of studies. The timing of Montag's recommendation of a program of this kind was excellent because the concept of community or junior colleges in this country was taking hold. World War II had created new technology and with it a new worker, the technician. A technical nurse educated at the associate degree level fit well into this new educational model.

The speed with which associate degree programs were accepted could not have been predicted. The movement became a national phenomenon. In 1976 there were 642 associate degree programs, as compared to 390 diploma programs and 341 baccalaureate programs.[6]

Montag's work related to associate degree nursing was highly specific. The new nursing program would educate a **nurse technician** who would perform the following functions:

- assist in the planning of nursing care for patients
- give general nursing care with supervision
- assist in the evaluation of nursing care given[7]

It was expected that baccalaureate programs in nursing would continue to grow and prepare professional nurses and that diploma programs would quickly decline. In actuality, baccalaureate programs did increase in number, but nowhere near the growth experienced at the associate degree level. Diploma programs began to decline, but not at all quickly.

During the period from 1970 to 1977, 101 junior college programs opened, 55 university/college programs were established, and 82 hospital schools closed. By 1980 the graduates from these three types of programs numbered 75,523. Of these, 24,995 were baccalaureate prepared, 36,034 held an associate degree, and 14,495 were diploma graduates.

For more than twenty years, through the 1960s and 1970s and into the 1980s, three different educational programs prepared three types of practitioners (based on the educational outcomes of those programs). These graduates were all eligible to take the **registered nurse licensure exam,** an exam developed to test minimal or safe nursing knowledge and skill. Although both Montag and Brown had envisioned two different types of nurses, prepared in two different types of educational programs for two different types of practice, the licensing exam, rather than the educational outcome, was used as the criterion for practice. This resulted in the development by boards of nursing of one (not two) legal scope of practice for graduates of ADN, BSN, and diploma schools. The very slow response of diploma programs to close or translate into associate or baccalaureate degree programs resulted in three (not two) educational pathways to practice.

It is little wonder, then, that the dilemma of defining professional and technical practice has continued so long. The emergence of the licensed practical nurse programs in the 1940s did not help this complex situation. Although boards of nursing at this time did develop a second legal scope of practice for the LPN, this was not at the associate degree level, as Montag has envisioned.

Clearly, the American Nurses' Association (ANA) 1965 position paper[8] was meant to clarify and bring to closure the ongoing technical/professional nurse debate.

The position paper stated that entry into professional nursing practice would be at the baccalaureate level and technical nurses would be prepared in schools offering an associate degree in nursing. The position paper did not close the subject of professional and technical nurses. However, it did signal the start of 20 years of discussion, debate, and some research, all attempting to define and differentiate the technical and professional nurse.

DIFFERENTIATING PROFESSIONAL AND TECHNICAL NURSING PRACTICE

Following publication of the 1965 ANA position paper, nursing literature began to fill with articles discussing technical and professional nursing. Clarification of the abilities of each type of practitioner were commonly described by educators who based their differentiation on the educational outcomes of each program. However, practice clarification continued to elude the profession.

In 1965 Waters stated, "If both professional and technical nurses are required for direct service to patients, clear distinctions as to their respective competence must be made as rapidly as possible, so that each group may be recruited, educated, and used efficiently, effectively, and economically."[9]

In 1966 Johnson commented, "Perhaps the most noticeable difference between the technical and the professional nurse is the difference in their knowledge."[10]

Many studies have been and are being done in the area of differences in the practice of nurses from various nursing programs. Because many clinical settings have one job description for nurses with different educational backgrounds, studies that looked only at what nurses *do* often found little or no difference in their practice.[11] However, studies that focused on knowledge base and patient outcomes often found differences in the practice of nurses from baccalaureate and associate degree programs.[12-14]

The flurry of activity throughout the 1970s culminated in the development of competencies of associate and baccalaureate graduates by the National League for Nursing (NLN) in 1978 and the ANA in 1980. This was followed by individual states, specialty nurse organizations, boards of nursing, and others developing their own competence statements in the ongoing effort to clarify differences between the two types of nurses.[15] (For examples of competence statements, see Appendix A.)

Throughout this "clarification" period, graduates of all three programs, diploma, associate degree, and baccalaureate degree, were hired into clinical positions in which there was only one job description and where the expectation of the setting was not differentiated by educational background.

SUPPORT FOR BACCALAUREATE ENTRY INTO PROFESSIONAL PRACTICE

The ANA followed their 1965 position paper with continuous reaffirmation of the goals stated in that document. In 1978 the ANA House of Delegates charged the association with developing competence statements for the two categories of nursing practice. In 1982 the ANA Commission on Nursing Education decided that "attempting to define nursing practice from a competency base instead of an educational base has not served to clarify two kinds of nursing practice."[16] In 1984 and 1985 the ANA reaffirmed the educational bases and established titles for two categories of nurses in the future.

Throughout 1985 and early 1986, support for the position of two categories of nurses began to develop and was reflected in public statements made by major nursing organizations. In 1985 the National Federation of Licensed Practical Nurses reaffirmed statements made in 1984 that endorsed two categories of nurses, educated at the associate degree and baccalaureate degree levels. In 1986 the NLN board of directors supported the concept of redefined levels of nursing practice, professional and technical. The American Association of Colleges of Nursing reaffirmed their support for the baccalaureate degree as entry into professional practice in 1986. And in October 1986 the American Organization of Nurse Executives (AONE) affirmed its belief that the baccalaureate in nursing should be the basic preparation for professional nursing practice. The AONE also supported the concept of two types of preparation for nursing practice, the baccalaureate and associate degrees in nursing. A list of organizations supporting the baccalaureate degree as the educational requirement for professional practice is found in Appendix B.

The move from four categories of education and practice to two categories seemed to be gaining momentum, although there were still a number of unanswered questions to be addressed, particularly those that dealt with the transition period.

At the 1987 ANA delegate assembly, the *Scope of Nursing Practice* was approved by the delegates. This document identified the differences between the technical and professional practice of nursing. It says in part, "the depth and breadth to which the individual nurse engages in the total scope the clinical practice of nursing are defined by the knowledge base of the nurse, the role of the nurse, and the nature of the client population within a practice environment. In the future, these same characteristics will differentiate the professional and technical practices of nursing."[17]

DELINEATION OF PROFESSIONAL AND TECHNICAL PRACTICE

The momentum that was building toward change in definitions of types of nurses needed for the future prompted numerous groups and individuals to begin to describe the differences between professional and technical nursing practice of the future.

A project funded by the W.K. Kellogg Foundation from 1983 through 1986 to the Western Interstate Commission for Higher Education (WICHE) had as its outcomes the development of competencies of associate degree and baccalaureate degree nurse graduates. This project, The Preparation and Utilization of New Nursing Graduates,[18] used a consensus-building multiple team approach to ultimately describe the differences between the two types of nurses. From these descriptions of ability, model job descriptions were formulated.

The WICHE project was successful in the consensus activity providing nursing with abilities and job descriptions of two types of nurses that were agreed upon by nurse educators, practitioners, and administrators. The project did not, and was not expected to, test the project outcomes in the clinical setting. However, differentiated demonstration sites were the appropriate next step.

Again the W.K. Kellogg Foundation funded a project through the Midwest Alliance in Nursing, titled "Defining and Differentiating Nursing Competencies."[19] This project developed differentiated competencies for associate and baccalaureate education curricula and job descriptions for graduates of such programs, and assisted in creating demonstration sites in hospitals in the Midwest, where differentiated practice could be observed and tested. Units functioning under these job descriptions demonstrated that differentiated practice "will work."

In October of 1986 the ICON (Integrated Competencies of Nurses) model of nursing practice was introduced at Yale New Haven Hospital.[20] This model integrates the basic competencies that nurses bring from their academic preparation (associate and baccalaureate degree graduates) into delivering the nursing process effectively and economically. The competencies have been used to develop differentiated job descriptions. This project has nurses functioning under the ICON model in several units of the hospital.

The continuing development of differentiated practice sites is a critical step in the ongoing process of change in the profession. In 1987 the National

Commission on Nursing Implementation Project provided the leadership and encouragement for several differentiated practice sites to be opened in various institutions across the country.

In the demonstration sites, nurses practice in job descriptions of the two types of nurses that are consistent with the outcomes of nursing education, as described by associate and baccalaureate degree educators. The major differences in practice that appear to be emerging are the following.

Professional nurses assume the responsibility to assist individuals, families, and groups to attain their maximum health potential and are accountable for their own actions in the care, coordination, and management of patient care and for coordination and direction of others in the nursing care environment. **Technical nurses** care for selected individual patients with well-defined health problems and are accountable for their own actions in the care of patients within the context of the total plan of care, which is coordinated by a professional nurse.

The professional nurse is characterized as care giver, case manager, and problem solver for individuals and groups of patients. Technical nurses care for individuals with common health or illness problems that have predictable outcomes.

Professional nurses are case managers, coordinating the care between the patient and existing health care services, adjusting plans for the delivery of health care services, obtaining informal support systems, and processing necessary support resources. Technical nurses organize the individualized care of patients, prioritize client needs, and implement care effectively, using personal and technological communication to interact with their clients and to document care.

Professional nursing knowledge incorporates all aspects of nursing service, as well as other disciplines, including theory, methods, processes, and analysis of nursing phenomenon. Technical nursing knowledge includes a circumscribed body of established nursing skills and knowledge relevant to a problem solving orientation for the health care of individuals and their families who experience common health disruptions.

Impacts on the Nurse, the Consumer, and Society

THE NURSE

Throughout the years of debate, questions that related to the impact of change from four educational categories of nurses to two often centered on what would happen to the nurses already in the system. Fears about loss of licensure or loss of prestige continued to confound the discussion. Because of these highly emotional issues, focusing on and restructuring the future were met with resistance, since many of the plans for the future did not spell out ways to proceed through the transition years. It is clear that transitional plans must address the use of the present nursing population, the ongoing need for all nurses in the system, and the methods to be used for change to take place. Although most proposals set forth by national and state groups stated that all licensed nurses would remain licensed at the level they are presently practicing or higher throughout their professional careers, such pronouncements were either not believed or not accepted.

Clarification of the scope of practice of two categories of nurses for the future were developed by the American Nurses' Association Task Force on Scope of Practice in 1986 and prepared for the House of Delegates in 1987. Generally it is believed that national consensus on scope of practice statements for technical and professional nurses will move the profession closer to its stated goals.

As the move toward two categories continues, nurses in practice will be affected. They will be expected to perform effectively in the newly created job descriptions that nursing service must design to utilize two categories of nurses to their highest abilities. This reorganization of the nursing delivery system will be a transitional one, over a period of several years, just as the restructuring of the nursing educational system will take time to complete.

Meanwhile, all nurses in practice will be needed to assure a continuing supply of practitioners for the community. More importantly, the changes recommended for the nursing profession that have been discussed for 25 years will also have an effect on the consumer of nursing services.

Ultimately, as the scope of practice of two categories of nurses are defined, nurse practice acts in each state will have to be rewritten. Licensing exams will also need to be revised to reflect the new practice and new educational outcomes.

This process of change on a state-by-state basis will require the involvement of nurses, consumers, other health care professionals, and legislators. A national plan for this step-by-step process is needed and a massive educational program for nurses and nonnurses is needed to clarify the need for change and the benefit to the community.

Titling.   One issue that has slowed the process to clarify two categories of nurses has been that of **titling,** or the determination of a descriptive name. While it is difficult for the nonnurse population to understand the emotionalism that surrounds titling, those within the profession are well aware of the prestige and pride associated with the title RN for over 50 years. Therefore, suggestions for nurses of the future to have a title other than registered nurse, whether that is the professional or technical nurse, is met with stiff resistance.

At the 1985 ANA convention, delegates voted to title the associate degree nurse, associate nurse (AN) and the baccalaureate degree nurse, registered nurse (RN). The following months did see progress in defining differentiated scopes of practice for the two types of nurses. However, the titles of AN and RN were still hotly debated.

It is believed by many that the differentiated practice and educational issues can continue to be developed without resolution of titling. However, titling must ultimately be settled and must be done in a way that will not further divide the nursing community.

In March 1987 the Tri Council in Nursing, a group made up of the presidents and executive directors from the American Association of Colleges of Nursing, the ANA, the American Organization of Nurse Executives, and the NLN, developed a discussion document on titling and licensure. That document described the consensus that was emerging in nursing that there will be two categories of nursing personnel, one prepared at the baccalaureate and one at the associate degree level. The document also stated that recommended titles for the professional nurses were registered nurse or registered professional nurse and for the technical nurse, associate nurse or registered associate nurse.

During the ANA Delegate Assembly in 1987, the delegates received a board information report called *Activities Around Implementation of the Baccalaureate*. This report included the Tri Council document on titling and licensure, thus recognizing some variability around titles.

At the 1987 NLN Convention, several resolutions were presented to the membership from the board of directors that reflected the thinking of the board regarding NLN's next steps in titling and licensure. The response of the membership to the resolutions on this subject was a parliamentary procedure to postpone indefinitely. In parliamentary terms this means that the issue cannot be brought up again at the meetings of that convention. The move to postpone does not prevent the board from continuing to address this issue. And, of course, the subject can be brought to the membership again at the next convention.

THE CONSUMER

The changes that have been proposed to clarify the practice of technical and professional nurses is expected to have a profound impact on clients. It is they who will benefit most from this clarification. When the consumers of care know what nurses can do for them and their families, they will be in a better position to select nurses to meet their needs and to evaluate the services that nurses provide.

Consumers do know a great deal about nurses now. A 1985 ANA national survey[21] of 602 adults showed that 68 percent of those surveyed believed that nurses are trained to play a larger role in providing health care services than they are presently allowed to do. Eighty-three percent expect to hear ideas from nurses about the ways nurses should expand their current responsibilities, as well as ways of containing health care costs. Sixty percent of the respondents answered "yes" to the question: "Would you be in favor of a measure requiring all newly registered nurses to have a four-year college degree?"

While the ANA survey suggests that consumers know that nurses have a great deal to offer in the way of health care, the survey also indicates that consumers are not aware of all the services available from nurses. Therefore, further clarification of nurses' roles would benefit all who seek or receive nursing care.

SOCIETY

Clearly, a change in the basic system of education for professional and technical nurses will have an effect on the present and future health care system. Initially, the nursing care delivery system will be different. Traditional systems such as hospitals and nursing homes will develop new job descriptions based on the preparation and skill of the nurse. Because the present system uses all nurses in the same manner, no matter what their educational background, nurses are often asked to function beyond their preparation, while others are constrained from practicing at the level of their preparation. This system is costly and can result in less than quality care.

As nursing delivery systems change to describe nursing practice at the level of each practitioner, a more efficient and high-quality system can emerge. All nurses will be utilized to their highest ability. All nursing care delivery systems will be able to define the type of care provided, the type of nurse giving the care, and the types of clients serviced.

Whether nurses practice in group settings or as employees in institutions or agencies, each will be accountable for a type of practice defined by their education and experience and for which they are licensed.

This change in defining practice more clearly will not only affect the nursing care delivery system. Because nurses work with other professionals, the role of the nurse and the relationship of the nurse to others will also change. One aspect of the nurse's role will not change. That is, in the future, as now, all nurses will be accountable for their own actions. The change that is expected to occur is that nurses, with practice clearly defined, will be a more effectively utilized resource by other professionals. It is also expected that the professional nurse, particularly the advanced practitioner with graduate preparation, will become a competitor for clients with other health care providers. Such competition in an economy such as that of the United States is considered healthy and advantageous to the consumer. Both the clarification of nurses' roles and the potential for competition will place nurses in a different position with physicians, social workers, and physical therapists. The role delineation suggests new skills for nurses such as negotiation and self-promotion.

There is still another expected influence on the health care system caused by the differentiation of practice of two categories of nurses. That is, the cost of health care is expected to be affected. With nursing care being provided by the most appropriate provider, a high-quality, cost-effective system is expected to result. In addition, because the care provided is more clearly delineated, the effectiveness of the care can be evaluated and priced appropriately rather than in aggregate costs by time of service or length of stay, as is presently done.

The health care system continues to change. Therefore, nursing must change with it to assure the community of an adequate supply of the appropriate nurse providers at the time the service is needed. The delineation of professional and technical nurses as defined by education and skill is the way to accomplish that.

Future Considerations

The cost of health care in the United States continues to escalate. In 1986 health care expenditures equaled 10.8 percent of the gross national product. This translates into more than $400 billion annually. It is expected that by 1990 the annual per person expenditure on health care in the United States will exceed $2,400.

Although there are a number of steps that must be taken by government, health care providers, and consumers to bring these costly expenditures under control, one suggestion often advanced is to offer incentives to consumers to seek out alternate health care providers, particularly for health promotion and maintenance and rehabilitative service. As more nurses are directly reimbursed for the care they provide to consumers, the consumer needs to understand what a nurse is and what nurses do.

In the future, when four educational categories have been changed to two, and the graduates of these programs are identified as practitioners with specific skills and knowledge, the consumer as well as the employer of nurses will be better able to select the kind of nurse for their particular needs. Nurse practitioners with graduate degrees in nursing will also be identified by knowledge base, role, practice environment, and the nature of the clients they serve.

Such a system is not only clearer for the consumer, but cost effective as well. It offers consumers the opportunity to select a provider of care for their specific need. Because of that direct relationship to the nurse, consumers also have the opportunity to evaluate the effectiveness of service they receive.

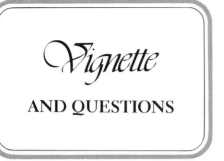

Vignette

AND QUESTIONS

The local hospital in which you are working has determined that development of job descriptions for professional and technical nurses is a step they are interested in taking. You are responsible for assisting in the implementation of a differentiated practice unit. The hospital has many nurses with varying educational backgrounds, all of whom are highly valued. Discuss the approach you would take to begin the process of changing the practice parameters for nurses in this hospital.

1. What resources would you use to begin this process?

2. Who would be involved in the planning?

3. How will you develop support for change?

4. What kinds of opposition do you expect to meet and how will you handle them?

INFORMATION SOURCES

American Nurses' Association
  2420 Pershing Road
  Kansas City, MO 64108

National League for Nursing
  10 Columbus Circle
  New York, NY 10019

American Association of Colleges of Nursing
  One Dupont Circle, NW
  Washington, DC 20036

American Organization of Nurse Executives
  840 North Lake Shore Drive
  Chicago, IL 60611

Western Interstate Commission for Higher Education
  P.O. Drawer P
  Boulder, CO 80302

Midwest Alliance in Nursing
  1226 W. Michigan St. 108BR
  Indianapolis, IN 46223

Appendix A: Examples of Competence Statements

These examples were collected by the staff at the National Commission on Nursing Implementation Project in 1986. The statements represent a range of national, regional, and state groups' efforts to define competencies that characterize nurses prepared at the Associate and Baccalaureate Degree Levels. The complete Working Paper from which these samples have been drawn is documented in Reference #15 of this chapter.

COMMUNICATION

BSN establishes and modifies communication systems.
ADN works within the context of established communication systems.

BSN uses communication networks to modify health care delivery.
ADN uses established communication networks to implement an effective health care plan.

NURSING PROCESS

BSN assesses health status of individuals, families, and communities.
ADN assists in identifying nursing problems of individuals.

BSN systematically establishes a data base with or without predesigned tools.
ADN collects data using established protocols or formats that are available in the immediate environment.

BSN implements a plan of care for clients, families, and groups in a variety of care settings.
ADN implements a plan of care for clients and families in a structured care setting.

BSN continually evaluates the responses of the nursing care to individuals and groups and initiates change based on the evaluation.
ADN participates in the evaluation process using established criteria with patients, families, and members of the nursing team.

Appendix B: Organizations Supporting the Baccalaureate as the Educational Requirement for Professional Nursing Practice*

American Association of Colleges of Nursing

American Association of Critical-Care Nurses

American Association of Nephrology Nurses and Technicians

American Association of Neuroscience Nurses

American Association of Nurse Anesthetists; Council on Accreditation of Nurse Anesthesia Educational Programs/Schools

American Association of Occupational Health Nurses

American Organization of Nurse Executives

American Public Health Association/Public Health Nurse Division

American Society of Post Anesthesia Nurses

Association of Operating Room Nurses

Association of Rehabilitation Nurses

Emergency Nurses Association

National Association of Pediatric Nurse Associates and Practitioners

National Federation of Licensed Practical Nurses

National League for Nursing

National Intravenous Therapy Association

National Student Nurses' Association

*This list includes only national nursing/specialty organizations. It does not include state boards of nursing. This list may be incomplete.

Nurses Association of the American College of Obstetricians and Gynecologists

Oncology Nursing Society*

Society for the Advancement of Nursing

Southern Regional Education Board; Council on Collegiate Education in Nursing

REFERENCES

1. Nutting MA: Educational Status of Nursing. US Bureau of Education. Nos. 7 and 475, Government Printing Office, 1912

2. Goldmark J: *Nursing and Nursing Education.* New York, National League for Nursing, 1922

3. Brown EL: *Nursing for the Future.* New York, Russell Sage Foundation, 1948

4. Lysaught J: *An Abstract for Action.* New York, McGraw-Hill, 1970

5. Montag ML: *Community College Education for Nursing.* New York, McGraw-Hill, 1959

6. Waters V: *Distinguishing Characteristics of Associate Degree Education for Nursing.* New York, National League for Nursing, 1978

7. Burnside H: *Perceived need for technical specialists* in *nursing care of hospitalized patients.* New York, League Exchange, 1974, 102

8. Position on education for nursing. Am J Nurs 63:95, 1965

9. Waters V: Distinctions are necessary. Am J Nurs 65:101, 1965

10. Johnson D: Competence in practice; technical and professional. Nurs Outlook 14:9, 1966

11. Kohnke MF: Literature versus practice in nursing education. Dissertation Abstracts, 33, 3481-A, 1973

12. McKenna ME: Differentiating between professional nursing practice and technical nursing practice. Dissertation Abstracts, 31, 4157-B, 1971

*The Oncology Nursing Society supports the baccalaureate, provided that baccalaureate programs are "accessible, flexible, affordable, and innovative."

13. Chamings PA, Teevan J: Comparison of expected competencies of baccalaureate and associate degree graduates in nursing. Image 11(1):16, 1979

14. DeBack V, Mentkowski M: Does the baccalaureate make a difference?: Differentiating nurse performance by education and experience. Nurs Educ 25:7, 1986

15. Content Analysis of Associate Degree and Baccalaureate Degree Competencies; A Working Paper. Unpublished manuscript. Milwaukee, National Commission on Nursing Implementation Project, 1986

16. Summary of Proceedings; 1982 Convention. Kansas City, MO, American Nurses' Association, p 96

17. *The Scope of Nursing Practice.* The American Nurses' Association, 1987

18. *The Preparation and Utilization of New Nursing Graduates.* Denver, Western Interstate Commission for Higher Education, 1986

19. Primm PL: Entry into practice; competency statements for BSNs and ADNs. Nurs Outlook 34:135, 1986

20. Rotkovitch R: ICON: A model of nursing practice for the future. Nurs Manag 17:54, 1986

21. Delegates hear survey results; people trust nurses to do more. Am Nurse, Sept. 1985, 3

ANN H. CARY, RN, PhD, MPH

CHAPTER 3

Credentialing: Opportunities and Responsibilities in Nursing

Background and Overview

There is a social contract between society and the professions. Under its terms, society grants the professions authority over functions vital to itself and permits them considerable autonomy in the conduct of their own affairs. In return, the professions are expected to act responsibly, always mindful of the public trust. Self-regulation to assure quality in performance is at the heart of this relationship. It is the authentic hallmark of a mature profession.[1]

The American Nurses' Association (ANA) publication, *Nursing: A Social Policy Statement*, reflects the contemporary perspective on the impact of credentialing on nurses, consumers, and society. Since 1903, when four states—North Carolina, New Jersey, New York, and Virginia—enacted the first nurse licensure laws in this country, the concept of both voluntary and statutory credentialing has been a hallmark of the profession of nursing. The philosophical approach to the regulation and recognition of nursing has not been without recurrent debate and political activism, both within and outside of the profession. However, it is these activities that have allowed the evolution of regulation to be responsive to the contemporary demands of consumers. Nursing can anticipate more, rather than less, in the way of dynamic interplay and collaboration between its professional societies and the demand exercised by society as a whole in the future.

CREDENTIALING PROCESSES

There are four methods of **credentialing,** or establishing the fact that one has the right to hold a position of authority, which influence registered nurses. In this discussion, references to the nurse mean registered nurses (RN) and exclude the licensed practical (vocational) nurse, unless otherwise noted. The process of credentialing includes licensure, certification, registration, and accreditation. Each contributes to a dimension of the quality assurance perspective used by the contemporary nursing profession.

LICENSURE

Licensure is one of the oldest mechanisms regulating the practice of nursing. It is defined in a 1971 Public Health Service (PHS) report as the process utilized by a government agency to grant permission to individuals to perform activities in a profession or occupation by ascertaining that the licensee has obtained a minimal degree of competency necessary to ensure the protection and safety of the public's health.[2] Each state implements its own legislative process for licensure of nursing within the specified limits of the state's statute. While licensure can exist for both individuals and institutions, discussion is limited herein to individuals.

All of the original, initial licensure laws for nurses were classified as permissive or voluntary. However, by 1987, all 50 states indicated that their licensure laws were mandatory or compulsory.[3] **Mandatory licensure** requires that all individuals practicing nursing must have a current nursing license. **Permissive licensure,** prevalent in the initial nurse licensing movement in the states, has allowed individuals to practice nursing without a license if the title *registered nurse* is not used and the individual does not profess to hold licensure.[3,4] The 1986 Health Occupations Revision Act for the District of Columbia indicates that the licensure law for nurses may qualify as being a permissive law.* It is possible that in those states more

* *Health Occupations Revision Act,* s^s 2-3301.3(d). Washington, D.C.: Dept. of Consumer and Regulatory Affairs, Occupational and Professional Licensing Administration, 1986, p 12. "Nothing in this chapter shall be construed to require licensure for or to otherwise regulate, restrict, or prohibit individuals from engaging in the practices, services, or activities set forth in the paragraphs of this subsection if the individuals do not hold themselves out, by title, description of services, or otherwise, to be practicing any of the health occupations regulated by this chapter."

recently changing the eligibility requirements for licensure, there are nurses who are licensed who do not meet the criteria under the mandatory licensure law, since these individuals are generally required to be "grand-fathered" under the contemporary law if they held valid licensure at the time of the licensure change. An example would be the states' requirement to have courses in their educational preparation in psychiatric nursing. For those nurses who graduated from programs not having the psychiatric preparation and holding valid licenses, their licenses would not have been declared invalid. Since nursing practice acts and licensure law requirements change, nurses should seek additional coursework in continuing education and formal academic credits to update their preparation congruent with the changing demands imposed by licensure.

Licensure laws vary among the states; however, they essentially contain the core components of the following:

- definition of the scope of nursing practice
- eligibility requirements for licensure
- exception clauses from licensure
- creation, functions, and qualifications of the licensing board and members
- grounds for revoking a license
- penalties for practicing without a license

Scope of Nursing Practice.   In defining the scope or domain of nursing practice in each state, the legal responsibilities of nurses are clarified. Often these definitions are intentionally broad, since specificity about functions and activities may imply limitation. With nursing practice and the health care field changing so rapidly, an "activity list" approach would be staggering in length and would require continual amendments to the law as new technology produced additional procedures that could be safely performed by nurses. Both the ANA and the National Council of State Boards of Nursing (NCSBN) have presented model legislation for nursing practice.[5,6] Although the two are quite different in structure and content, thereby offering states diversity in modeling, neither model appears to be enthusiastically utilized by the states. It is apparent that individual state diversity in nurse licensure laws is the rule rather than the exception.

The way in which states regulate the definition and activities of advanced nursing practice is germane to the issue of broad definitions of nursing practice. Forty-three states have included advanced nursing practice in their statutory or regulatory reforms.[7] In some cases the definitions allow for the coverage of advanced nursing practice through broadened interpretation or minor changes by state boards. This results in state statutes remaining essentially intact as written. Another approach utilized by states is to construct new definitions of nursing concerning advanced practice as well as typical nursing practice. This may entail prolonged legislative lobbying and political know-how on the part of nurses, as the road to achieving acceptance of overall definitions of the expanded role of the nurse is often fraught with dissention between nursing and medicine. A third approach is the promotion of regulations that guide nurses in the performance of their advanced practice.[8] Typically these authorizations come from joint (medical and nursing) licensure boards or a single professional board.

Eligibility Criteria.   Graduates seeking their initial licensure should contact the state board of nurse examiners in the state where they intend to be licensed. Graduates from schools of nursing are typically assisted in their application process by their schools. Nurses from other countries must meet the qualification for licensure by the states. They are expected to initially take the Commission on Graduates of Foreign Nursing Schools (CGFNS) qualifying examination in their own country to determine their proficiency in nursing and English comprehension. After obtaining the CGFNS certificate, the applicant must fulfill all licensure requirements of the state of application, including a passing score on the state board exam (NCLEX-RN).

Generally the requirements for licensure include the following:

- completion and degree from a state board of nursing approved school of nursing (Some states do not require that the student have completed nonnursing courses.)
- a passing score (NCSBN recommended score of 1600) on the NCLEX-RN examination, which is given in every state
- evidence of "good" moral character (may also include good physical and mental health)
- payment of required fee

Typically, states issue temporary licenses for graduates from state approved schools until the results of the first licensing exam are available.

The NCLEX-RN is a **criterion-reference** examination (a form of evaluation that determines what a person does or does not know in relationship to predetermined standards) initiated in July 1982. In contrast to the earlier **norm-referenced** (a form of evaluation that is interested in one's performance relative to the performance of others in a well-defined group), sectioned exam, the passing score on the NCLEX-RN is predicated on expert-generated criteria representative of acceptable nursing practice. Only one score is given, so the entire exam must be repeated if a failing score is received.

Once the license is received, it must be renewed in accordance with the licensure requirements in the state issuing the renewal. The requirements include a fee payment, the provision of demographic and occupational data, answers to questions concerning revocation and convictions of offenses since last renewal, and, in some states, evidence of the mandatory number of continuing education (CE) hours necessary for renewal. The CE emphasis is a reflection of the expectation that nurses maintain competence and currency in practice. The criteria for the issuance of CE units is set by a certifying agency, eg, ANA. CE credits can be issued for a variety of forms of education—formal academic courses, at-home programmed instructional materials, audiovisual learning formats, challenge exams, staff development programs, preparation and publication of articles and research, and grand rounds. While the mandatory nature and number of CE units varies among states (some require none), the nurse must not waiver in maintaining a documentation file for evidence of attendance. Participating in CE processes where the nurse's attendance is not documented or where there is no receipt of credit for CE units may constitute a lack of evidence to verify completion. This can be easily avoided with accurate documentation.

Personal mobility among locations is rarely hindered by the state licensure process for nurses. The utilization of a national standardized exam has made the **endorsement** or approval of nurses licensed in other states a simplified process. The requirements of the state licensure law in which the nurse is seeking licensure by endorsement must be met. There must be proof that the state of licensure has not revoked the nurse's license. In states where the formal nursing preparation is not equivalent to the state's requirements, courses and the examination may be mandatory. In the case where requirements are met, the state board exam is not retaken. Licensure by endorsement has replaced the former process of licensure by **reciprocity,** which consisted of accepting licenses only if each state involved accepted the other's licenses.

Licensure Exemption.   State licensure laws typically specify who is exempt from licensure, and this will vary among states. Examples of exceptions to licensure may include anyone supplying nursing assistance in an emergency; basic students in nursing programs; anyone currently licensed in a state who may be caring for clients temporarily in another state; anyone employed by the US government as a nurse; a legally qualified nurse serving with the Red Cross during a disaster; anyone employed not as a nurse and performing family remedies or practicing in accordance with religious tenets of a church.[3] It is prudent to require that exemptions from licensure be received in writing from the state board rather than relying on assurances from instructions or individuals from whom employment or volunteer status is sought.

Licensing Bodies.   The board of nursing examiners, created to administer and enforce the state nursing laws, may be known by many names (health professions board, state nursing occupation board, etc). The responsibilities of the state boards entail the oversight activities necessary to assure that the nursing practice act is followed. This is accomplished through setting minimum standards and establishing rules and regulations to implement the law. In addition, demographic and occupational data are collected on the constituency and collaboration is maintained with other state and professional boards. Typical responsibilities include the following:

- approving minimum standards for programs of nursing in the state
- evaluating applicants for licensure eligibility
- issuing licenses
- invoking sanctions against those who may not practice within minimum standards or who violate the law
- issuing limitations for licensure for identified individuals
- mandating activities required to demonstrate competency and currency for licensure renewal

Most boards of nursing have consumer and other health professional representation in their board membership.

Revocation and Penalties. The **revocation** or cancellation of a nurse's license is a serious process. Grounds for revocation are discussed in each state's nurse practice act and may vary among states. Activities constituting grounds for revocation may include the following:

- practicing while impaired by biochemical substances, physical or mental disabilities
- practicing negligently or outside the scope of practice
- aiding others to illegally practice nursing as specified by law
- fraudulently obtaining a license
- practicing while license is suspended or revoked
- being convicted of a felony or a crime of a vile nature
- demonstrating unprofessional conduct

This last condition is purposefully vague in state laws so as not to prevent the inclusion of activities that may have been overlooked. Activities that may fall under this condition include the following:

- violating confidentiality of clients
- demonstrating unsafe nursing practice through inappropriate judgment
- failing to follow policies and procedures to insure client safety
- inflicting abuse—physical or mental—on clients
- failing to supervise others for whom responsible

- falsifying documentation
- failing to report factual data of incompetent/illegal practices of licensed health professionals

While state laws and judicial interpretation in the courts may not include or be limited to these examples, they guide the nurse in areas of concern for licensure revocation. The *Code of Ethics* for nurses can be a source of guidance for the adherence to professional expectations for licensed nurses.[9]

In the event that charges for a violation of the state nursing practice act are raised, the nurse is accorded due process under the constitution. The state board will receive a field report and is mandated to investigate it. The nurse must be notified of the charge and allowed time to summon a defense. Hearings are held by the board or a state judicial officer, at which the evidence of the plaintiff and defendant is presented. The outcomes of the hearing may be that charges are dismissed; that the individual may be reprimanded or censured; and/or that the individual's license is suspended or revoked. Reinstatement or reissuance of the license is the judgment and responsibility of the board. Once licenses are suspended or revoked, penalties for practicing without a current license are the same as for those holding no license. Penalties can vary from fines to imprisonment.

The licensure of registered nurses is considered mandatory in every state. It serves as the minimum entry requirement for being employed as a registered nurse. Since licensure conveys the legal authority to practice as a licensed registered nurse in the state of licensure, its power, enforcement, and penalties for violation cannot be underestimated. All nurses should have a current copy of the state nurse practice act for review.

Sunset laws provide the regulatory structure for requiring the intermittent reevaluations of licensing agencies to determine if board changes or activities need to be implemented. Most state nursing boards have reevaluated their practice acts to reflect changes in society and practice.[10] These new or amended laws may contain differences from previous regulations that require nurses to be knowledgeable of the content of the current act. Since the sunset laws in the states that have adopted them will mandate continued examination of the boards and their practice acts, nursing may expect that the state practice act will continue to evolve to reflect movements of the health care industry, its consumers, and the science of nursing.

CERTIFICATION

In contrast to licensure, **certification** is generally viewed as a voluntary mechanism that contributes to the professional credentialing system for nurses. It is also defined in the PHS report as a process instituted by a professional association or agency (nongovernmental) that awards recognition to individuals distinguished by meeting the predetermined criteria set forth by the organization.[2] Methods for qualification may be specified academic achievement levels (graduation with specific degrees), length of employment in the specialty field, and/or performance outcomes on examinations. Usually letters of reference and endorsement must be supplied for those seeking certification. Certification opportunities for nurses are sponsored by professional organizations, institutions, or the state of practice.

Professional Certification. Certification in nursing differentiates the distinguished practice of a nursing specialty from the implied general practice knowledge base indicated by the licensure process. It creates the opportunity for nurses who have developed a specialized knowledge base and practice to earn a measure of distinction for that specialization.

The ANA established its certification program in 1973. This has remained a voluntary program for nurses to demonstrate their "qualifications, practice and nursing knowledge."[11] From 1975 to 1986 more than 40,000 nurses received and are holding ANA certification. The general eligibility requirements are that the applicant hold a current license to practice as a registered nurse and meet specific eligibility requirements of the particular area of the specialty. There is a fee required for application, as well as for the examination. Testing sites for the examination are in every state, Guam, and the Virgin Islands. Currently there are 17 areas in which certification is awarded. In 1988 a school nurse certification was added. Table 3-1 specifies the certification practice areas and designation initials to add to RN.

The issue of currency in certified areas is addressed in the fact that the certification is confirmed for a period of five years. Options for renewal include the submission of evidence of continuing education (number of units specified) during the five-year period of valid certification or achievement of a passing score on the examination again. Those opting not to recertify at the end of the five-year period may apply at a later time.

For nurses seeking certification recognition, obtaining a copy of the current certification catalogue is the initial step. Information in the catalogue will assist in determining if the eligibility requirements for the area of certification can be met. There are unique requirements among specialty areas that demand a careful matching of the applicant's preparation, professional positions, responsibilities, supervision, and length of job position with those described in the catalogue.

Nurse anesthetists are certified through a national exam administered by the Council on Certification of Nurse Anesthetists. Eligibility for certification is based on graduation from a school for nurse anesthetists accredited by the Council on Accreditation. Both councils are independent bodies of the American Association of Nurse Anesthetists (AANA).

TABLE 3-1

ANA Certification Practice Areas and Designations[11]

Generalist Certification—RNC—Registered Nurse, Certified
  Medical Surgical Nurse
  Gerontological Nurse
  Psychiatric and Mental Health Nurse
  Maternal and Child Health Nurse
  Child and Adolescent Nurse
  High Risk Perinatal Nurse
  Community Health Nurse
  School Nurse
Practitioner Certification—RNC—Registered Nurse, Certified
  Gerontological Nurse Practitioner
  Pediatric Nurse Practitioner
  Adult Nurse Practitioner
  Family Nurse Practitioner
  School Nurse Practitioner
Specialist Certification—RNCS—Registered Nurse, Certified Specialist
  Clinical Specialist in Medical Surgical Nursing
  Clinical Specialist in Adult Psychiatric and Mental Health Nursing
  Clinical Specialist in Child and Adolescent Psychiatric and Mental Health
    Nursing
Nursing Administration Certification
  Nursing Administration—RNCNA—Registered Nurse, Certified in Nursing
    Administration
  Nursing Administration, Advanced—RNCNAA—Registered Nurse, Certified in
    Nursing Administration, Advanced

Nurse-midwives are certified by a national certification program for nurse-midwives administered by the American College of Nurse-Midwives (ACNM). A separate body within the ACNM approves educational programs for nurse-midwives.

Nurse practitioners may be authorized to practice by certification and in some states by licensure. A nurse practitioner is a registered nurse who has successfully completed a formal program of study designed to prepare him/her to deliver primary health care, including the ability to: a) assess the health status of individuals and families through health and medical history taking, physical examination, and defining health and developmental problems; b) institute and provide continuity of health care to clients; c) provide instruction and counseling to individuals, families, and groups; and d) work in collaboration with other health care providers and agencies. Other terms used to indicate credentialing are *approval, registration, authorization,* and *recognition.*[8] (See Table 3–2.)

Institutional Certification. Academic, commercial, or health care agencies sponsor certification programs for nurses in specialty areas. In fact, the development of the nurse practitioner as a specialty was initially and predominantly instituted through the institutional certification process in the 1970s.[17]

Standards for the certification process are at the discretion of the sponsor and are likely to vary across institutions in content, length, standards for admission and completion, method of competency verification, and cost. Certification by one institution may have limited recognition by another institution or on a state or national level.

While the institutional model for certification may fulfill an immediate, localized need for specialty preparation, the endorsement for specialty practice preparation is heavily weighted toward the master's degree and professional certification model.

TABLE 3-2

National Organizations Sponsoring Certification Programs for Nursing Specialization[3,11,12]

American Nurses' Association (18 areas by 1988)
American Association of Critical Care Nurses Certification Corporation
American Board of Neurosurgical Nursing
American Association of Nurse Anesthetists
American College of Nurse-Midwives Division of Examiners
American Urological Association, Allied
Association of Operating Room Nurses Certification Board
Association for Practitioners in Infection Control
National Intravenous Therapy Association
NAACOG Certification Corporation
    Ob/Gyn nurse practitioners
    Inpatient obstetric nurses
    Neonatal/ICU nurses
    Neonatal nurse practitioners
American Board of Occupational Health Nurses
Board of Nephrology Examiners
Emergency Nurses Association
National Board of Pediatric Nurse Practitioners and Associates, Rehabilitation
    Pediatric nurses
    Practitioners and associates

State Certification. A regulatory structure for obtaining certification for specialty practice is through the state boards of nursing in states that require a legal endorsement. This process was initiated in the mid-1970s as nurse anesthetists, nurse practitioners, and nurse-midwives sought additional legal endorsement for specialty practice beyond the basic license. More than half the states have a legal endorsement for advanced practice. State certification requirements vary and may include the following:

- certification from a recognized professional organization
- state examinations
- approved educational programs
- continuing education documentation

State certification is viewed by some as increasing the recognition and defining the specialty practice, and controlling the activities of the practitioners through legal sanctions. Additionally, it impacts on the reimbursement outcomes and malpractice insurance avenues for these nurses.[18]

Due to differences in state certification requirements, this process may limit professional mobility and encourage nonstandardized criteria for entry into specialty advanced practice. The ANA supports voluntary national professional certification rather than mandatory state certification.

In 1977 the PHS—DHEW (Public Health Service—Department of Health, Education and Welfare; currently Health and Human Services) recommended that a national certifying commission be established to certify the certifying organizations. The functions recommended for this national commission were[13]:

- to develop and evaluate criteria and policies to recognize certifying organizations and to monitor their compliance with the criteria
- to participate in the development of national standards of credentialing health occupations
- to provide consultation and technical assistance to certifying organizations

The National Commission for Health Certifying Agencies is the current body of certifiers setting uniform standards and guidelines for allied health professionals.

Nurses can obtain certification through three vehicles—professional organizations, academic and/or health care agencies, and state boards of nursing. Contact with the professional, institutional, and licensing organizations that may represent nurses can determine the availability of certification opportunities.

REGISTRATION

The term *registration* is linked in the PHS definition of certification, "Certification or Registration."[2] There is no alternate definition given. However, in the nurse credentialing study, the term is defined differently. **Registration** is a process of documenting past and current competency and achievements of an individual. Membership on the registry consists of nurses who are assessed and assigned a status based on the assessment data.[14] The ANA catalogue on certification does not use the term in conjunction with certification.

ACCREDITATION

Accreditation is a credentialing term that applies to agencies and organizations rather than individuals. It is a process by which an agency or organization evaluates and recognizes an institution or program as meeting specified criteria and standards. This approach is voluntary in nature and is awarded by a nongovernmental organization.[2,15]

The accreditation process allows an agency/program/institution to examine its strengths and limitations through an in-depth peer review process. The National League for Nursing (NLN) has had an accreditation program for schools of nursing education since 1949 (under the title of National Nursing Accrediting Service) and for community nursing and home health agencies since 1966. Application for accreditation includes the creation of a self-study report, an on-site review by peer visitors to amplify, clarify, and verify the documentation, and the payment of a fee. The accreditation status is valid for a specified amount of time, after which the process must be completed again. State boards of nursing approve basic nursing programs in their respective states as an adjunct to their graduates being eligible to take state licensing exams. Licensure eligibility for nurse graduates and federal funding for nursing are intimately bound with accreditation by the State Board of Nurse Examiners and the NLN respectively.

The accreditation model is an organizational program approach that is common to health care and educational institutions. The Joint Commission for the Accreditation of Hospitals (JCAH) accredits hospitals and is anticipating offering its accreditation process to home health care agencies by 1988.[16] Regional associations of colleges and secondary schools accredit colleges and schools containing nursing programs.

The nursing profession has access to credentialing opportunities on both the individual and organizational level, from both legal/mandatory, voluntary, nonfederal sources, and for different levels of standards (entry to advanced specialist). Nursing can reflect on both the strengths and weaknesses in their credentialing system among other health professionals. Marching in step with the changing health care scene and incorporating consumer and professional concerns about the regulation of nursing practice can augment nursing's history of credentialing leadership among professionals.

Impacts on the Nurse, the Consumer, and Society

THE NURSE

Credentialing poses both opportunity and responsibility for nurses, consumers, and society. For nurses in particular it offers the means of establishing a licensed or specialization credential whereby minimum standards for each are apparent, attainable, and recognizable to peers and society. Since the criteria for the credentials are standardized nationally (licensure exams, national organization criteria), and are predominantly consistent from state to state, the nurse's credentials may not be imperiled by interstate mobility.

Professional regulation and recognition are opportunities afforded by credentialing. The establishment of professional qualifications and the ability of nurse peer regulation through the construction of nurse practice acts, licensure laws, state boards of nursing, and the continual revision of nurse practice acts set the tone for the nursing profession to respond to consumer demands, evolutions in practice, and the demarcation of responsibilities among other professionals. Nurses are the most knowledgeable about their professional preparation and subsequent utilization by consumers. They must continue to educate employers, consumers, and society about the capabilities, limitations, and realistic expectations of nurse professionals. Professionalism can be enhanced through nurses actively participating in the regulation of their professional scope of practice.

The opportunity offered to nurses in recognition of distinction in a practice specialization is critical. The acknowledgment of competence among professional peers can provide both psychological and monetary rewards. With the body of scientific knowledge rapidly advancing, there comes a time where today's information quickly yields in accuracy to tomorrow's discoveries. Nurses who maintain the leading edge of new knowledge and proficiency have the opportunity to be recognized for their professional achievement.

The responsibilities imposed on nurses by credentialing are not to be considered lightly. Violations of licensure laws may have legal sanctions and may result in criminal and civil penalties. Nurses must actively participate in the updating of the nurse practice acts and encourage peers to maintain the scope of practice. The nurse has an ethical and, in some states, a legal obligation to report violations of legal practice. For the profession of nursing to maintain self-regulation, the profession must continue to hold its members accountable to the standards. Nursing is not "they"; it is "we." Nurses must contribute to standard setting, monitoring, and currency of practice regulation in order for the professional regulations to be successful.

Professional growth is the responsibility of nurses who are licensed. It can only be through continued knowledge and skill acquisition that nurses maintain a currency and depth of professional practice. The employment of nurses reflects areas of increasing specialization as scientific and technical knowledge accelerate. This may forebode that nurses must know more and develop greater competencies in specific rather than general areas. It is the responsibility of nurses to validate and assert their qualifications, knowledge, and practice so that efficient utilization of their skills can be implemented in the health care delivery system. Certification facilitates the recognition and responsibility of that achievement of distinction. Nurses with expertise must continue to participate in the setting of standards, criteria, and essential content of the certification process.

The efforts to improve professionalism through the dynamic activities involved in credentialing can insure consumers and nurses that nursing is committed to the quality of nursing practice. Effective self-regulation is the underpinning of peer and consumer trust.

THE CONSUMER

The credentialing process for nurses deeds opportunity and responsibility for consumers as well. Clients and employers of nurses have the opportunity to screen them, based on their licensure status, as having demonstrated minimum standards of competency in nursing knowledge. This licensure exam does not judge the applicants' correct demonstration of nursing activities—only the knowledge of these activities. The program from which the student graduates is responsible for having provided supervision of the correct performance of activities, which should be reflected partially in the academic grades. Because a licensed nurse is regulated by the provisions of the nurse practice act and licensure in a state, consumers can expect that they will not be harmed while under the care of the licensed nurse. The legal basis for this expectation can form the critical element of trust between the consumer and the nurse that there will be adherence to the letter and spirit of the law. With the practice of nursing being regulated by the states, the consumer can expect a higher level of nursing competency through the licensure process than from an unlicensed caregiver. This expectation is particularly valid when the nurse has achieved certification credentials in addition to the licensure designation, RN.

Consumers should require competent nursing services from individuals possessing the credentials. They must report perceived discrepancies in nursing care to the institutional nurse administrator and/or the state board of nursing. Complaints need to be factual and documented with evidence when possible. Nurses are responsible for assessing their need for professional development, while employers have the responsibility of offering staff development to keep nurses current and proficient. Licensure credentials must be checked for currency and violations corrected.

With the inclusion of consumers on many of the state boards of nursing, there is opportunity for consumers to add to their knowledge and to participate in the monitoring of nursing practice in their state. Consumers must act responsibly to contribute to the maintenance of current standards for nursing practice. Their active participation can reduce the concern that the regulatory board may promote professional self-interest to the detriment of consumer safety and concern for quality of care.

The connection between the credentialing of nurses and quality of care for consumers can be strengthened. Licensure is predicated on the attainment of minimum standards, certification is based on the assessment of knowledge, professional achievement and recognition of peers, and accreditation is awarded based on structural and process criteria. This connection can be greatly strengthened through the inclusion of outcome standards for credentialing. For example, in institutional accreditation, in addition to examining the organizational structure for its necessary components and the ratio of licensed nurses to clients/acuity, outcome indicators of mortality rates, consumer satisfaction scores, length of stay, readmission rates, and acuity differentials between admission and discharge might be monitored. The outcome indicators give a clearer picture of the results of the health care resources utilized for consumers and how the standards impact on the clients. Outcome standards for credentialing may be a stronger link to the quality of care conclusion than the current methods. Many organizations are clearly moving to develop this methodology for field testing.

SOCIETY

Societal values dictate the expectations for professionals. The profession of nursing as one of the oldest health professions remains a valued commodity of the US health care system. This is reflected in the monetary support for preparation, the legal sanction for nursing practice, and the dominant numbers of nurses as compared to other health professionals. The value for nursing can be maintained as long as nurses continue to fulfill unique functions and services demanded by contemporary society.

Credentialing contributes to the credibility of nursing that is valued by society. It promotes the adherence to minimum standards, recognizes professional achievement and advancement of knowledge, and conveys legal and professional concern for the safety of nursing services consumed by clients. Additionally, it acknowledges the expansion of nursing practice in the health care system in a supportive and regulatory manner.

Credentialing offers society an opportunity to judge the adequacy of professional performance and self-regulation. Society incurs the responsibility to support actions that benefit the nursing care consumption of its members and to clearly indicate when changes in the nursing profession are warranted by consumers. With credentialing as the process of communication between society and the nursing profession, consumers and nurses have a vehicle through which to convey their values.

Future Considerations

The credentialing opportunities for nurses do not exist without questions about the current mechanisms. Concerns about the validity of the licensure process have to do with the promotion of professional self-interest and access to practice, the nature and extent of enforcement for infractions, the theoretical limit to mobility imposed by the state licensure process, inconsistent national criteria for the renewal of licenses, and the limitation imposed on the use of personnel by health care systems. The inclusion of consumers on boards of nursing and the sunset laws requiring intermittent evaluations of licensing boards have broadened the consumer input and mandated that regulations and practice acts reflect the current scope of practice. The nursing profession must strive to determine the best ways to utilize consumer and other professional input in mandating the scope of practice. Consumers will continue to demand protection from harm in the consumption of health care services and will expect that the licensure laws protect the public interest.

With the growth of the multicorporation health care systems in the 1980s and 1990s, it is conceivable that the concept of institutional licensure may be rejuvenated to take advantage of the corporate philosophy of control of employees and positions as a cost-effective management strategy. The debate over a system of institutional vs. individual professional licensure was signaled in the 1971 *Report on Licensure and Related Health Personnel Credentialing by DHEW* (now HHS).[2] This was a proposal in which health care facilities would be responsible for the professional regulation of the people they employed by virtue of the institution's state license to operate. In this system of licensure it might be possible for health care personnel to float among job classifications, depending on the job descriptions, staff development education, and institutional experiences. The economic advantages for the general use of personnel in this manner are apparent. Institutions could substitute lesser qualified and less costly personnel for nursing activities.

Federally funded demonstration projects concluded that the concept was not practically feasible without major adjustment. Professional response to this proposal has resulted in flagrant opposition by the ANA, NLN, and AMA. Although promotion for the concept was miniscule by the late 1970s, there have been subsequent attempts to pass state legislation on behalf of institutional licensure, although none have succeeded to date. In the continuing push for cost containment in the health care system, more rather than less emphasis on institutional licensure of health professionals would be expected.

The debate over the state vs. federal regulations of licensure for nurses stems from the inconsistencies among state licensure requirements. Eligibility requirements vary, as do the requirements for renewal of licenses. The status quo poses the consideration of whether national licensure standards might improve the comparability of licensed professional nurses and therefore the safety for consumers of health care systems in different regions. The administration of a national licensing exam has been one move toward consistency. Nurses, legislators, and professional organizations will continue the debate as political and consumer pressures ebb and flow.

Another area of inconsistency under challenge is the continuing education (CE) requirements for licensure and certification renewal. While a number of states require continuing education, enforcement and monitoring is a problem. Should continuing education be mandated more consistently on a national or state level, teaching and screening mechanisms for enforcement would need to be strengthened. The question of which organizations would be capable of certifying the CE and what modes of learning would be required (knowledge, skill demonstration, attitudes) need to be addressed. This may be an area where something is better than nothing in the states to demonstrate currency for renewal until a valid model has been field tested and criteria have been established. It is possible that a licensure and adjunct certification model for renewal is a viable option to judge proficiency in current nursing knowledge and practice.

The system of credentialing can be only as strong as the system of monitoring and enforcement for compliance. The expenses involved in these processes may need to be escalated as the procedure becomes tighter in the attempt to make the method successful. As consumers become more knowledgeable and assertive, complaints concerning professional nursing infractions may escalate. The profession has the responsibility to investigate the dispute vigorously in an attempt to determine the true situation. Professionals must consider objective yet firm actions for those in violation of the self-regulatory nature of the credential process if it is to be successful. Professional rehabilitation and probation can be critical supports for those who qualify. The credentialing system in nursing must aggressively protect the public's consumption of nursing as safe, competent, and ethical if it is to enjoy continuing societal support in the future. Consistent peer regulation is the only alternative if the survival of nursing as a profession is to be maintained.

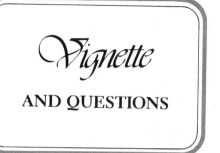

Vignette

AND QUESTIONS

Two senior students from the school of nursing are meeting with two representatives from the school of pharmacy, the school of physical therapy, and the school of social work to discuss professional quality assurance mechanisms in a health professions seminar course. After hearing from the other school representatives, the students ascertain that professional credentialing is common to all. Nursing has a legal mechanism directed by individual states to direct the entrance and exit from the profession in the form of current licensure. In addition, the renewal process for licensure may have additional eligibility requirements (CEU) in accordance with some state laws. The nursing practice act guides the scope of nursing practice in the state. The state boards of nursing are the bodies empowered with administering the standards, hearing complaints and recommending disposition, and approving the educational process at the schools of nursing in the states. The voluntary mechanism in credentialing is through professional certification, which acknowledges the individual's knowledge, professional achievement, and peer recognition in an area of specialization. The remaining mechanism is the process of voluntary accreditation of health care institutions and educational nursing programs. This type of credentialing is earned by organizations rather than individuals. The credentialing process in nursing is provided through legal, professional, group, and individual entities and can be viewed as addressing professional quality assurance at a number of levels.

1. Read the nurse practice act in your state. Can you develop a job description of a nurse from the act? Share the job description with your peers.

2. What new recommendations would you make to the state board of nursing regarding the eligibility and renewal criteria for licensure in your state?

3. Debate the advantages and disadvantages of institutional licensure vs. individual licensure for nurses.

4. What might be the advantages and disadvantages of a national credentialing system for nurses?

INFORMATION SOURCES

American Nurses' Association (ANA)
    Certification Registrar
    2420 Pershing Road
    Kansas City, MO 64108

American Journal of Nursing (AJN)
    Directory Issue—Listing of International, National, State and
    Regional Organizations

National League for Nursing (NLN)
    10 Columbus Circle
    New York, NY 10019-1350

Joint Commision on Accreditation of Hospitals (JCAH)
    840 N. Lake Shore Drive
    Chicago, IL 60611

National Council of State Boards of Nursing (NCSBN)
    625 N. Michigan Ave., Suite 1544
    Chicago, IL 60611

National Commission for Health Certifying Agencies (NCHCA)
    1011 Connecticut Avenue, N.W., Suite 700
    Washington, DC 20036

American Association of Nurse Anesthetists (AANA)
    216 West Higgins
    Park Ridge, IL 60068

American Association of Critical Care Nurses (AACN)
    One Civic Plaza, Suite 330
    Newport Beach, CA 92660

American Board of Neurosurgical Nursing (ABNN)
    7500 Old Oak Blvd.
    Cleveland, OH 44130

American College of Nurse-Midwives (ACNM)
    1522 K. Street, N.W.
    Suite 1120
    Washington, DC 20005

American Urological Association, Allied (AUAA)
6845 Lake Shore Drive
P.O. Box 9397
Raytown, MO 64133

Association of Operating Room Nurses (AORN)
10170 E. Mississippi Ave.
Denver, CO 80231

Association for Practitioners in Infection Control (APIC)
505 E. Hawley St.
Mundelein, IL 60060

National Intravenous Therapy Association (NITA)
87 Blanchard Rd.
Cambridge, MA 02138

NAACOG Certification Corporation (NCC)
645 N. Michigan Ave., Suite 1058
Chicago, IL 60611

Emergency Nurses Association
230 E. Ohio, 6th Floor
Chicago, IL 60611

American Association of Occupational Health Nurses, Inc.
50 Lenox Pointe
Atlanta, GA 30324

National Association of Pediatric Nurse Associates and Practitioners
1000 Maplewood Dr., Suite 104
Maple Shade, NJ 08052

Public Health Nursing/American Public Health Association
1015 Fifteenth St., N.W.
Washington, DC 20005

REFERENCES

1. *Nursing: A Social Policy Statement.* Kansas City, MO, American Nurses' Association, 1980

2. US Department of Health, Education and Welfare: *Report on licensure and related health personnel credentialing.* DHEW Publ. No. (HSM) 72-11, 1972, p 7

3. Kelly L: *Dimensions of Professional Nursing*. NY, Macmillan, 1985

4. Pinkerton S: Legislative issues in licensure of registered nurses. In McCloskey, J, and Grace H. (Eds), *Current Issues in Nursing*. Oxford, England, Blackwell Scientific Publication, 1981

5. American Nurses' Association: *The Nursing Practice Act: Suggested State Legislation*. Kansas City, MO, The Association, 1980

6. *The Model Nursing Practice Act*. Chicago, IL: National Council of State Boards of Nursing, 1982

7. LaBar C: *The Regulation of Advanced Nursing Practice as Provided for in Nursing Practice Acts and Administrative Rules*. Kansas City, MO, American Nurses' Association, 1983; and LaBar, C., *Boards of Nursing, Composition, Membership Qualifications, and Statutory Authority* Kansas City, MO, American Nurses' Association, 1985

8. Lang NM: Nurse practice acts: The advanced practitioner. *In Patterns in Specialization: Challenge to the Curriculum*. NY, National League for Nursing, 1986, pp 67–76

9. *Code for Nurses With Interpretive Statements*. Kansas City, American Nurses' Association, 1985

10. Grobe S: Sunset laws. *Am J Nurs* 81:1355, July, 1981

11. *American Nurses Association 1987 Certification Catalogue*. American Nurses' Association, 1986, p 2

12. Cipriano PF: Certification: Self-regulation for specialty practice. *Patterns in Specialization: Challenge to the Curriculum*. NY, National League for Nursing, 1986, p 77

13. US Department of Health, Education and Welfare: *Credentialing Health Manpower*. DHEW Publ. No. (OS)-77-50057, 1977, pp 7–17

14. *The Study of Credentialing in Nursing: A New Approach*, vol 1. The Report of the Committee: Milwaukee, 1979

15. Lenn MP: Accreditation: The state of the art. In *Patterns in Specialization: Challenge to the Curriculum* NY: National League for Nursing, 1986, p 41

16. *Hosp Weekly*, 29:19, 1986

17. Sultz HA, Henry OM, Kinyon LJ, Buck GM, Bullough B: A decade of change for nurse practitioners. Nurs Outlook, parts 1-3. 31-137, 216, 266, 1983

18. Third Party Reimbursement, Pennsylvania Nurse 42:5, 3, 1987

SUSAN B. GANTZ, RN, MSN

Entrepreneurial Nurses: Where Did They Come From? Where Are They Going?

CHAPTER 4

Background and Overview

A familiar dialogue:

"You're a nurse? What hospital do you work in?"

The enlightened dialogue:

"You're a nurse? What field do you specialize in?"

The futuristic dialogue?

"You're a nurse? What do you do?"

For a small but growing number of nurses, today's answer is:

"I operate an adult day care center with support classes for family care takers."

"I manage a brokerage firm that matches corporate clients with a health promotion program that meets their needs."

"I manufacture and distribute toys that stimulate newborns' ability to develop neurologically."

"I conduct seminars and workshops for nurses who want to establish independent practice."

54

"We provide *total* home care to anyone requiring health management services."

"I design software to support efficient interdisciplinary case management."

"I am a therapist in private practice, specializing in women's health."

These are actual examples. What do these nurses have in common? They own and operate businesses. These nurses are addressing areas of concern and interest to nursing, and are practicing within existing social and legal constraints. Many nurses see the small business as a means to achieve economic independence, autonomy, control of practice, and personal satisfaction. Such nurses have successfully combined two distinct bodies of knowledge: nursing and business.

As part of learning and practicing new things, many people have these thoughts—about school, work, or projects:

I could do this better.

I have a really good idea. I know I could sell it.

I want more for myself than this.

Yet, it is difficult to act on these ideas. Such action requires initiative, commitment, persistence, knowledge, and optimism to institute change. What makes the difference between the dreamers and the doers? Does it take a certain personality? Are you born with business sense? Peter Drucker,[1] a leading expert on entrepreneurship, says no. Is creating a nursing product or service something that everyone can do? Probably yes. Is it something every nurse should do? Definitely not.

A nurse pursuing entrepreneurial activity must be willing to face risk and, possibly, failure. New products or services created by entrepreneurs are notable for their unpredictable success. Who could have predicted the economic return on plastic sweatsuits, hulahoops, sugarless gum, sawdust bread, bee pollen for arthritis, and electrolyte drinks for athletic prowess? Even more puzzling, why are day care centers and hospices struggling to survive when there seems to be unlimited need? Consumers do not always make rational investments with their health care dollars.

This chapter looks at the following:

- a perspective on past, present, and future nurses who are entrepreneurial (Who are they? What drives them? What contributions do they make to nursing?)
- a consideration of enabling strengths and restraining limitations on entrepreneurial activity for nurses, imposed by existing health care delivery systems, laws, patient expectations, and personal characteristics
- a discussion of trends offering promise for potential entrepreneurial nurses

- the impact on society and traditional nursing practice by nurses who
  pursue entrepreneurial activity
- the future for entrepreneurs in nursing

BACKGROUND: WHO ARE ENTREPRENEURS?

There is currently, in nursing, a fascination with nurses who are entrepreneurs sparked by professional, economic, cultural, and technological trends. The term "nurse entrepreneur" appears frequently in current nursing literature, yet it describes neither job content nor job context. The term is an attempt to incorporate and recognize the contributions made by nurses to the profession by those who choose innovative business endeavors as effective ways to impact the definition and delivery of nursing services. However, other professionals conduct entrepreneurial activity without designation as "attorney entrepreneurs," "accounting entrepreneurs," or "engineering entrepreneurs." The confusion comes partly from the linking of two nouns: nurse and entrepreneur. Clarity is gained by using an adjective to further describe the noun: the entrepreneurial nurse.

Webster's Third International Unabridged Dictionary [2] defines **entrepreneur** as "the organizer of an economic venture who owns, manages, and assumes the risk of a business with the intent to generate a profit." The American Nurses' Association (ANA) currently defines an entrepreneur as an individual who is self-employed, is generating income through direct reimbursement for services, and is engaged in activity related to nursing. However, this definition excludes individuals such as Lillian Wald, founder of the Henry Street Settlement House in New York, who was an employee of a charity, and who expanded the role of nurses through innovative services to new markets. Today, it also excludes creative clinical nurses who innovate within existing agencies because they are salaried.

In *The Entrepreneurial Life,* [3] A. Silver identifies the word "entrepreneur," as first used by the French in the sixteenth century, to describe men engaged in leading military expeditions. Silver credits Joseph Schumpter, a German economist at Harvard, for defining the criterion of entrepreneurship as innovation, doing things in a new way, shaping subsequent events and outcomes. Silver's analysis of entrepreneurial activity highlights three elements: creativity/energy, focus/intensity, and frustration. He identifies the entrepreneur as someone dissatisfied with his or her career path (though not with the chosen field) who decides to make a mark on the world by developing and selling a product or service that will make life easier for a large number of people.

Riccardi and Dayani, authors of *The Nurse Entrepreneur,* [4] identify the entrepreneur as an innovator of a business enterprise who recognizes opportunities to introduce a new product, a new production process, or an improved organization, and who raises necessary money, assembles the factors of production, and organizes an operation to exploit the opportunity.

Peter Drucker, in the opening chapter of *Innovation and Entrepreneurship*,[1] develops the concept that entrepreneurial activity is systematic, managed, purposeful innovation. For Drucker, to be entrepreneurial an enterprise has to have special characteristics over and above being new and small. It must create something new, something different; it must change or transmute values; and it must create a new market and a new customer. He emphasizes that the entrepreneur always searches for change, responds to it, and exploits it as an opportunity. This is the vision and challenge for nurses who wish to be entrepreneurs.

In further refining the characteristics and activities of entrepreneurs, Gifford Pinchott III[5] introduced his analysis of the entrepreneurial potential *within* organizations and developed the concept of "intrapreneuring." The **intrapreneurs** have many of the same drives and skills that entrepreneurs possess, but choose to work within existing organizations, according to Pinchott, because they want access to corporate resources, rewards, recognition, technology, and credibility.

Intrapreneurs effectively delegate a number of tasks to stay focused on doing what they do best. They may be cynical about the system, but are confident about their ability to use it for their own purposes. Intrapreneurs understand marketing both within and outside of the organization, and see advantages to sharing and purchasing needed resources among affiliated organizations. They are salaried employees—for example, university faculty who develop practice centers, staff nurses who implement commercial research product testing for fees, or hospital nurses who develop day-care centers for children with special medical needs.

Entrepreneurial nurses create innovative business ventures that are within nursing. This definition excludes nurses involved in businesses that are not innovative (eg, nurse registry for private duty) and nurses who may be involved in innovative ventures outside nursing (eg, shopping and errand services for the busy executive). Finally, it also excludes nurses who leave nursing to work in other professions such as medicine, ministry, and law. They bring a nursing perspective to those professions, but owe first allegiance to another discipline.

In summary, entrepreneurial nurses innovate, provide new services or products, or create new markets for traditional services. They are legally and financially accountable for activities and responsible for the acquisition and allocation of resources. Entrepreneurial nurses operate with the intent to make a profit, expand, or grow, and manage all aspects/functions contributing to development, distribution, and reimbursement/remuneration of their innovation. They assume responsibility for risks and reap rewards of success while earning income from their business activities. Some entrepreneurial nurses own their business and some have intrapreneurial agreements with employers.

HISTORICAL PERSPECTIVE ON ENTREPRENEURIAL NURSING

In the United States entrepreneurial nursing has roots in the innovative practice of Lillian Wald at the Henry Street Nurses Settlement (1893), the creation of visiting nurses associations in Boston, Philadelphia, and Chicago in the 1880s, the establishment of private duty registries, and the founding of Mary Breckenridge's Frontier Nursing Service in 1928. However, between 1930 and 1965, nursing practice became increasingly supervised, regulated, and structured by those outside nursing practice: physicians, administrators, educators, and public officials. Three major restrictions on innovation emerged.

First, medicine dominated the health care arena with the development of sophisticated diagnostic technologies and advances in pharmaceuticals. Lives saved by surgery and antibiotics gave tremendous power to the specialized practitioners who controlled access to these desirable products and services.

Second, nurse practice acts were developed at nursing's request to set quality standards and definition for entry into practice. Surprisingly, this often was done by boards with no nursing representation. Many of the nurse practice acts were written to exclude untrained nurses from practice, but were rigidly prescriptive. As health care changed and roles were expanded consistent with advanced training, those acts were used to limit nursing actions. Many of the acts remain to be rewritten in terms consistent with existing practice and health care policy.

Third, hospitals became the centralized site for the delivery of medical and health care services, and, over time, became the largest employers of nurses. Before this period most nurses were in private practice in community settings where they delivered many of the supportive-educative services now associated with advanced (baccalaureate) preparation.

By 1965 the demands for specialized care, the medicalization of health, the use of complicated technology within hospitals, and the development of effective, complex drugs all served to reinforce professional dominance of the physician and the hospital as the source for health care.

The 1970s, however, brought significant changes for potential entrepreneurial nurses.

- The feminist movement raised a variety of gender issues. Although it had some adverse effects on traditionally female occupations such as teaching and nursing, the message was heard.[6]

- Increasing costs of care, awareness of iatrogenic illness, a nostalgia for putting mind and body back together, and readily available health information together gave momentum to self-care and an interest in the consumer's point of view.
- Lifestyle and person-inflicted deaths (homicide, suicide, accidents, heart disease, etc) replaced nature and disease as leading causes of death for all ages.
- Some associations (ANA, NLN, and nurse specialty organizations) and government agencies (first HEW, then HHS) saw promise in supporting expanded roles, including the nurse practitioner and other arenas in primary care.
- Lucille Kinlein,[7] credited as the first modern nurse in independent practice, hung out her shingle, surviving the challenges of peers, patients, and payment.
- Increasing numbers of nurses obtained bachelor's degrees and experienced the reality shock of the work environment. With determination they sought the responsibility, accountability, achievement, growth, and recognition promised them with university preparation.

Impacts on the Nurse, the Consumer, and Society

THE NURSE

The character of nursing in the decades ahead will closely reflect deliberate career choices, since virtually all options are available to women. Few have studied the role of men in nursing, and it is almost impossible to predict changes that would occur with a truly gender neutral profession. Many of the following statements, therefore, address changes that are related to women's roles in professional nursing.

For many young women in the 1950s and 1960s, the goal was to "get married." Young women in the 1970s sought to "get a job." The young women of the 1980s seek to "develop a career." For women of the 1990s, it may well be to "start a business." Advancement in the business world as an entrepreneur holds promise.

Women are moving into more responsible positions in business, but according to a University of Michigan study in 1985 (reported in *The Wall Street Journal*), only 2.6 percent of all corporate executives at or above the rank of vice president were women. One option available to those who want to move up the corporate ladder but are held back, may be to start their own business. Women own nearly 25 percent of all small businesses, according to latest census data (1982), and are starting businesses at three times the rate of males.

For a number of years, nursing has lost creative practitioners to real estate, insurance and stock brokerage firms, law, medicine, management, and small business. Today recruitment and retention provide major challenges for schools of nursing, hospitals, and nursing homes. New roles for nurses as case managers, independent contractors, private practitioners, and health advocates are constantly evolving.

Today's Entrepreneurial Nurse.   In reviewing the publications of entrepreneurial nurses and interviewing a small sample (ten), similarities were striking. The majority exhibited the following traits:

- products of university preparation in the activist 1960s
- attracted to the possibilities made visible in the 1970s
- frustrated in their earlier jobs
- experienced nurses (eight to ten years of practice) with specific expertise, eg, cardiac rehabilitation, diabetes chronic care, enterostomal therapy
- children of middle-class families where one or both parents were self-employed
- highly self-confident
- known as "rebels" and initiators of change in their traditional jobs

It is possible that these nurses are the product of a unique series of events. The majority are between the ages of 30 and 45 and many chose nursing because it offered an acceptable career in the 1960s. A few even admitted that they would not choose nursing today, but none regretted the choice of their youth. It is not as clear if nursing continues to attract individuals with characteristics associated with current entrepreneurial nurses.

The literature supports the fact that entrepreneurial nurses are typical of other successful entrepreneurs. Shapero[8] identifies four factors facilitating entrepreneurial success as follows:

- displacement—time to move on indicated by situational crisis
- propensity to want to be in control of one's life, to make one's own rules (internal vs. external locus of control)
- credibility derived from self-esteem, family support, feedback from co-workers, clients, supervisors
- resources—money and its management

Winston,[9] in *Entrepreneurial Women*, agrees and notes in addition the importance of role models, a willingness to take calculated risks, and the motivation to accomplish one thing particularly well. A strong sense of guilt and a positive experience with overcoming personal adversity are two additional traits documented by Silver,[3] in his assessment of several hundred entrepreneurs. Literature that attempts to identify characteristics of successful entrepreneurs describes them as action-oriented risk takers, thriving on change and diversity, impatient, opinionated, independent, and interested in making an idea happen and deriving profit from the effort.

In contrast, nurses are known for their practical, problem solving skills; attention to detail and defined tasks; compassion and caring; willingness to work within systems; and orientation to service. There is also a stereotype of nurses as patient, dependent, willing to compromise, and complacent individuals with high needs for security and affiliation. In general, the characteristics that seem to best describe nurses may be at odds with those that are the hallmark of the entrepreneur.

Motivation for Entrepreneurial Nurses.   What motivates the nurse who starts a business? Is it possible that you have what it takes? Neal's book, *Nurses in Business*,[10] is a collection of essays by nurses who agree that they: 1) have a desire for independence, control and autonomy, the support and encouragement of family and friends, and demonstrated ability in decision making and problem solving; 2) have a specific area of expertise and derive satisfaction in creative endeavors; and 3) have secure resources, were frustrated with their jobs, and were committed to a good idea or mission. Nurses, and others who have shared personal stories in many articles, have had to overcome fears about failure, anxiety about financial management, lack of business expertise, dependence and affiliation needs, demands of competing roles (eg, spouse, parent, employee), and socialization to roles that traditionally have been devalued.

Those who publish and are members of support organizations such as the Nurse Consultants Association are visible. Those who have chosen to do entrepreneurial activities within organizations are less so. In addition, there is a growing sophistication within hospital units that nursing has beneficial potential for certain industries—ones that rely on nursing's product testing, referral to services, and creative ideas.[11] Improved sleep apnea monitors for home use, stuffed toys with casts and braces, and decubitus care dressing products are three commercial examples that resulted from nursing's communication of patient needs to industry.

Choosing the Entrepreneurial Life: Opportunities and Constraints.   Nurses bring needed assessment and intervention skills to the hospital setting. Increasingly, these skills may serve consumers in other settings. Recognizing trends, identifying needs, and having the vision to fulfill the entrepreneurial challenge go hand in hand. There is a complex interrelationship between nursing's potential impact on society and society's ability to articulate what it wants. Nurses choosing entrepreneurial paths will be supported by the following trends:

- There are more resources for learning about business accessible to nurses than ever before. Classes, seminars, support organizations, and consultants provide guidance for novice efforts.
- Care that was previously provided in hospitals under direct control of MDs is planned and delivered in many settings under less restrictive conditions.
- Need for nursing services is stimulated at both ends of the age spectrum by increasing numbers of elderly with impairment and chronic disease, and many newborns who survive low birth weight and congenital problems pose complex long-term care needs.
- There is growing interest and commitment to health promotion and wellness for all ages. This is driven in part by high costs of medical interventions and crisis orientation, and in part by recognition that personal decisions impact quality and quantity of life.
- The mixed blessing of sophisticated medical technology and related ethical and economic issues provide a new forum for support services.
- Expanded roles created by consumer interests, Preferred-Provider Organizations, Health Maintenance Organizations, DRG's, and quality assurance.
- Venture capital, loan programs, and payment options and incentives are increasingly available, as are small business incubators that provide a range of support services for the fledgling business.
- A complex, fast-paced world demands reliance on experts and consultants, creating fragmentation, dehumanization, nostalgia for comfort and caring, and simplicity.
- Computers have enormous impact on data collection, information management, and analysis.
- Marketing as a process and skill has moved into prominence and acceptability in the nonprofit and service arenas.[12,13]
- With the demographic projections about Acquired Immune Deficiency Syndrome (AIDS), we face an epidemic that will challenge the best of education, nursing, and medicine.
- Nursing research supports the cost effectiveness of nursing interventions on both the quality and quantity of life.

Some of the persistent obstacles that restrain nurses in their pursuit of autonomy and achievement are as follows:

- Practice acts, licensing and certification requirements and regulations protect the status quo.[14]
- Nursing services may not be clearly understood and may be undervalued, thus creating reimbursement issues in both third-party and fee-for-service arenas.

- Malpractice and liability fears abound, fed by enormous jury awards and the enjoining of all professionals and organizations involved in the potential misdeed.
- The image of nurses has not immediately expanded as their roles have; it is a major job to educate potential markets.[14]
- Peers are sometimes threatened, providing neither support nor referral.
- The complexity of organizing and managing the demands of a business may cut into time available for providing services.
- Appropriate accepted methods to promote services and advertise products are still in process.
- Education typically provides no foundation for independent aspects of being an entrepreneur.
- Home care, day care, respite care, hospice, health promotion support, and disease prevention/intervention are not typically covered by insurance and may be closely regulated if they gain coverage.
- Shortage of nurses in tertiary care is accompanied by increasing competition from physicians, psychologists, therapists, health educators, social workers, and other health professionals for the financially secure potential patient.

Nurses who have vision to search newspapers and reports and to listen attentively to consumers will seek opportunity in the seven categories of opportunity identified by Drucker[1] as follows:

- the unexpected success, failure, or outside event
- the incongruity between what is and what could be
- the process need—there must be a better way
- changes in industry or market structure
- demographic changes understood as projections
- changes in perception, mood, meaning—when facts do not change, but the meaning given them does
- new knowledge, both scientific and nonscientific

There are three general classes of potential entrepreneurial endeavors: product development, service delivery, and management. In each case the entrepreneurial nurse conducts marketing research and chooses one or more of the following options based on assessment of consumer desires, competition, and her/his own internal organization:

- provision of a new product/service to usual clients
- provision of a new product/service to new clients
- provision of an old product/service to new clients
- provision of an old product/service to usual clients in a new "package"

Identifying new products might include software for nursing research, interactive videos for education, and health/self-assessment tools adapted for consumer use. Service delivery might include brokering,[15] the matching of clients and services for a fee, chronic disease management in diabetes care centers, and training seminars for consumers in techniques of medical self-care. A final example would encompass the administration of services actually delivered by others, for example, home care, staffing, needs assessment, and program evaluation.

In each case, the entrepreneurial nurse needs to be familiar with the marketing process, writing a business plan, and obtaining financial backing, as well as being comfortable with a particular area of nursing expertise. Technical assistance, financial support, and a variety of printed materials are available to assist the fledgling entrepreneur who is well advised to learn from the efforts of others.

THE CONSUMER AND SOCIETY

Are nurses who initiate entrepreneurial activities out of step with trends?

- In the 1980s, for the first time, more than 50 percent of physicians were *salaried* employees.
- Competition for health care dollars is fierce; nurses stand to gain by studies of costs, but also to be visible and therefore vulnerable.
- Uncertainty as to what government, consumers, insurance, and industry want to invest in prevails: is basic health care a right? And if it is, what is it? How do we allocate scarce resources? To what extent do we commit to wellness and sustaining health?
- Consumers (all those who might potentially purchase nursing services, including individuals, corporations, hospitals, elderly) struggle to understand the concept of the nurse in business. Is she/he still a nurse?

For nurses who wish to add business skills to their areas of professional expertise, who are willing to be entirely open to possibilities, and who are committed to change, the future holds exciting possibilities. Nurses must devote as much time and energy to understanding the marketplace as they do to understanding their own needs for autonomy and professionalism.[16]

First, marketing and selling are not the same thing. The nurse practitioner, for example, who wishes to market professional skills to a day care center must focus on how these skills enhance the center's goals, and not just on how the relationship would meet personal needs to deliver a service. The nurse must ask: Why should they add a service to their center? Would their clients pay enough to make it feasible? Will nurse practitioner services enhance the business the day care center is in? The advantage of autonomy and practice unrestrained by corporate bureaucracy is attractive to the nurse. Is it equally attractive to the customer? Yes—if it is skillfully marketed.

There are a number of service industries that have had a major economic impact. They all offer a well-defined product—completed tax returns, clean windows, oil changes—which clearly meet a well-defined consumer need/want. Much remains to be understood about the cost of nursing, who values services, what the return on investment will be, and who can provide these answers. A refocusing of analysis is called for, one which attends to a thorough understanding of contracting. This, then, will have impact on education, practice, and positioning of nurses.

Second, a nurse may use entrepreneurial skills within traditional settings. As a transitional step, intrapreneuring may be better than entrepreneuring. Pinchott[5] suggests working within the corporation when you meet the following criteria:

- have an idea about improving the company business
- want to do new things, but simultaneously want the friendships and security of belonging to an organization
- can develop capital for your idea inside the organization
- can utilize the company name or channels to provide an increased chance of success
- want to practice creating a business inside before risking your own funds outside
- want to let someone else deal with hassles (space, utilities, insurance, taxes) while you create

Third, if nursing focuses on the needs of various markets (physicians, industry, elderly, children, hospitals, indigent, etc) can we assess, measure, and document the advantages for them to buy services from independent agents?[17] If these benefits cannot be communicated or do not exist, can entrepreneurial ventures in nursing succeed?

Fourth, is third-party reimbursement really the force that restrains the market? Only in health care have we come to expect the security blanket of insurance and public assistance. Consumers do not purchase other goods and services through third-party mechanisms. The question of who buys services and from whom and under what circumstances needs to be carefully studied.

Many of those who have significant needs that could be addressed by nursing will never be covered by any but total national health care insurance. It is also unclear how many people are restrained from health promotion and disease prevention actions by lack of coverage. Many interventions are personal decisions that could be made on the basis of readily available resources and knowledge.

It is undeniable that small business growth is an important factor in the economy of the United States. It is also clear that many small businesses fail because they attempt to compete with the established niches of large corporations. Notable successes, however, have been achieved where entrepreneurs satisfy the desires of their clients for new products, new services, and better ways to meet existing needs.

Nurses who dream, plan, and listen may completely reshape the health care delivery system to respond to market analysis. The possibilities are there for those who recognize who the customers are and understand how to satisfy them.

Future Considerations

Nursing must combine inwardly turned self-analysis with outwardly directed attention to the marketplace. Of great importance will be a clear understanding of who the consumers of nursing products and services are, who they might be in the future, as well as the complexities of financial management.

Nurses today have role models, skills, technical assistance, and knowledge that will contribute to increased willingness to start innovative businesses. Both consumers and financial administrators are increasingly aware that care delivered through hospitals may be neither the most cost effective, nor the best, in a given situation. Educated consumers stand to gain through lowered costs and improved health status.

The nurses who succeed as entrepreneurs will occupy a unique niche, satisfy customers, and find and document better ways to provide needed services. Their skills in understanding patients' needs, their awareness of political and legal process, and their creative responses to both will contribute.

As well-defined arenas provide visible, reimbursable, lucrative profit centers, (eg, home health services, day care for children with chronic illness, work-site health promotion), they will attract regulation and licensing. Nurses will need to document the efficacy and effectiveness of their care, and to use political representation to insure legislation supportive to the best interests of consumers.

Research will support the cost effectiveness of nursing intervention, and choices to sustain status quo will be more difficult to make. Some of this research may be financed by industry as well as public resources. As a knowledge base develops, nurses will be increasingly willing to make conclusions and recommendations, not just to assess and gather information for other decision makers.

As a result of political activism, changes in laws and practice acts will allow nurses to incorporate with other professionals and open new channels for collaborative practice. The delivery of health care will become both increasingly complex with the proliferation of small, specialized businesses and centrally controlled with a parallel trend to large conglomerates with subsidiaries and contract networks. New structures will offer opportunities for nurses to engage in independent activity, varying from the management and operation of self-care centers to the contracting for nursing services in every imaginable setting.

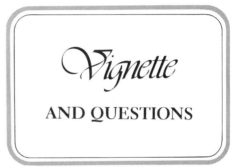

Lisa is frustrated in her role as a staff nurse on a diabetic unit because there never seems to be enough time to provide the teaching, support, and guidance that would help her patients adapt the demands of chronic disease to their life styles. She hates all the paper work required on her unit. She is thinking about starting her own business to offer services she thinks are needed and that she knows how to provide.

Lisa's father owns the only drugstore in their relatively small town. He thinks her idea has merit. Many of his customers who have diabetes seem confused and overwhelmed about their treatment, testing, medication, exercise, and dietary restrictions. He offers to lend her some of his business experience, and together they begin to list what she must do before she quits her hospital job. They choose a "who, what, where, how" format:

Who does she want to provide services for? Who is serving them now? Do they want the proposed services, and are they willing and able to pay for them? How will she find out? Do they see nurses as a desirable source of these services?

What services will she offer? Are there legal restraints to her practice? How will her services be competitive, better, valuable to the client?

How will she target and attract customers? How will she promote her services? Can she set up a referral system—will doctors and other nurses be supportive? What funds will be needed? Where will they come from? How will they be managed? This begins to seem very complex to Lisa. She wonders if maybe she could talk her hospital into setting up a practice for her. They could handle the administrative details and free her to educate and support her patients.

1. Is the business Lisa is proposing entrepreneurial?

2. Does Lisa understand how to find out what her potential clients want, or is she clearer when it comes to the services she wants to provide?

3. What are Lisa's chances for success, based on the enabling and restraining forces that appear to be at work?

4. Given an aging population, advances in treatment and monitoring technology, and her knowledge of diabetes, what innovative opportunities are available for Lisa?

INFORMATION SOURCES

American Nurses' Association, Inc.
  Center for Research
  2420 Pershing Road
  Kansas City, MO 64108

  Will provide lists of contacts identified as entrepreneurs.

American Entrepreneurs Association
  2311 Pontius Ave.
  Los Angeles, CA 90064

  Prints *Entrepreneur* magazine; offers phone counseling, reduced rates on manuals and reports.

(The) Center for Entrepreneurial Management
  83 Spring Street
  New York, NY 10012

  Offers technical assistance, materials, and books.

Nurse Consultants Association, Inc.
  P.O. Box 25875
  Colorado Springs, CO 80936

  Association of nurses not involved in direct care. Offers business meetings, seminars, newsletter.

Nurse Entrepreneur Exchange
    4286 Redwood Highway, Suite 252
    San Rafael, CA 94903

    Provides newsletter, forum for idea exchange.

Nurses in Business Association
    420 Taberwood Way
    Rosewell, GA 30076

    Local organization, willing to share support model with states.
        Provides workshops and seminars.

Small Business Association
    1441 L Street NW, Room 100
    Washington, DC 20416

    Catalogue lists materials including: Checklist for Going into Business,
        Business Plan for Small Service Firms.

REFERENCES

1. Drucker PF: *Innovation and Entrepreneurship, Practice and Principles.* New York, Harper & Row, Pub, 1985

2. *Webster's Third International Dictionary.* Springfield, MA, G & C Merriam, 1961

3. Silver AD: *The Entrepreneurial Life.* New York, Wiley, 1986

4. Riccardi BR, Dayani EC: *The Nurse Entrepreneur.* Reston, VA, Prentice-Hall, 1982

5. Pinchott G: *Intrapreneuring: Why You Don't Have to Leave the Corporation to Become an Entrepreneur.* New York, Harper & Row, Pub, 1983

6. Vance C, Talbott S, McBride A, Mason D: An uneasy alliance: Nursing and the women's movement. Nurs Outlook 33:281, November/December 1985

7. Kinlein L: *Independent Practice with Nursing Clients.* Philadelphia, Lippincott, 1979

8. Shapero A: Have you got what it takes to start your own business? Savvy 4:33, April 1980

9. Winston S: *Entrepreneurial Women.* New York, Newsweek Books, 1979

10. Neal ME (ed): *Nurses in Business.* Pacific Palisades, CA, NURSECO, Inc, 1982

11. Kotler P: *Marketing for Non-Profit Organizations*. Englewood Cliffs, NJ, Prentice-Hall, 1982

12. Kotler P, Conner RA: Marketing professional services. J Marketing 41:71, January 1977

13. Urquhart AL, Wooding GA, Budinger KM, Henry BM: Perspectives on nursing issues and health care trends. JONA 16:17, January 1986

14. Felton G, Kelly HD, Renehan K, Alley J: Nursing entrepreneurs, a success story. Nurs Outlook 33:276, Nov/Dec 1985

15. Eisenhaer LA: Health care brokering—a career option for changing times. Nurs Health Care 7:417, October 1986

16. Holtz H: *How to Succeed as an Independent Consultant*. New York, Wiley, 1983

17. Neal ME: Starting your own business, In del Bueno DE (ed): A *Financial Guide for Nurses*. Boston, Blackwell, 1981, pp 71–86

ANDREA O. HOLLINGSWORTH, RN, PhD

CHAPTER 5　　*The Evolvement of Faculty Practice*

Background and Overview

In recent years the nursing profession has begun to examine the role of faculty and its relationship to nursing practice. Just what are the expectations of a nurse with advanced academic preparation who chooses to teach nursing? Should this individual be primarily an academician and required to fulfill the role of all university faculty? Or should this person be primarily a practitioner of nursing and develop clinical expertise in the area in which he/she teaches? The more challenging question perhaps is: should they be both? This leads to an even more intriguing question: must they be both?

Historically, nurses who taught in the early hospitals' educational programs were both teachers and practitioners of nursing. They were skilled, experienced nurses with little in the way of academic training. As nursing began to shift into higher education, a dichotomy arose between the role of the bedside nurse and the faculty member. The focus of nurse educators' attention was directed toward the mastery of the academic skills of curriculum development teaching-learning methods, research, and publication.[1]

Bellinger et al[2] believe that another significant factor that contributed to the split between education and service was the "constraints placed on nursing service departments by hospital administrators which hindered hospital based nurses from evolving roles with greater degrees of independence. Thus, more highly educated nurses sought greater freedom and less bureaucratic restraints by entering the academic field."

As nurse educators developed more skill in curriculum planning and implementation and attempted to meet the demands of an academic appointment, they spent less time in clinical practice. As educators spent more time concerned with matters of doctoral study, promotion, and tenure, they placed less emphasis on maintaining and developing clinical skills. Nurses in practice viewed them not as nurse educators, but as being separate from the practice of nursing. Practitioners believed that faculty had lost their clinical expertise and could not educate students for the reality of practice. The gap between education and practice widened.

Today nurse faculty are returning to practice roles and developing new roles to allow them to meet the demands of both education and practice. In other words, faculty are attempting to unify practice for the benefit of patients, students, and the profession as a whole.

These new roles are commonly referred to as **faculty practice.** This title reflects the educator's need to be identified as a member of an academic group, but at the same time sharing in the practice of the nursing profession. By taking on this role, the faculty member maintains and increases clinical skills. By doing so, the educator serves as a role model for students in the clinical areas. However, it is more than a simple matter of maintaining clinical expertise. Faculty practice should have an impact on the entire profession. The need for nursing faculty to practice is not a momentary trend. It is a mature recognition of the accountability of the discipline to the profession of nursing; it is evidence of an understanding of our nature, purpose, and destiny as a clinical discipline, a professional discipline, and an applied discipline.[3]

MODELS OF PRACTICE

Though the need for faculty to practice is clear, it is also apparent that there is no uniform policy throughout the profession that facilitates this practice. Bellinger et al[2] surveyed National League for Nursing (NLN) accredited baccalaureate programs in the United States and "found that the majority (number of respondents = 82, 70%) of schools had no policy governing faculty practice. The format of practice policies varied widely at the 35 schools where there was a policy." Without uniform policies and widespread support, many faculty may not be able to practice. In addition to not having policies to guide them, faculty may also find that they are not given release time, less responsibility, or lighter teaching loads to facilitate them in the accomplishment of their practice-oriented goals.

However, some models for faculty practice have been established. Nursing faculty, individually and collectively, are seeking effective methods of incorporating practice and teaching. Different modes of faculty practice have been identified, such as dual appointments in practice and education, private practice, development of a practice within a nursing college, and others.[4]

Dual appointments in practice and education vary from institution to institution. In some instances a model has been developed for an entire faculty to follow. An example of such a model is Rush-Presbyterian University in Chicago. There, Christman[5] has developed the role of the **practitioner-teacher.** Every faculty member has an appointment as a practitioner in the hospital, as well as faculty responsibilities. This model is implemented at all levels of nursing administration.

This type of model with dual appointments for faculty may not be applicable at many colleges and universities. Therefore, other institutions search for a model that allows for joint faculty practice appointments. Another example of a model is the one developed at the University of Pennsylvania. Fagin[6] describes a faculty appointment known as the clinician-educator. **Clinician-educators** are fully credentialed faculty members who are expected to engage in scholarly activities, including publications, and their teaching is likely to be practice-oriented. They hold a joint appointment with the university and a clinical agency. Clinician-educators have all rights and privileges of other faculty in the school of nursing, except voting on tenure and compensation of tenured faculty. "Therefore, they have the collegiability and protection of an academic environment but will have a contract to perform in a specified clinical role."[6] This type of role allows a faculty member to practice while experiencing the benefits of a faculty position.

Some faculty have chosen to maintain a **private practice** while fulfilling an academic appointment. An example of this is again taken from the University of Pennsylvania School of Nursing. Dr. Margaret Cotroneo maintains a practice in family therapy while holding a standing faculty position at the School of Nursing in the Psychiatric-Mental Health Section. She sees clients in her practice for approximately 20 hours per week. The Clinical Practice Group of the University of Pennsylvania acts as the administrator of her practice in return for a percentage of her income.

Dr. Cotroneo involves graduate students in her practice by preceptoring them as they work with families and by allowing them to participate in her research with families. This arrangement allows her an extended amount of time to earn tenure in her standing faculty position. She believes that this faculty practice model allows her to maintain her therapist role, which at the same time enhances the learning experience of her students.[7]

Another type of faculty practice situation is a **clinical practice** run by a faculty group from one institution. A good example of such a practice is the Yale Nurse-Midwifery Practice. This practice was established at the Yale University School of Nursing in November 1975.[8] Currently, the practice consists of three nurse-midwives, all full-time university faculty. They maintain a caseload of about 50 deliveries per year, plus well-woman gynecology and family planning services. Nurse-midwifery students are involved in the practice.

"At this School of Nursing, faculty practice is required for academic promotion and tenure. Thus this practice helps meet this requirement for the participating faculty."[8] The faculty in this practice believe that besides maintaining a high level of clinical competence, they are also role models for the students and an important link between the community and the university.

Another example of a faculty practice within a school of nursing is at the Creighton University School of Nursing. "The School of Nursing set up its own home health agency, Creighton Home Health Care (CHHC) in July, 1982. A fully-certified Medicare/Medicaid provider of nursing services, CHHC also offers social services and speech and physical therapy through contracts with these allied health professionals."[9] The core staff includes a nurse-director and three nursing and support staff members. Four members of the community health/community mental health course group and their students also provide care and services through the agency.[9] "It is the belief of this School of Nursing that faculty members be first and foremost competent and confident professional nurses and leaders of the health care team."[9] This type of practice allows faculty to reach these goals and at the same time provides student experiences and allows the faculty to meet the demands of their faculty positions.

Kruger[4] describes yet another type of **joint faculty/practice position**. She worked with a pediatric unit to develop a parent education program and a parent support group. At the same time, she was a faculty member of a nursing department of a university. "After the program began, she involved specially selected nursing students in the implementation of the programs. The educator and practitioner roles were thus combined."[4]

Though this last example may not be significantly different from other joint faculty appointments, it does illustrate the potential for creativity and flexibility in these joint appointments. It is also an excellent example of how undergraduate students can also benefit from combining education and practice. The students in this group felt that their learning had been enhanced by their instructor's involvement with the hospital nursing staff.

The models mentioned here are certainly not an inclusive list of all types of joint faculty/practice appointments. Each institution must develop the type of practice models that best meet the needs of their faculty and best represent their mission and philosophy. What is common to all, however, is that the models provide practice opportunities that are related to the teaching and research interests of the faculty. In addition, the practice settings allow for the involvement of students, whether graduate or undergraduate. In this way, students are given excellent learning opportunities with faculty who are strong role models and who have close working relationships with staff.

Faculty practice, however, is not entirely free of difficulties or problems for the nurses who choose this role. Although the nursing literature contains many examples of faculty practice models, there has been little research done on the subject.[10] Nurses who choose to do both roles may experience role conflict. This could occur when the demands of one of their roles is excessive, leading them to believe that they may be neglecting the other role, or the roles themselves may bring them into conflict with either their practice or educational settings. Support and understanding from administrators and colleagues is essential if an individual is going to be successful in dual or shared roles.

In addition, from the faculty viewpoint, a dual appointment or joint position can present difficulties when the faculty member applies for promotion or tenure. "Faculty have not only not been rewarded for faculty practice, they have been penalized. The rewards traditionally available in academia—tenure and promotion—are difficult or impossible to obtain."[11] Thus, it can be seen that many faculty might be reluctant to take on a faculty practice position, for fear of role duplicity and the barriers that such a position may impose to their efforts for career rewards.

Impacts on the Nurse, the Consumer, and Society

THE NURSE

The benefits of faculty practice positions can be shared by faculty, staff nurses, and students alike, and therefore the entire profession of nursing will be improved. Nursing remains a practice profession and the continuing gap between service and education can only be to its detriment. Practice is the heart of the profession. Research, education, and scholarship basically all have one goal: to improve nursing practice through increased nursing knowledge.

For the faculty member, a practice position gives more than just an opportunity to maintain and develop clinical skills. Obviously, it does achieve this goal, but it also provides potential clinical sites for research and stimulation for research questions. "Clinical research can be facilitated by the presence of the nurse researcher in a practice position. Practice models which recognize the essential role of research in faculty practice are an important development in nursing's maturity."[6]

In addition to the faculty member benefiting, the student experience will also be enhanced. All of the models that are represented in this chapter provide clinical learning experiences for students. However, this type of clinical experience gives the student much more than the routine clinical setting. In faculty practice settings, students see their instructors as strong role models. They benefit from the collaboration and cooperation that exists between staff and faculty. Students may also have closer contact with the staff because of the established working relationships between faculty and practitioners. Kruger[4] quotes a student who evaluated such a learning experience: "It is very valuable to have someone who is very familiar with the medical center and I think we (students) are accepted more readily."

However, the benefits of such positions are not limited to faculty and students. Staff nurses can also gain from collaboration with the faculty members in a practice setting. Staff can benefit from the expertise of the faculty members and utilize them as a resource. If the faculty are involved in research, it may provide the staff with opportunities to participate in the development of research questions. If the faculty and staff are willing to work as a group, they may even carry out a research project together. This allows the staff to value research in a way that may have been previously unavailable to them.

THE CONSUMER

The consumer will also benefit from faculty practice. As was seen from the group practices, consumers were provided with services that might not otherwise exist. In addition, a faculty practice such as the midwifery group gives the public an alternate mode of health care. Young childbearing families have the opportunity to choose midwifery care over routine obstetrical care. Without the support of the school of nursing, this consumer choice may not have been possible.

Besides offering the consumer an alternative mode of health care, a faculty practice can offer affordable, high-quality care. The example of the community-based faculty practice at Creighton University supports this concept. Ryan[12] gives some "assumptions which underlie this particular faculty practice: 1) that high-quality, affordable care includes minimal services necessary to achieve desired outcomes using minimum resources; 2) that nursing is a service that the consumer will pay for; and 3) that nursing is therefore income generating."

Nursing must realize its ability to be its own profit center as it demonstrates its own high-quality impact on practice. "The profession must demonstrate that nursing is an economical and efficient alternative to institutionalized and technologized care modes."[12]

SOCIETY

Primary care as provided by nurses can offer the American consumer health care with a focus on health promotion and disease prevention. Profound changes are needed in the health care delivery system of this country, and with this focus nurses could lead the way for future models of care. As Sheila Ryan clearly states:

> Nurses need to be defining their future roles, and faculty are logical problem solvers, role models, and independent care providers in the ambulatory, community, home, and industrial arenas. Faculty practice can support curriculum relevance. Academic institutions can set the pace and the approaches for new health delivery alternatives.[12]

Future Considerations

Models for faculty practice continue to develop and evolve as faculty in various college and university settings strive to meet academic and practice demands. The models developed to-date may meet the needs of many faculty and institutions, but creativity and receptivity on the part of faculty and administrators are needed to develop additional and different models. The nursing literature supports the concept of faculty practice, presenting models that can be replicated and offering support and suggestions for future developments. There seems to be no debate as to the need for faculty to have the opportunity to practice as part of their academic role.

As this trend continues, some thought must be given as to how faculty practice will affect nursing education and the delivery of nursing services.

Reports thus far have demonstrated that students have responded positively to clinical experiences with faculty who are in practice roles.[4,13] The students report that their acceptance into the clinical setting was enhanced by their instructor's clinical role. They also felt the overall learning experience to be a positive one. If the faculty practice models continue to develop, this can only be viewed as a positive trend for nursing education. The models, thus far, seem to enhance the learning experiences of students. Thus, the student no longer will view the instructor as "teacher" only, but will have a role model of practitioner and teacher. Since the heart of the nursing profession is practice, this is an appropriate trend.

However, another important aspect of the faculty practice model is that faculty must still meet the demands of an academic position. These demands may include research, publication, and participation in professional/community service. A joint position between academia and practice can enhance a faculty member's ability to carry out clinical research. Identification of research problems and the sharing of research ideas can be enhanced by a faculty member being a staff member of a clinical setting. It may also provide opportunities for collaborative research projects between nursing faculty and nursing staff members. Research that is carried out with the involvement of the members of nursing service may have more immediate applicability to nursing care in that institution.

In addition to benefiting nursing education, faculty practice models can also provide alternative methods of delivery of nursing and health care. Some of the models cited in this chapter serve as examples of alternative methods, particularly the nurse-midwifery practice. Another example is the development of a **group practice** within the outpatient department of the University of North Carolina at Chapel Hill Medical Center.[14] This practice, staffed by the nurse practitioner faculty with physician backup, offers complete health assessments, screening, and lifestyle counseling. After the clinic was established and running smoothly, it was used as a clinical site for graduate students.

The teacher-clinicians at this clinic offered preventive services at a reasonable fee and they were very satisfied with the growth of their clinic population. However, they reported that marketing their services was an important part of the development of their practice.[14] Nurse faculty practice settings can offer the public many health care services at reasonable cost and, in doing so, offer alternatives to the present health care delivery system. However, the practitioners have to include the education of the public and the marketing of their services as part of their practice. Nurses have a valued service to offer the public, and nurse faculty are often in the best position to be the providers of such services and information.

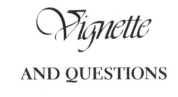

Vignette
AND QUESTIONS

Dr. Martin is a faculty member at a school of nursing at a large research university. She has a master's degree in pediatric nursing and has just completed her doctorate. Her appointment to the faculty is as an assistant professor in the department of Maternal-Child Health. Her primary responsibility is the implementation of the undergraduate clinical course for the care of acutely ill children. The university is affiliated with a nationally known children's hospital, where Dr. Martin supervises students in their clinical experience.

After one year Dr. Martin realizes that she is losing touch with the concerns of the nurses in the clinical setting. Even though she works in the hospital's per diem pool, she believes that she is not actively involved in nursing practice. With the assistance of the Dean of the School of Nursing and the Administrator for Nursing Service at the hospital, she explores the possibilities for changing her role at the hospital and school.

Her goal is to be actively involved in nursing practice at the hospital, while meeting the requirements of her academic appointment. She is particularly interested in pursuing collaborative research with some of the clinical specialists and physicians at the hospital. At the same time, she is worried about meeting the demands of her university appointment and giving sufficient time to a practice appointment.

1. What type of role or appointment might be most appropriate for Dr. Martin in an acute care setting with teaching responsibilities for undergraduate students? Considering that she has both clinical and teaching expertise, how could these skills be best utilized?

2. What type of supports will she require from the dean of her school and from the nursing administrator of the hospital?

3. What advantages will there be from this appointment: For the nursing students? For the staff nurses? For the patients? For Dr. Martin?

4. Might there be any disadvantages for all these same groups or individuals?

INFORMATION SOURCES

Annual Symposium on Nursing Faculty Practice, Kansas City, MO, American Academy of Nursing, 1983–present

National League for Nursing Publication 15, 1831, 1980

REFERENCES

1. Spera J: Faculty practice as one component of faculty role. In *Cognitive Dissonance: Interpreting and Implementing Faculty Roles in Nursing Education.* New York, National League for Nursing, 1980

2. Bellinger K, Reid J, Sanders D: Faculty practice policy. J Nurs Educ 24:214, 1985

3. Algase D: Faculty practice: A means to advance the discipline of nursing. J Nurs Educ 25:74, 1986

4. Kruger S: The demonstration of a joint faculty/practice position. J Nurs Educ 24:350, 1985

5. Christman L: The practitioner-teacher. Nurse Educator 4:8, 1979

6. Fagin C: Institutionalizing faculty practice. Nurs Outlook 34:140, 1986

7. Cotroneo M: Personal correspondence. April, 1987

8. Nichols C: Faculty practice: Something for everyone. Nurs Outlook 33: 85, 1985.

9. Ryan S, Barger-Lux M: Faculty expertise in practice—A school succeeding. Nurs Health Care February: 75, 1985

10. Lambert C, Lambert V: A review and synthesis of the research on role conflict and its impact on nurses involved in faculty practice programs. J Nurs Educ 27:54, 1988

11. Roncole M: Faculty practice: Making it work, In *Perspectives in Nursing*. New York, National League for Nursing, 1985

12. Ryan S: Faculty practice: A community linked model. In *Annual Symposium on Nursing Faculty Practice* 2:722, 1985

13. Harmon Y: A nursing faculty practice in a Veterans Administration medical center: An asset to service and education. J Nurs Educ 25:81, 1986, 81–84

14. Nettles-Carlson B, Friedman B: Group faculty practice. Nurs Outlook 33:170, 1985

ANN MARRINER-TOMEY, RN, PhD, FAAN

CHAPTER 6 *Assignment Systems: The Delivery of Nursing Care in the Acute Care Setting*

Background and Overview

The assignment of activities associated with the delivery of nursing care has undergone a number of changes throughout history. **Case method,** the earliest recognized mode of nursing care delivery, was done in the early part of the twentieth century by private-duty nurses in the homes of affluent patients. There essentially was nothing that could be done in a hospital, at that time, that could not be done in the home. Consequently, most nurses worked 12-hour shifts, six or seven days a week, in the homes of their patients. Caring for the one patient was the nurse's total assignment.

Patients without the resources to be cared for at home received care given predominantly by nursing students in hospitals. Typically, the director of nursing and head nurses were the only graduate nurses employed by the hospitals. Students gave total care to the patients to whom they were assigned while they were on duty.

During the depression nurses were less able to find work in the homes of affluent patients and, as a result, began to return to hospitals to earn room and board. Student enrollments decreased and the case method of care by graduate nurses became common. As the economy improved and technology advanced, the case method of care was reimplemented for affluent patients in hospitals by private-duty nurses until intensive care units became common. Intensive care nurses, however, often have implemented the case method to meet the needs of their patients. Primary nursing, a more recent method of assignment (which will be discussed in greater depth later in the chapter), is a version of the case method that includes 24-hour responsibility for the patient instead of responsibility only while on duty in the hospital. With the current focus on early discharge from hospitals to the home, it appears that the case method may be regaining popularity.

The case method of patient-centered care did not prove to be a compatible mode of nursing care delivery in the bureaucratic institution called the hospital. As a result, during the 1920s, hospitals adopted Taylor's scientific management through **functional nursing,** which flourished until after World War II.

World War II had a dramatic effect on the delivery of nursing care. Many nurses who had been working in hospitals in the United States joined the armed forces to care for the wounded. Techniques in medical science were advancing rapidly, resulting in increasing demands upon nurses. Due to the war effort, there was a dearth of graduate nurses. Consequently, other levels of personnel, including volunteers, nurses' aides, and practical nurses, were recruited. These new personnel were unable to provide total patient care, so the functional method of assigning responsibility for specific tasks to each worker, depending upon his/her ability, became increasingly useful. Volunteers could escort patients, pass mail, and deliver flowers while nurses' aides could do housekeeping chores, deliver meals, help feed patients, and, in some ambulatory cases, even bathe patients. Practical nurses typically bathed patients and did some treatments, leaving the registered nurses to pass medications and do the remaining treatments. The division of labor was based upon specialization and the nurse in charge was responsible for delegating the tasks according to the nature of the task and each worker's status and expertise. One individual did the same task for numerous patients, which resulted in various health workers parading through the patient's room, each providing a piece of the care.[1,2]

No one person was responsible for the total care of the patient. Because of each worker's specialization, a great deal of work was completed in a short period of time. Even today, functional nursing is observed in some agencies, especially on the evening or night shift, when a few nursing personnel care for many patients. Unfortunately, the care delivered by way of functional nursing proved to be fragmented and depersonalized, accountability was difficult to establish, and job satisfaction was questionable. Tasks could get repetitious and boring, and become automatic, which could lead to mistakes.

The employment of the less skilled workers continued even after the war ended because of the shortage of nurses. Although many of the same tasks associated with patient care were still prevalent, the variety of skill levels needed by nurses necessitated another reorganization in the delivery of nursing care. That reorganization led to **team nursing,** which was developed in the 1950s. Team nursing fostered hierarchy and classical management techniques. It was designed to organize personnel with different skill levels under the direction of a more skilled team leader. The team leader coordinated and supervised a team of health care providers, who cared for a group of patients. The objective was to make optimal use of personnel by matching the worker's preparation with the patient's need.

The team leader would accompany the physician on his patient rounds, transcribe the physician's orders, administer medications, monitor parenteral fluids, and assist team members as necessary. Registered nurses were assigned the most critically ill patients. Practical nurses typically were assigned the bathing, feeding, and changing of dressings on the less critically ill, while aides were expected to help ambulatory patients with bathing and grooming. Written care plans were used to keep the team informed of changes in patients' conditions and team conferences were utilized as a method of problem solving and care planning. Unfortunately, the matching of worker talents with the assignment, team conferences, and care planning often were omitted because of the time that it took to coordinate these activities. Fragmented care resulted. As with functional nursing, accountability was difficult to assess.[1,3]

Primary nursing was instituted during the late 1960s and early 1970s by professional nurses who were unhappy with fragmented care and a lack of direct patient care. It was characterized by autonomy, authority, and accountability, as the primary nurse had 24-hour responsibility for the four to six patients in his/her caseload from the time of admission to discharge.[4] Ideally, the primary nurse was a registered nurse who admitted the patient, assessed needs, planned and coordinated the care, and implemented and evaluated that care. The primary nurse delegated the direct care to an associate nurse when the primary nurse was not in the hospital. Primary nurses typically worked 40-hour work weeks, but consulted with associate nurses by telephone at other times. The associate nurse implemented the primary nurse's plans for care. Primary nursing was designed to place the registered nurse at the bedside, giving patient care. However, it takes large numbers of well-qualified registered nurses to implement primary nursing. Because of the difficulty in obtaining an all-registered nurse staff, the system has been modified to make primary nurses predominantly planners who delegate much of the direct care to others, even when they are on duty. In some cases, less qualified personnel have been called primary nurses, but they usually lack the background to do in-depth assessments and planning of care. While primary nursing was designed to increase professional satisfaction and quality of care and to decrease costs, research findings have shown diverse results.

Modular nursing was a modification of team and primary nursing. It was sometimes used when there were not enough registered nurses to practice primary nursing. Patients were divided by geographical location into small groups of six to twelve patients, called modules. Nurses were assigned to modules and each module was staffed by at least one registered nurse. The module leader had 24-hour responsibility for the patients, but functioned much like a team leader while on duty. By assigning the same staff to the same module, continuity of care was fostered. Duties were arranged so that staff within the module assumed work activities for each other when someone was off duty. It was intended to save staff time by focusing care on a localized group of patients and to foster continuity of care. It followed the same principles as team nursing.[5-7]

Impacts on the Nurse, the Consumer, and Society

THE NURSE

Functional Nursing.   Functional nursing is considered a cost-effective and efficient way to get the job accomplished, particularly during periods of staff shortage or instability when many part-time and float staff are being utilized. It is a job- or task-oriented mode of assignment, which centralizes all decisions to the head nurse and discourages nursing care planning and goal setting. Workers can become highly skilled, due to the repetitiousness of this mode of assignment, with some personnel liking the repetitiveness and others finding it boring.

The head nurse plans and assigns appropriately prepared staff to specific components of care, such as medication administration, treatments, admissions, discharges, physical hygiene, ward maintenance, and inservice conferences. The head nurse also assesses the patient's needs, plans nursing interventions, coordinates the medical plan of care and evaluates the care, supervises the nursing care given by staff, receives reports from staff members, and evaluates the completeness of the assignment of each staff member.

Staff members review written assignments and clarify their assignments and responsibilities with the head nurse. They report patient progress, problems, or changes in patient conditions to the head nurse.

Team Nursing.   Team nursing is an effective method of utilizing several levels of nursing personnel. It delegates authority to provide total nursing care for a predetermined number of patients to a team nursing staff with a professional nurse as the team leader. The team leader tries to match the patients' needs with the nursing skills of each team member. There is group involvement in planning, implementing, and evaluating care through the use of team conferences and care plans.

The delegation of work to team members is carried out by the team leader, who usually has less managerial experience and education than the head nurse (who did the delegation when using the functional method). Some team leaders carry out tasks themselves that they should delegate. This tends to occur because team leaders are uncomfortable with delegation and the increased amount of time spent coordinating the delegated work and checking on the workers.

However, there may be an increased satisfaction of staff and patient needs with team nursing because of the esprit de corps of team work and of the fostered development of personnel. Because of the small number of staff and patients, the team leader may be better able to match staff abilities with patient needs and may be able to provide more direction for the delegated work. In addition, nurses will find it easier to familiarize themselves with one-half to one-third of the patients on the unit rather than all of the patients on the unit.

The head nurse identifies the number of teams needed and assigns team leaders, team members, ward maintenance personnel, and team conference planners. In addition, the head nurse collaborates with physicians and communicates changes in health care to the appropriate team leader. The assignment of new patients to a team and the evaluation of patient care plans, the implementation of nursing care, and patient progress also are a vital function of the head nurse's role.

The team leader, by comparison, plans and assigns components of patient care to qualified team members. In addition, he or she assesses all new patients assigned to the team; supervises, assists with, and evaluates the care given by team members; plans and conducts daily team conferences to review and revise nursing care plans; maintains communication with the head nurse; and prepares the report for the next shift.

Team members review the written assignments and clarify them with the team leader. They complete their assignments; document the care given, the patient's response to it, and any new problems that have arisen; and attend team conferences to help revise care plans.

Primary Nursing. Primary nursing places the registered nurse at the patient's bedside. The primary nurse is responsible for a small number of patients for 24 hours a day from the time of admission until discharge. Admitting the patient, assessing the patient's needs, planning and coordinating the care, and implementing and evaluating that care are the responsibility of the primary nurse. Associate nurses are responsible for instituting nursing measures delegated by the primary nurse. The nurse who has the greatest amount of contact with the patient is the one who makes the key decisions about his or her nursing care. This increases the nurse's authority, responsibility, and accountability[8] and, consequently, should increase job satisfaction. However, there are conflicting research findings on this matter. Ciske,[9] Kent,[10] Marram,[11] and Sellick et al[12] found an increase in job satisfaction; Collins[13] and Hegedus[14] found no significant differences, while Campbell[15] and Cassata[16] found reduced satisfaction. Betz[17] and Joiner, Johnson, and Corkrean[18] found an increase in turnover, while Campbell[15] found reduced turnover rates. Unfortunately, many of the studies have serious design flaws such as small sample size, absent reliability and validity data, undisclosed statistical tests, and lack of comparability among units. One could expect job satisfaction to vary according to the timing of the data collection. Job dissatisfaction is likely to be high during the initiation of the change to primary nursing. As a result, one could expect turnover to be high near the initiation of the change and then to decrease with a concomitant increase in reported job satisfaction.

The head nurse, on a primary nursing care unit, serves as the unit's nursing administrator and coordinator. He or she monitors the staff's assignments and tries to balance the work load through the assignment of primary nurses to patients upon admission. The head nurse monitors the system, refers physicians and others to the appropriate primary or associate nurse, selects new staff members, and evaluates staff on performance criteria. An increasing amount of the head nurse's time goes to the role of clinical consultant and to promoting the professional growth of the staff.[4]

The primary nurse assesses, plans, implements the plans, evaluates and changes the plans, and communicates and collaborates with others involved with the care of the patient. The primary nurse has 24-hour responsibility for a case load. The associate nurse reviews his or her assignment with the primary nurse, provides care to the patient in the primary nurse's absence, documents the care, and reports changes to the primary nurse.

Modular Nursing.   Modular nursing combines aspects of team and primary nursing, based on geographically defined units. A small group of personnel care for a small group of patients. One approach is to permanently assign nurses to 6 to 12 patients in a specific geographic location, with duties arranged so that staff within the module assume work activities for each other when one is off duty. The module leader has 24-hour responsibility for the patients and may rotate through all shifts. This allows for the use of less skilled workers under the direction of a registered nurse, while the more qualified nurse does the assessing, planning, teaching, and evaluating. The module may decrease pressure on staff and allow for more individualized care. It is designed to increase continuity of care by allowing nurses to consistently plan and implement care for each patient. As more registered nurses are available, the modules can break into even smaller modules.

The head nurse acts as a coordinator, identifies the number of modules, and assigns module leaders and members to each module. This can be quite difficult because of differing numbers of staff, odd numbers of patients, and differing patient acuity levels.

The module leader plans and assigns components of patient care to qualified module leaders. The leader assesses new patients assigned to the module; supervises, assists with, and evaluates care given; prepares the report for the next shift; and may be responsible for phone follow-up after discharge.

Module members clarify their assignments with the module leader, complete their assignments, and document the care given.[5-7]

THE CONSUMER AND SOCIETY

Functional Nursing.   With functional nursing, a variety of people perform the necessary functions to give complete care.[7] One nurse may take the patient's vital signs, another pass his medications, and still another do treatments. Consequently, no one is familiar with the patient's total needs and care may be fragmented and lack continuity. It is difficult to know who to ask for what help, as responsibility is difficult to fix. Because care is divided among several nurses, it is easy for each person to shirk responsibility for omissions or mistakes. The functional method is best designed to use different levels of skill and to do large amounts of work quickly and economically in times of emergency or during nursing shortages.

Team Nursing.   Because staff members do many tasks for a limited number of patients, there is an increased likelihood of errors over the functional method where one person does a single task for many patients. Continuity of care is not fostered, as patients are not assigned to the same staff all of the time and in reality care plans and team conferences are often omitted. Individualization of patient care is difficult because of large assignments. Because of the number of people involved with each patient's care, accountability can be difficult to fix. Team nursing is probably the most expensive mode because of the amount of coordination needed. Staff talent is limited to fewer patients. Less educated staff may have more down time when they cannot do what needs to be done. When teams are changed frequently, the economy of familiarity with the patients is lost.

Primary Nursing.   Primary nursing was designed to improve quality of care, increase continuity of care, foster individualistic and completeness of care, and, consequently, increase patient satisfaction while decreasing costs. However,[19] Mills[8] found no differences between team and primary nursing regarding continuity, individualization, and completeness of care. Hamera and O'Connell[20] found no significant difference in the number of contacts with patients or the amount of time spent with patients. Some research studies found increased patient satisfaction[14,21,22] and others found no differences.[8,13,23] Some research studies reported an increase in quality of care,[10,13,24-27] while others found no difference.[3,14] There are also conflicting findings about the effect of primary nursing on cost of care from decreasing costs[5] through no differences[13] to an increase in costs.[3,17] Once again, there are flaws in the research designs that cast doubt on the findings.

Modular Nursing.   The principles of modular nursing are the same as team nursing. The difference is primarily one of size. A little more efficiency is lost because staff mobility is even less than in team nursing. However, there can be closer monitoring of each case, with an opportunity to identify patient needs and reduce errors. Consequently, continuity and quality of care can be fostered. Accountability is easier to place.

Future Considerations

Second generation primary nursing, or **case management,** enhances professional nursing through the locus of accountability. It fosters the development of a culture that integrates the realities of delivering care with the evolution of professional nursing. The primary nurse or case manager establishes a working relationship with the client and family, makes ongoing nursing assessments, plans and coordinates care, teaches, and evaluates the outcomes. The care tasks can be done by technical or associate nurses, but the primary nurse or case manager is accountable for the outcomes of the care. The care givers can be interchangeable within and between shifts, but primary nurses are not.

Twenty-four hour accountability does not mean 24-hour availability. Availability by phone and during scheduled off time is very disruptive to one's personal life. Such availability should not be necessary, since nurses usually work in ready-made group practices. With role clarity and realistic expectations, the care can be delegated to associate nurses in the primary nurse's absence.

The primary nurse or case manager is responsible for a caseload of clients. Case management is a decentralized role that requires a good clinician to assess, plan, implement, and evaluate care and a good manager to coordinate the care provided to clients and their families by other health care providers. Because the case manager is accountable for outcomes, even though other health care providers participate in the delivery of care, short-term and outcome goals are important parts of the nursing process. The outcomes are the expected results of the nursing care. They are the consequences of the nursing interventions that were planned from the assessment and diagnoses. The outcomes are observable and measurable, and can be directly related to costs. They are used to evaluate the effectiveness of the nursing care.

Case management requires professional nurses who possess clinical and management skills and a desire for lifelong learning. Professional nurses have a spirit of inquiry and can identify their own learning needs and seek out learning opportunities. Case management fosters a culture that focuses on outcomes, encourages research about the effect of nursing interventions on client outcomes, develops product pricing, restructures formal evaluation of case managers to emphasize outcomes, and markets utilization of primary nurses by such means as clear identification of who the primary nurse is, use of business cards, patient contracts, and telephone follow-up after discharge.[28]

Primary nursing developed as a philosophy of care that integrated nursing theory and process with technical skills and practice. It brought about changes in patterns of communications between nurses and physicians that fostered mutual trust and respect and can evolve into interdependent and collaborative practice. **Joint practice** is the collaboration of nurses and physicians working together for the welfare of their shared patients. It is enhanced by primary nursing, encouragement of nurse decision making, joint practice committee, integrated patient records, and joint record review. Collaborative or joint practice is a progressive mode for the future.[29,30]

The research findings about modes of nursing service delivery do cause one to ponder the possibility that the individual nurse's performance may be more influential to quality of care than the mode of nursing service delivery. A well-educated and skilled nurse may give excellent care, no matter what the mode of delivery, while another nurse may not do well under any circumstances. A nurse needs more education and experience now than ever before in the history of nursing.

With a focus on controlling costs, we can expect the continued increase in ambulatory services, increased acuity in acute and critical care settings with short-term stays, and a continued increase in home care. Because of the aging population, we can expect a continued increase in chronic disease and long-term care. To help control costs, health promotion with groups of people is particularly important.

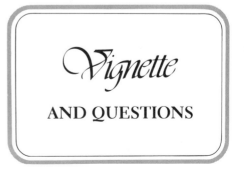

Ms. Smith is a baccalaureate-prepared head nurse on a 60-bed critical care unit. The unit has two wings, with 30 beds on each wing. On the day shift, she has two baccalaureate-prepared nurses, two associate degree–prepared nurses, and six licensed practical nurses. What mode of nursing service delivery would you recommend she use to organize the unit?

Modular nursing, which combines aspects

of team and primary nursing, could be used on this unit that has two wings with 30 beds on each wing. Each wing could be divided into two modules, with one baccalaureate degree-prepared and one associate-degree prepared nurse serving as module leaders on each wing. Three licensed practical nurses could be assigned to assist each module leader.

1. What might the head nurse do if she could replace the licensed practical nurses with registered nurses?

2. What might the head nurse do during a critical nursing shortage after two registered nurses and two practical nurses left the institution and were replaced with nurses' aides?

INFORMATION SOURCES

Joiner C, Marram van Servellen G: *Job Enhancement in Nursing: A Guide to Improving Morale, Productivity, and Retention.* Rockville, MD, Aspen Systems Corporation, 1984

Kron T, Gray A: *The Management of Patient Care: Putting Leadership Skills to Work.* Philadelphia, Saunders, 1987

Marram GD: *Primary Nursing.* St. Louis, CV Mosby, 1974

Marram G, Flynn K: *Cost-Effectiveness of Primary and Team Nursing.* Wakefield, MA, Contemporary Publishing, 1976

REFERENCES

1. McLennan M: Nursing care delivery systems: What is the most effective means of assigning patients for nursing care? Nurs Leadership 6:72, 1983

2. Kroemeke GT: Functional nursing vs. primary nursing in a hemodialysis unit. Nephrol Nurse 3:18, 1981

3. Shukla RK: All RN model of nursing care delivery: A cost benefit evaluation. Inquiry 20:173, 1983

4. Sovie MD: The primary nursing system contributes to the quality of burn nursing care. J Burn Care Rehabil 4:43, 1983

5. Ferrin T: One hospital's successful implementation of primary nursing. Nurs Adm Q 5:1, 1981

6. Hartshorn J: Team nursing to modular nursing: A planned change. SCNA News 8:6, 1981

7. Pearson A: Accountability in nursing: Primary nursing. Nurs Times 79:37, 1983

8. Mills ME: A comparison of primary and team nursing care systems as an influence on patient and staff perceptions of care. Unpublished doctoral dissertation, Johns Hopkins University, Baltimore, 1979

9. Ciske K: Will primary nursing survive in the 80s? Nurs Adm Q 5:79, 1981

10. Kent LA, Larson E: Evaluating the effectiveness of primary nursing practice. J Nurs Admin 13:34, 1983

11. Marram GD: The comparative costs of operating a team and primary nursing unit. JONA 6:21, 1976

12. Sellick KJ, Russell S, Beckmann JL: Primary nursing: An evaluation of its effects on patient perception of care and staff satisfaction. Int J Nurs Stud 20:265, 1983

13. Collins VB: The primary nursing role as a model for evaluating quality of patient care, patient satisfaction, job satisfaction, and cost effectiveness in acute care settings. Dissertation Abstracts International 36:1655B. (University Microfilms No. 75-22,117), 1975

14. Hegedus, KS: Primary nursing: Evaluation of professional nursing practice. Nurs Dimensions 7:85, 1980

15. Campbell SD: Primary nursing: It works in long-term care. J Gerontol Nurs 11:12, 1985

16. Cassata, DM: The effect of two patterns of nursing care on the perceptions of patients and nursing staff in two urban hospitals. Dissertation Abstracts International 34:5534B. (University Microfilms No. 74-10,492), 1973

17. Betz M: Some hidden costs of primary nursing. Nur and Health Care 2:150, 1981

18. Joiner C, Johnson V, Corkrean M: Is primary nursing the answer? Nur Adm Q 5:69, 1981

19. Altman J, Thielbar S: Educational efforts to support primary nursing. J Nurs Staff Dev 1:119, 1985

20. Hamera E, O'Connell K: Patient-centered variables in primary and team nursing. Res in Nurs and Health 4:183, 1981

21. Daeffler RJ: Patients' perceptions of care under team and primary nursing. JONA 5:20, 1975

22. Watson J: Patient evaluation of a primary nursing project. Aust Nurs J 8:30, 1978

23. Blair F, et al: Primary nursing in the emergency department: Nurse and patient satisfaction. J of Em Nurs 8:181, 1982

24. Erichhorn ML, Frevert EI: Evaluation of a primary nursing system using the quality patient care scale. JONA 9:11, 1979

25. Felton G: Increasing the quality of nursing care by introducing the concept of primary nursing: A model project. Nur Res 24:27, 1975

26. Steckel SB, Barnfather J, Owen M: Implementing primary nursing within a research design. Nurs Dimensions 7:78, 1980

27. Binnie F: Primary nursing—a practical possibility: One method of implementing and maintaining primary nursing. NZ Nurs J 75:7, 1982

28. Zander, K: Second generation primary nursing. JONA 15:18, 1985

29. Anderson DJ, Finn MC: Collaborative practice: Developing a structure that works. Nurs Adm Q 8:19, 1983

30. Coluccio M, Maquire P: Collaborative practice: Becoming a reality through primary nursing. Nurse Adm Q 7:59, 1983

SUE POPKESS-VAWTER, RN, PhD

CHAPTER 7   *Nursing Diagnosis:*
Its Development
and Future

Background and Overview

"The ground swell of enthusiasm engendered by nursing diagnosis suggests that this movement may have a significant impact on the profession. It seems all the more incumbent on us, then, to raise critical questions, to tease apart the nuances, to promote serious discussion among colleagues, and to refine, change, and grow."[1] Shamansky and Yanni[1] disputed that nursing diagnoses in their present form limited nursing practice, created obstacles to clear communication among nurses, and constrained nursing inference and intuition. Such debates stimulate clarity of expression among nursing professionals who support the nursing diagnosis movement. Numerous issues have surfaced as a result of the creation of a nursing diagnosis taxonomy.

    The purpose of this chapter is to provide background information about the historical evolution of nursing diagnosis and a discussion of the major impacts that nursing diagnosis has had on the profession, other professions, and the consumer and society. Future considerations include the refinement of the existing nursing diagnosis listing, enhancement of professionalism, reimbursement, and computerization. Finally, a vignette will be presented to exemplify the major points in the chapter, and discussion questions will be posed to stimulate dialogue.

HISTORICAL EVOLUTION OF NURSING DIAGNOSIS

Nursing diagnosis gained national recognition in 1973, when the First National Nursing Diagnosis Conference Group gathered to articulate more clearly what nurses have to offer for patients' specific problems.[2] This need was recognized in the literature long before the words *nursing diagnosis* were first used by Fry.[3] In reviewing the literature from 1950 to the present, a variety of terms were used to express the focus of nursing diagnosis. For example, Abdellah[4] posed "nursing problems" as the content that patients and families presented. Durand and Prince[5] emphasized that nursing diagnoses are the conclusion of recognition of patients' patterns, while Chambers[6] spoke of patients' specific needs that require nursing action. It seemed apparent that there truly was a need to articulate the nursing focus more clearly. Over these years, many historical events in the profession were occurring concurrently. Nurses were learning physical and psychosocial assessment skills, applying nursing process, participating in the problem-oriented medical record movement, and doing research that contributed to the nursing body of knowledge. The influence on the development of nursing diagnosis on each of these historical events will be incorporated into the forthcoming discussions.

Nursing Diagnosis Defined. The definition of nursing diagnosis has evolved to more clearly address what it is and how it differs from other professional diagnoses. In 1973 the first National Conference Group defined nursing diagnosis as the conclusion that occurs as the result of nursing assessment.[2] This succinct definition supplied the missing part of what was currently called nursing process—the missing link between assessment and planning. Gordon, one of the frequently cited experts in nursing diagnosis, presented this commonly used definition of nursing diagnosis in 1976: "Nursing diagnoses, or clinical diagnoses made by professional nurses, describe actual or potential health problems which nurses by virtue of their education and experience are capable and licensed to treat."[7] This definition speaks to three important points. First, she differentiated between actual and potential health problems, drawing attention to the preventive responsibilities of nurses as well as care for immediate problems. Second, she noted how nurses should be professionally prepared and experienced in order to treat the diagnoses once they are made. Finally, she included the legal aspects of diagnosing, which should prompt nurses to analyze their states' nurse practice acts to be assured that they were adequately "covered" to make nursing diagnoses.

Much struggle and debate have occurred among nurses when trying to define the essence of nursing. Through the clouds of confusion and debate came this short, clear definition of nursing from the American Nurses' Association (ANA), which incorporated nursing diagnosis in the definition, "nursing is the diagnosis and treatment of human responses to actual or potential health problems."[8] In the preceding years, ANA also published Standards of Practice,[9] incorporating nursing diagnosis throughout nursing process. Thus the professional organization recognized and committed itself to the use of nursing diagnosis as a means to carry out nursing practice.

It seems that the Social Policy Statement definition of nursing has clarified how nursing diagnoses differ from other professional diagnoses. If nursing diagnoses are viewed as human responses to actual or potential health problems, it becomes quite clear that the focus of nursing is with human beings and their responses to health and illness concerns. Note the latter part of the previous sentence—health and illness concerns. It was the belief of the Diagnosis Development and Testing Committee of the Mid-America Nursing Diagnosis Conference Group[10] that nursing diagnoses include both health-oriented as well as illness- or problem-oriented nursing diagnoses. Therefore this more encompassing definition was proposed: **nursing diagnoses** are conclusions that describe human responses to actual or potential health concerns and practices. Similarly, Carpenito[11] defined nursing diagnosis to include both a health state and an actual or potential alteration in an individual's life processes.

Types of Nursing Diagnoses. As Gordon presented in her definition, two types of nursing diagnoses include actual or potential health problems. Within the broader definition, actual or potential human responses are the conclusions from the nursing physical and psychosocial assessment data base. Objective and subjective signs and symptoms or defining characteristics are clustered to indicate that a health or illness concern exists. Further analysis of the data base may reveal an etiological or related contributing factor to express the nursing diagnosis in a two-part statement. Equally as important, nurses are responsible for collecting cues to detect potential illness and concerns. Actual human responses are planned and cared for while potential human responses are planned for in order to support and perpetuate health concerns and prevent illness concerns.

Some authors differentiate between **potential and possible nursing diagnoses.** Potential nursing diagnoses are those concerns that are high risk or probable, and possible concerns are those that have not been verified or validated.[12] In the practice world, probable, possible, and potential have little relevant difference. If students, upon conclusion of a holistic nursing assessment, can differentiate between actual and potential human responses, holistic care planning will result. The additional subcategory, possible, only complicates the decision-making and diagnostic process without directing nurses in different actions other than direct intervention (actual concerns) or preventive care (potential concerns).

In fact, this author believes that instead of potential problems, "at risk for" presents nurses with more substantial direction for nursing action than potential. For example, a 35-year-old obese male who smokes, has a strong family history of myocardial infarction, and has been diagnosed with borderline hypertension is in the "at risk for" heart disease category. An individualized nursing diagnosis using this category would be knowledge deficit regarding high risk for heart disease related to lack of health teaching. Another example for an immobile patient would be at risk for skin breakdown related to impaired mobility. By using the at risk alternative, nurses are required to summarize risk factors that were detected in the holistic assessment process. The summary of risk factors should lead to diagnostic categories and in turn lead to individualized two-part diagnostic statements.

Approved List of Nursing Diagnoses. Nurses would understand more clearly the limitations of the present North American Nursing Diagnosis Association (NANDA) listing of approved nursing diagnoses if they had participated in the first five national conferences. Most nurses misunderstand that the listing is a finished list that should be applicable to any patient or nursing care setting. The NANDA listing has been approved for testing only—most diagnoses have not been empirically tested to be substantiated, refined, and in the form usable in practice.

Beginning in 1973, 100 participants at the first National Nursing Diagnosis Conference were divided into ten groups and ironically generated 100 nursing diagnoses. Using participants' experiential backgrounds, they developed diagnoses using ten physiologic systems as a guide while considering developmental, environmental, sociological, and psychological points of view. Diagnoses were also considered from preventive, acute, long-term, and rehabilitative care aspects. The same inductive group process was used to generate nursing diagnoses at the second through the fifth conferences. The diagnoses list from the previous conference was mailed to participants so that they might prioritize the three to five diagnoses that most interested them. At the next conference, they were grouped according to chosen diagnoses and worked to refine existing statements and sometimes to develop new statements. At each conference the group process became more sophisticated, participants were more informed about nursing diagnoses, and more empirical literature was available to develop accurate statements. The PES (problem, etiology, and signs and symptoms) format used in later conferences gave an improved structure in order to make clearer and more practical diagnoses (see Table 7-1).

At the close of each of the first five conferences, members voted to accept or reject individual diagnoses proposed by the conference work groups. "Acceptance" meant that diagnoses were ready for clinical testing; it did not mean that these diagnoses were finished and in final form. Some

TABLE 7-1

Example of PES Format[31]

PROBLEM: Mobility, Impairment of

ETIOLOGY:

Imposed limitations of movement within the environment; etiological factors
may include:
therapy, pain, fatigue, trauma, lack of required physical support,
environmental factors, psychosocial factors

SIGNS AND SYMPTOMS (DEFINING CHARACTERISTICS):

Inability to move
Reluctance to attempt movement
Perceived inability to move
Goals incongruent with abilities
Altered perception of position/presence of body part(s)
Alteration in coordination of movement
Limited active range of motion
Decreased muscle strength and/or control
Imposed restrictions of movement

---

diagnoses were named "TBD," or to be developed, meaning that all parts of
the PES format were not complete. Even so, these labels were listed at the
end of each conference alphabetical listing.

The sixth conference,[13] when the small group process was eliminated,
was the first official NANDA conference. Since that time, the diagnosis
submission and refinement process has been accomplished through
NANDA committees.

Up to the time of the seventh conference, the listing of accepted
nursing diagnoses was in alphabetical order. At the seventh conference in
1986, the NANDA membership voted on a taxonomic structure other than
an alphabetical listing. The proposed organizing structures were the Unitary
Human framework[14] and Gordon's 11 patterns.[15] Unitary Human framework uses the following patterns: exchanging, communicating, relating,
valuing, choosing, moving, perceiving, knowing, and feeling. Although
many of the members discussed the ambiguity of the nine patterns within
Unitary Human framework, the majority vote was to accept this framework
as an organizing taxonomy for present and future nursing diagnoses. In its
present form, there are four levels of abstraction within this taxonomy,
going from abstract to concrete as the levels go higher. Existing diagnoses
are categorized within the framework, and the actual framework structure

suggests additional diagnoses that should be named in order for each subcategory of Unitary Human to be described.[16]

STRENGTHS AND LIMITATIONS OF EXISTING LISTS OF NURSING DIAGNOSES

Actual lists of nursing diagnoses did not exist until the first nursing diagnosis conference in 1973. Campbell[17] in 1978 published the first text that listed nursing diagnoses. After the proceedings of the first conferences were published, other texts and articles included a listing of conference-generated diagnoses as well as additional diagnoses from authors' experiences and research. A PES format has been adopted by most authors as a clear means of presenting nursing diagnoses. (Refer to resource listing at the conclusion of this chapter for texts that include listings of nursing diagnoses.)

Existing lists share several strengths and limitations. The first strength common to nursing diagnosis listings is the applicability to medical-surgical nursing, under which most patients are categorized. Although medical-surgical nursing is a subspecialty, the human responses and health concerns are far-reaching for most other nursing subspecialties. Therefore, a major strength is the relevance of the lists for the majority of patients and clients. For example, physiologic problem categories, including airway clearance, bowel elimination, breathing pattern, cardiac output, fluid volume deficit, gas exchange, alteration in nutrition, sexual dysfunction, skin integrity, tissue perfusion, and urinary elimination, reflect the usual concerns for patients with medical or surgical problems. On the other hand, patients and clients in maternal, child, community, and even psychological nursing share these concerns. The psychosocial categories listed in most references (communication, coping, diversional activity, fear, grieving, home maintenance management, knowledge deficit, mobility, noncompliance, parenting, rape trauma, self-care deficit, self-concept, sensory perceptual, sleep pattern, spiritual distress, thought processes) are medical-surgical predominant; however, again, practice in other nursing care areas and settings involves these diagnoses as well.

The second strength is that most texts have followed suit in using NANDA's PES format to organize and present each diagnostic label, including a definition, etiologies, and defining characteristics (signs and symptoms). Definitions of labels are the least consistent part not always listed in nursing diagnosis texts. However, if texts list etiologies and defining characteristics, nurses will be guided adequately in assessment so that nursing diagnoses can be made. Variations of PES format include etiologies further divided into pathophysiological, situational and maturational sub-categories,[11] diagnostic divisions (general taxonomic category of diagnoses),[18] and nursing diagnoses based on identified etiologies (most frequently used two-part diagnostic statements).[19]

There are three limitations of the existing lists of nursing diagnoses. First, if texts and articles refer only to the conference lists, inappropriate labeling often will occur. Numerous inpatient settings have restricted nurses to use only the NANDA listing. By doing so, patients are forced into labels that are not appropriate for their health/illness concern. In turn, care planning is inappropriate for their original area of concern. There are many other labels not included in the NANDA lists that exist in nursing practice. Some authors have added labels to the NANDA list that are equally suitable for testing and temporary use.

Second, most diagnoses originated from a medical model rather than a nursing model. Until recently, schools of nursing patterned their curricula after a medical model, since most faculty in their generic programs used the physiologic systems to guide nursing education. As previously listed, numerous physiologic nursing diagnoses resulted, reflecting only the physical part of individuals. Nursing models are holistic in the way that they emphasize the biopsychosocial elements of human beings and thus guide nursing diagnoses to express the human responses to physical and psychosocial concerns. The most recent nursing diagnosis research, articles, and texts are beginning to emphasize nursing models and reflect holistic or biopsychosocial nursing diagnoses.

Finally, not all practice areas are represented in the existing nursing diagnosis labels. Nurses in major divisions and subspecialty areas have expressed a lack of existing labels in their areas of practice. As discussed earlier, most labels express concerns for adult, medical-surgical patients and are rarely reflective of psychiatric, community, well-baby and child, maternal, and well-adult areas of nursing practice. At the seventh NANDA conference, 21 new diagnoses were accepted that included more diagnoses reflecting psychosocial and well-baby and child areas.[20] Eventually, subspecialties and unrepresented nursing practices are becoming active in generating labels that express patients' and clients' concerns in their practice areas.

Impacts on the Nurse, the Consumer, and Society

THE NURSE

Three types of nursing care include independent, interdependent, and dependent nursing care. **Independent nursing care** refers to actions that are totally left up to the nurse to assess, diagnose, plan, intervene, evaluate, and revise without reliance upon other health care professionals' input or intervention. **Interdependent nursing care** refers to the same steps of nursing process with the input, assistance, and collaboration with other health care professionals. Finally, **dependent nursing care** refers to nursing process as directed by and relying upon another health care professional's input and intervention. Nursing diagnostic categories that might exemplify each of these types of nursing care would include alteration in skin integrity (independent), immobility (interdependent), and decreased cardiac output (dependent).

Although these three types of nursing care have varying degrees of dependence upon other health care professionals, communication among nurses regardless of type is enhanced through nursing diagnoses. Functional nursing care planning emphasizes the tasks of nursing care and does not reflect the patient-orientation or their human responses. Patients and clients are outsiders to care given rather the recipients of the care because it is not patient-oriented. Nursing diagnoses, on the other hand, explicitly name not only individuals' healthy responses and responses to the alterations in health, but the related factors (etiologies) that should direct nursing care planning and interventions.

Approximately ten years ago nurses would come to work and receive report that focused on medical diagnoses, medications and treatments ordered, and the functional nursing tasks to carry out orders. Little recognition was given to the nurses' independent care planning and intervention. In fact, rarely were interdependent nursing care plans generated. Predominantly dependent nursing care planning occurred. Today there are growing numbers of nurses making nursing diagnoses from the admission assessment and throughout the inpatient and outpatient processes. Now upon receiving report from a nursing diagnosis framework, nurses can determine how patients and clients are responding to the disease or health concerns happening in their lives. When written appropriately, nursing diagnoses direct outcome criteria and interventions simply through reading the two-part diagnostic statements.

As nurses discover greater independence through emphasis on human responses rather than medical diagnoses, a different variety of nursing diagnoses will be generated. These diagnostic labels will more clearly describe what nurses do to help patients' specific problems, which addresses the original purpose set forth by the first National Nursing Diagnosis Conference Group. The nursing diagnosis taxonomy will serve as a common means of communication among nurses to focus not only caregiving practices but administrative, educational, and research activities.

It appears that the more separated from the acute care setting, the easier it is for nurses to make independent and interdependent types of nursing diagnoses. Hospitals today contract with physicians to administer to their clientele. In most hospitals, nursing care is still categorized under the room charges. Dependent nursing care tends to cause nursing to remain in the room charges and does not readily allow for expansion into the interdependent and independent nursing care. Eventually, if institutions contracted for nursing care with nursing corporations directly, a more balanced distribution of dependent, interdependent, and independent nursing care could be given. Nevertheless, all three types of nursing care must continue in the current structures of inpatient and outpatient care settings. Holistic nursing assessment through the entire nursing process will assure balance among the three types of nursing care.

Kim[21] and Guzzetta and Dossey[22] explain the difficulty that nurses in acute care settings (especially intensive care units) have in dealing with medical diagnoses and dependent nursing diagnoses. They suggest that emphasis on patients' physiologic responses eliminates the risk of "practicing medicine," since physiologic principles and terminology are for the use of any profession. Most states' nursing practice acts specify that nursing diagnoses be separate from medical diagnoses; thus nurses are accountable to differentiate clearly between medical and nursing diagnoses. This professional charge requires nurses to have in-depth knowledge of anatomy and physiology, which assists them in knowing the alteration in body function. Such knowledge assists in the generation of nursing diagnoses that emphasize physiologic responses rather than reiteration of medical diagnoses. Some might argue that nurses are only changing the name; however, physiologic responses guide nursing caregiving, while medical diagnoses do not. An example to clarify might be the medical diagnosis myocardial infarction. One of the major human responses to myocardial infarction is decreased cardiac output. Patients have numerous responses to decreased cardiac output such as fear, anxiety, decreased mentation, confusion, restlessness, breathlessness, fatigue, and arrhythmia. Notice how the human responses become the first part of a two-part diagnostic statement and the decreased cardiac output becomes the etiological second part of a statement to which the first part is related—confusion related to decreased cardiac output or fatigue related to decreased cardiac output. As demonstrated by these examples, myocardial infarction does not direct nursing care, but the variety of human responses direct patient outcome criteria and the related etiology or etiologies direct nursing interventions.

Traditionally, nurses care for patients according to physicians' directives and patients' basic human needs. In the early 1970s, nursing process and nursing assessment skills were being taught in schools of nursing and inservice programs throughout the United States. Partly due to the advent of critical care units, where life-threatening situations were common, nurses were required to develop more in-depth assessment skills, which provided them with greater understanding of the human body and its responses to disease. Nursing histories and physicals were beginning to appear as a permanent part of patients' records.

Two major flaws in the application of nursing process and assessment skills were the lack of holistic assessment (complete biopsychosocial data base) and the omission of the intervening step between assessment and planning, nursing diagnosis. As nurses carved out their roles in acute and critical care areas, they developed a pseudo-security in believing that they were giving independent nursing care. Physicians were trusting nurses' judgments and actions so completely, that they were in attendance less. Therefore, many nurses believed that their nursing roles were independent, while in reality they were practicing as "junior doctors." This false autonomy only served to strengthen the use of the medical model and medical diagnoses as an outcome of nurses doing physical assessment.

As critical care nurses became skilled at physical assessment, nurses in inpatient and outpatient settings began to learn physical assessment skills and apply them in their areas of practice. Often critical care nurses were the teachers of assessment skills. Since critical care emphasizes the life-threatening physical assessment measures, assessment tended to omit the psychosocial areas of individuals. Additionally, when students and nurses begin to learn new skills, emphasis is placed on physical attainment (the "how-to skills") rather than interpersonal skills. Thus the psychosocial portion of holistic assessment was not recognized until later, when the physical skills were mastered. Unfortunately, some nurses still have not expanded their assessment skills to include interpersonal interchange as an important part of nursing care.

Although nurses became very proficient in doing histories and physicals assessment, they often leaped into care planning without summarizing what was found in their assessments. Therefore, a connection was not evident between the data base and care plan, and consequently care plans were not individualized with specific assessment information. If there was a relationship between the data base and care plan, it was not complete and all of the pertinent conclusions were not prioritized and included in care planning. It could be that nursing diagnoses did not gain recognition among nurses until assessment skills were considered part of nursing care. This would explain why the conclusions of nursing assessment, nursing diagnoses, were omitted.

Now most nurses practice holistic assessments so that nursing diagnoses flow from the data base to become the focus of nursing care planning and to guide the remainder of nursing process. The ANA Standards of Practice[9] demonstrate clearly how nursing process incorporates nursing diagnoses. Those standards are a model for minimum nursing care to assure that, regardless of the care setting, nursing is administered through a systematic, organized approach.

Numerous books have been written about the decision-making, scientific diagnostic process that occurs when going from assessment data base to conclusive statements about individuals' statuses.[23,24,15] While collecting data, many nurses think in terms of needs because of the influence of

Maslow[25] and Henderson.[26] Others think in terms of problems, not only stemming from the medical model, but from Weed's problem-oriented medical record.[27] Only recently have nurses begun to think in terms of the existing nursing diagnoses to describe the actual or potential health problems. It is important for nurses to go one step further to define the precise human response and include the etiologic statement to make a two-part diagnostic label, which in turn directs outcome criteria and nursing interventions. To illustrate, after assessing a 68-year-old patient with COPD who has developed pneumonia and is hospitalized in the respiratory intensive care unit, nurses must not stop with the diagnostic category of ineffective breathing pattern. Ineffective breathing pattern, or breathlessness, has numerous additional human responses subcategorized.[28] Although the pathology is of primary concern to the intensive care nurse, the patient's stressful response to breathlessness is only aggravating an already compromised blood gas picture. Clearly, intervention for breathlessness could improve gas exchange and reduce energy expenditure, both allowing more rapid response to treatments and in turn promote recuperation. A more accurate nursing diagnosis label to express this human response would be fear of dying related to breathlessness. The important point here is for nurses not to stop with the NANDA or any other listing of nursing diagnostic "labels." These listings are actually categories from which to chose expressions of human responses and etiologies that make up the two-part, individualized nursing diagnosis, or the conclusions of nursing assessment.

When broad diagnostic categories are identified, the thought process must continue to determine which is the most important human response for which to intervene and what are its related factors (etiologies) for which nursing care is planned. In the example given, breathlessness appeared to be a priority human response which if not controlled would impact negatively upon other diagnostic categories that the patient exhibited, such as fatigue and confusion. The human response (fear of dying) directs outcome criteria, "patient will express reduced fear on a scale of 1-10 eight hours after admission." Breathlessness, the etiological statement, is the focus of nursing intervention, or the means by which the fear may be reduced. Thus, if the nurse can effectively intervene for breathlessness, the fear should be reduced. After eight hours, the nurse evaluates whether the patient has reduced fear by asking him to tell how fearful he is now on a scale from 1 to 10. It should be apparent how this two-part statement guides nursing care differently from "nursing diagnoses" (categories) such as ineffective breathing pattern or impaired gas exchange.

Once the two-part label is used for care planning, the interventions, evaluations, and revisions flow directly and easily from the diagnosis. If outcome criteria are stated completely, nurses in the evaluation phase of process need only to review the outcome criteria and compare them to individuals' current states based on secondary or ongoing assessments. Outcome criteria should be patient centered, specific, realistic, measurable, and state the direction and time of change to occur.

Without the complete use of nursing process based on nursing diagnoses, nursing care is planned and carried out in a vacuum. With the inclusion of each of these steps, nurses are directed and assisted in caregiving.

Impact on Other Health Professions.   The true impact of nursing diagnoses probably began after the first national nursing diagnosis conference in 1973. In order to communicate openly among health professionals, the planners and conveners of the conference invited representatives from physicians active in classification of medicine, the American Hospital Association, the Joint Commission on Accreditation of Hospitals, and the American Medical Record Association.[2] These professionals did not attend the remaining six conferences as recognized groups, and consequently no organized effort was made to facilitate communications among these professions. As a result, confusion has resulted among health professionals regarding the purpose of nurses diagnosing. Just as assessment skills were misinterpreted by physicians, nursing diagnoses only added to the misinterpretation that nurses were trying to perform physicians' traditional tasks. At first, nurses were performing as junior doctors because they were modeled by physicians to learn assessment and diagnostic skills. Some nurses continue to practice along medical lines rather than being clear on the difference in purpose behind nursing assessment and diagnoses.

The purpose of nursing history and assessment is to provide information about patients and clients as a basis for nursing diagnosis and care planning. Nursing diagnoses are the conclusions of the nursing assessment data base or those that describe human responses to actual or potential health concerns and practices. Medical assessment and diagnoses direct physicians to cure and/or manage disease processes, whereas nursing assessment and diagnoses assist nurses to care for patients' or clients' responses to disease processes or health concerns. Unless nurses are able to clearly differentiate between nursing and medical processes, confusion will continue, collaborative efforts will be stifled, and patients and clients will suffer, as well as the nursing profession itself.

Along the same lines, the confusion described with the medical profession is similar to that with the dietary, pharmacy, and social work professions. When holistic nursing assessment is performed and holistic nursing diagnoses are made, nurses are accountable and responsible for the total person's biopsychosocial well-being. Holism also implies that nurses are accountable and responsible for all aspects of care, including nutritional, pharmacologic, and psychosocial welfare. In years past, these "turfs" have been disputed and argued among the professions and nursing diagnoses seem to have rekindled the flames of disagreement. Once again, the nursing profession must articulate clearly the purpose of nursing diagnoses to all health professionals and work toward collaborative care so that patients and clients are not made to suffer. If nurses could think of this collaborative effort as analogous to a concert orchestra conductor and the players, they could explain how nurses orchestrate all aspects of care. Some may believe that physicians are the orchestrators and nurses are the professionals being directed. It seems that because of the 24-hour accountability, primary nursing, and caseload management, nurses are in greater attendance with patients and clients than other professionals to determine the most appropriate timing to meet most or all of their needs.

When nurses help other professionals to understand the intent of nursing diagnosis, the enhancement of interdisciplinary health care should occur. When patients' total health care needs are identified by nurses, it becomes clearer how interdisciplinary relations can enhance patient care and appropriate referrals may be made. For example, a nurse would communicate to a surgeon the nursing diagnosis, fear of surgery related to father's intraoperative death. They can develop a collaborative plan of care to work through or manage the fear prior to surgery or even postpone surgery until the fear can be managed. The patient, with a diagnosis of nutritional deficit related to body image greater than actual body size, should be referred to the dietary professional who works collaboratively with a psychiatric clinical nurse specialist in developing a dietary plan. For a patient with diabetes who has a nursing diagnosis, noncompliance with self-administration of insulin related to poor vision and manual dexterity, nurses can collaborate with pharmacologic professionals to locate special syringes and insulin packaging to accommodate self-care. If this referral does not promote compliance, the social worker can be consulted to arrange for home care or visiting nurses to administer the insulin. These are all examples of interdependent nursing diagnoses.

Weed's[27] problem-oriented medical record (POMR) system assisted physicians to make more complete and explanatory documentation of care. Nurses patterned after and participated in POMR as well as most other health care professionals. A summative listing of patients' problems and concerns, as suggested by Weed, would assist increased communication among all health professionals involved in patients' care. Whether in inpatient or outpatient settings, the front pages of health care records could include each discipline's diagnostic statements to help professionals be more knowledgeable about collaborative efforts. Ultimately nurses could be responsible for orchestrating the collaboration and referrals among all professionals. The value of such a central listing is beyond explanation.

THE CONSUMER AND SOCIETY

Nursing diagnoses can be one of the most important means for nurses to inform the consumer and society in general about what the nursing profession offers. First, nursing diagnoses allow consumers to know precisely the focus of care given by nurses. Through unfortunate experiences and the mass media, consumers often have a very negative, stereotypical view of nurses. Superficial properties such as the bedpan or syringe seem to express what nurses do, or the movies' Nurse Ratchets convey the unfeeling self-centeredness that the profession would like to bury. Barnard[29] believed that through the ANA Social Policy Statement, nursing is the only health profession that made a formal statement about its practice to the public to affirm social accountability. The statement[8] maintains that nursing can be said to be owned by society, since the profession's interest must be to serve society's perceived interests. The public good must be nursing's overriding concern. It goes on to state that nursing has made a substantial contribution toward a health-oriented system of care; however, care of the sick remains a basic responsibility. The ANA's definition of nursing clearly states nurses' central focus and charge. Once consumers have experienced the true meaning of the nursing care, they become willing to pay for these services, which in turn promotes nursing as a profession. Word of mouth referrals from satisfied consumers is perhaps the best means to publicize what nurses can do. What type of care are consumers seeking and willing to pay for?—holistic, individualized care that focuses on balanced biopsychosocial human concerns and responses. Not all nurses who deliver this type of care use nursing diagnosis labels; but if their care were analyzed, specific human responses and etiological factors would be apparent. Ask satisfied consumers of nursing care what human responses and concerns were the focus of their care and it should become evident that nursing diagnoses, though not written as such, were actually present.

Second, nursing diagnoses permit quality of care to be readily measured because of the specific and individualized way in which they are written. When nursing care is given through functional tasks without attention to human responses, quality of care can be excellent, but it is often inappropriately directed and some human responses may be overlooked. Once again the ANA Standards of Care show how nursing process is implemented through use of nursing diagnoses and the quality measures are specified throughout the process.

Additionally, if time and motion studies could be done in care settings where nursing diagnoses are and are not used, most likely the setting where diagnoses are used would have less duplication of effort and greater continuity of care. By using a central listing of nursing diagnoses and caregiving interventions, nurses are able to build upon each other's previous plans and interventions. When conclusions about patients' human responses are not made, nursing becomes fragmented and the quality of care diminishes.

Future Considerations

REFINEMENT OF NURSING DIAGNOSIS LISTINGS

From 1973 to 1982 the National Nursing Diagnosis Conference Groups used the inductive group process to develop and refine the listing of nursing diagnoses. Over a period of usually four days, each group refined diagnoses using the PES format and at the end of the meeting, participants voted on the "accepted" diagnoses. At the seventh conference, diagnoses were submitted to the Diagnosis Review Committee and materials regarding proposed diagnoses were mailed to participants prior to the meeting so that discussion and voting could take place to "accept" the new labels for testing. The formal process for submission is outlined by the review committee in the Development/Submission Guidelines for Proposed New Nursing Diagnoses,[30] which continues through the intervening time between conferences.

Reports of research studies are increasing at every NANDA conference. For example, there were four research papers presented at the Third Conference and six papers at the Fourth Conference.[31] Whereas at the Seventh Conference, there were 17 research papers, including three on nursing diagnosis in general, one on research methodology, three on the process of making nursing diagnoses, three on implementation issues, and seven on specific nursing diagnosis labels.[32] Nurses in practice, administration, and education are increasing research skills and experiences so that the nursing body of knowledge is improving in quality and quantity. Nursing diagnoses labels serve as practical research topics. Most labels have not been researched to the extent that etiologies and defining characteristics have been sufficiently validated. It seems appropriate that validation studies of the variables that describe diagnostic labels should be the first step in research concerning nursing diagnoses. Once labels are validated and instruments or measurement techniques are developed to recognize labels in the practical world, intervention studies then can proceed. Without formal validation of labels, treatment or intervention studies seem premature. It is important that nurse researchers realize that the existing labels were mainly developed through the inductive small group process at the NANDA conferences; thus the tentativeness of most labels can be appreciated.

There seems to be an "ivory tower" stigma existing in the nursing profession today. In other words, many nurses believe that nursing research is being conducted in isolation from the real world. Research may have existed in this way in the past, but in the last five to ten years proliferation of research at the bedside, in academia, and in administration has occurred. Nurses are gaining confidence at all levels of academic preparation to conduct or participate in research studies that address problems in their areas of practice. Most nurses are not self-sufficient in their abilities to implement all areas of the research process. Chinn and Jacobs[33] believed that a single person is unable to effectively make significant contributions in all levels of theory development, which includes both quantitative and qualitative research methods. Collaborative efforts to conduct research should be encouraged among nurses. Nurses who have knowledge and skills in the content areas being researched, in the research process itself, and in statistical applications are only a few examples of the broad spectrum of expertise included in a total research project.

Most nursing diagnoses express problem areas that are universally important to the bedside nurse, the academician, and the administrator. All three want to learn more about diagnostic categories such as pain and knowledge deficit. Once again, collaborative efforts among nurses in these three roles can produce meaningful answers to clarify specific nursing diagnoses, as well as more global nursing care concerns.

Until recently there has been a lack of clear methodologies for testing nursing diagnosis labels. It appears that descriptive, exploratory studies are a beginning for new diagnoses that have little research base. A balance of qualitative and quantitative methods is being described in the literature that assist new researchers in choosing an appropriate methodology for a particular label. Among the most clearly described and practical methodologies presented at the Seventh NANDA Conference[32] for descriptive studies to validate nursing diagnoses are the following:

- Clinical Validation Model. Combination of use of an instrument to measure nurse-reported or self-reported information regarding the diagnosis and a semistructured interview technique to validate existing objective and subjective diagnoses data as well as additional data not found in the literature[34,35]
- Delphi Survey. Survey, usually in three or four separate mailings, to nurses who are in the area of practice related to the diagnosis being validated[36,37]
- Questionnaire to Field Experts. Structured or open-ended questionnaire or case study assignment given to a few specially qualified or nationally recognized experts in one or repeated mailings[36,38]
- Retrospective Comparative Record Audit. Nursing notes, laboratory findings, vital signs flowsheets, etc—are audited for incidence of objective and subjective data regarding actual or potential diagnoses[39,40]

Additionally, Clinton[41] explained three categories of research methodologies that would be helpful to further develop nursing diagnoses: 1) practical feasibility of the nomenclature in multiple settings throughout the country through pooled survey research; 2) reliability, specifically internal consistency, interrater, and intrarater, for nursing diagnoses and nurses making them; and 3) validity testing, specifically construct, external criterion, and discriminant validity testing to determine whether nursing diagnoses actually describe what they say they do. Each of these categories goes beyond the preliminary development accomplished through descriptive methodologies. Over time, nursing diagnosis research will reflect all of these methodologies, which eventually will validate the existing and future listings.

One important aspect to remember in developing methodologies to validate nursing diagnoses is obtaining both the nursing and patients'/families' perspectives. Educational research has shown that nurses frequently teach what they believe patients should know without seeking patients' and clients' input,[42-44] whereas patients and their families often have different needs to know. It is no wonder that patient teaching sometimes is not effective.

This same consideration is true for making and validating nursing diagnoses. Most diagnoses listed include both objective and subjective signs and symptoms of human responses. The objective signs can be validated through the nursing assessments and measurements. The subjective symptoms usually can be validated through patients' and families' verbal validation. However, some diagnoses, such as breathlessness, are totally subjective. Breathlessness is defined as the unpleasant feeling of difficulty to breathe based on individual's subjective perception of impaired ventilation.[45] Fatigue is another example of a diagnostic category that depends only upon individuals' subjective validation as a defining characteristic necessary to make the diagnosis.

When nurse researchers are thorough in testing both objective and subjective defining characteristics for all tentative diagnoses, data may be pooled and finally diagnoses can be called confirmed. Studies then can be designed to test interventions that are based on confirmed nursing diagnoses using the validated definitions, defining characteristics and etiologies.

ENHANCEMENT OF PROFESSIONALISM

Nursing has been described as an evolving profession because it does not meet all of the criteria for an established profession. Kellams[46] believed that all professions continually worked at meeting the criteria for a profession. Not long ago, nursing did not meet professional criteria; but today, all of the criteria noted by Bixler and Bixler[47] and Kellams[46] are met to some degree.

In fact, many of the criteria were not clearly focused until the nursing diagnosis movement.

Most of the criteria have been indirectly addressed throughout the previous sections in this chapter. Each criterion will be highlighted briefly again. The first criterion, satisfying a societal need, is clearly discussed in the Social Policy Statement.[8] Nurses are concerned with the public good and offer health and illness care to meet society's needs.

The second and third criteria include having a unique body of knowledge and increasing that body of knowledge. As reported in each of the NANDA proceedings, nursing diagnoses have assisted nurses in studying what nurses do and that research is steadily increasing as diagnoses are being clarified.

Criteria four and five require that professions have standards and control their own practices. Through the ANA Standards,[9] nursing states minimal standards from which individual states can base nurse practice acts. By doing so, nursing controls its practice. Included in the Standards and in many states' nurse practice acts are statements about the purpose of nursing diagnoses, which is to direct nursing process or nursing care.

The sixth criterion speaks to a code of ethics, which ANA house of delegates originally adopted in 1950.[48] The final criterion requires that professions educate its practitioners in institutions of higher learning, which has been supported by the ANA[49] and the National League for Nursing, the educational accrediting body for the nursing profession. It seems that presently nursing is reasonably meeting these professional criteria and the nursing diagnosis movement has served to direct the profession in this effort.

REIMBURSEMENT BASED ON NURSING DIAGNOSES

Nursing care has been included in the "room rent" for too many years. Nursing diagnoses begin to delineate precisely the profession's areas of concern. Although the current DRG system is based on medical diagnoses, it sets a precedence upon which to base research and acuity ratings to determine the cost of applying nursing process for combinations of diagnostic labels.[50] In a federally funded study completed in the state of New Jersey,[51] 28 nursing diagnostic labels were used. Not only did this study demonstrate what nurses do and how nursing diagnoses can facilitate delivery of nursing care, but the study provided justification for the need for various types of nursing care that could be reimbursed for services rendered.

Halloran, Kiley, and Nosek[52] studied 1294 adult patients in nonintensive care areas to determine the influence of nursing care complexity and DRGs on patients' lengths of stay. Nursing diagnoses were used to express nursing care delivered to patients in this sample. Nursing complexity (nursing diagnoses) explained approximately 20 percent more variation than did DRGs. Thus, they found that nurses play an important role in optimizing patients' lengths of stay through their caregiving.

Gebbie[53] addressed the participants at the seventh NANDA conference regarding fee-based reimbursement using nursing diagnoses. She believed that the reason why diagnosis-based reimbursement systems have not developed was due to the fact that nursing diagnoses are not yet fully established. Gebbie stated that satisfied consumers will be the ones who will allow nurses to be reimbursed. Before reimbursement can occur, nurses must document their practices, showing that nursing care is reasonable and necessary.

Once this type of evidence is supplied, a final step of being a profession can be met—that is, controlling the profession through fee for service. Cost analysis studies could support the acute, clinic, rehabilitative, and primary preventive phases of nursing care for almost every diagnosis that exists today. Because of the nursing profession's nurturing, handmaiden history, the profession has been backward about assigning dollar signs to what nurses do. Smalley[54] believed that nurses, through use of nursing diagnoses, will admit and refer individuals to primary, secondary, and tertiary care settings for nursing services and obtain third-party payment from the government and insurance companies for these services. Unless nurses make honest, concerted attempts at meeting this final criterion, the profession will die.

COMPUTERIZATION OF NURSING DIAGNOSES

In 1986 the Computers Committee of the Mid-America Regional Nursing Diagnosis Conference Group surveyed a random sampling of inpatient health care agencies ranging from 100 to 500 and greater beds listed in the American Hospital Association Directory.[55] The committee wanted to know what computer applications were being utilized to document implementation of nursing process and to what extent they were computerizing nursing care planning based on nursing diagnoses. The committee had a 49.6 percent return rate, receiving 228 responses from the 460 originally mailed. Among the findings, they found that the greater the number of beds, the greater the use of computerization of nursing diagnoses. The majority of computer use was for charging patients, ordering tests, tracking admissions, and discharging patients. Only 11.4 percent computer use was for planning and documentation of nursing care.

One of the undesirable aspects of nursing that nurses complain about is excessive documentation of nursing care and patient assessment progress. Although not evident in the above reported survey, many institutions and facilities are in the planning stages of computerizing nursing recordings.

Adaptation of the POMR format has assisted in short-cutting documentation, especially through use of the flowsheets for vital signs, procedures, treatments, and assessments. Although many nurses are reconsidering the use of soap-noting, the subjective, objective, assessment, plan, intervention, evaluation, and revision (SOAPIER) format has served as an effective means of documenting all steps of the nursing process. Also, use of standard care plans has increased in inpatient and outpatient care settings.

Each of the above described recordings includes numerous time-consuming communications. Through computerization, standard assessment forms that use decision-tree type of format can lead to all conceivable diagnostic categories as the outcomes of nursing assessment. For example, diagnostic categories for an individual who has right hemiplegia might include impaired physical mobility, self-care deficit, potential for injury, impaired verbal communication, disturbance in self-concept, and sexual dysfunction. Once the overall diagnostic category is given, defining criteria (signs and symptoms) and etiologies can be called up on the computer, which would assist in making individualized, two-part diagnostic statements for patients and clients. Entry of diagnostic labels as summary of nursing assessment then can be recorded as part of the permanent record, and standard care plans for each diagnosis can be called up to the screen for perusal. A lightpen can be used to indicate which portions of the standard care plan nurses would like to use. Entries of specific patient information into this "skeleton" plan tailor it to become an individualized care plan. Then a hard copy of the plan can be included in the permanent record. Once assessment and care planning are complete, a standard flowsheet format can be called on the screen and nurses can penlight standard assessments/treatments and add others appropriate for their patients and clients. A hard copy of the flowsheets would be placed in the permanent record after every shift or outpatient visit. For documentation of patient progress, standard entry formats can be called up on the screen and nurses can enter progress notes through word processing at the computer terminal.

One of the first computerized parts of nursing documentations was the drug record. Nurses can easily enter medications administered by using computer entry onto a standard medication computer form. Other records easily adapted are the discharge plan and summary, outpatient teaching protocols, and other creative, prescriptive interventions. By computerizing all of these records, nurses can readily obtain previous records categorized according to nursing diagnoses that can facilitate care planning and allow for continuity of care.

Grier[56] outlined the steps necessary for implementation of computerized nursing process, specifically nursing diagnosis. She enumerated barriers to computerization of nursing diagnoses, but also suggested ways to overcome them. She believed that for each nursing diagnosis, an algorithm that describes how to arrive at that particular label, desired outcome of care, nursing interventions to meet the outcome, and subsequent administrative decisions should be developed and coded for computer use. Although these are painstaking activities that take place over a long period of time, these very activities will cause nurses, as directed by Shamansky and Yanni,[1] to raise critical questions, tease apart nuances, promote serious discussion among colleagues, and to refine, change, and grow.

BSN student Valarie Bright was in her second week of coronary care rotation. Ms. Bright was caring for a 65-year-old male who had experienced an inferior wall myocardial infarction the day before. After morning care, she completed two soap notes for the nursing diagnoses, decreased cardiac output related to inferior myocardial infarction and impaired breathing pattern related to congestive heart failure. About

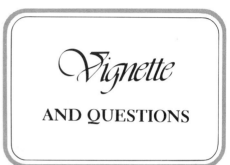

2 PM, Dr. Jones made his rounds and reviewed Ms. Bright's nursing notes written about his patient, which had not been cosigned by her instructor. Upon reading her two soap notes, he abruptly closed the chart and asked where he might find this student, Valarie Bright. Obviously upset, Dr. Jones accused Ms. Bright of making medical diagnoses for which she had no education. After listening respectfully, Valarie gained her composure and explained to Dr. Jones that she was new at making nursing diagnoses and she would consult with her instructor to revise the diagnoses to reflect nursing instead of medicine. Dr. Jones agreed that she should consult with her instructor immediately and requested that Valarie explain to him the difference between medical and nursing diagnoses later that afternoon. Valarie relayed the incident to her instructor and they proceeded to discuss why her diagnoses reflected medicine rather than nursing.

Consider the following questions:

1. What are the major differences between medical and nursing diagnoses?

2. What should the student say to Dr. Jones to explain the purpose of nursing diagnoses?

3. How can she stress to Dr. Jones how interdisciplinary caregiving can be improved if nurses use nursing diagnoses?

4. Rewrite her nursing diagnoses so that they reflect nursing instead of medicine.

INFORMATION SOURCES

Carpenito LJ: *Handbook of Nursing Diagnosis*. Philadelphia, Lippincott, 1984

Gettrust KV, Ryan SC, Engelman DS: *Applied Nursing Diagnosis: Guides for Comprehensive Care Planning*. New York, Wiley, 1985

Houldin AD, Saltstein SW, Ganley KM: *Nursing Diagnoses for Wellness: Supporting Strengths*. Philadelphia, Lippincott, 1987

Kim MJ, McFarland GK, McLane AM: *Pocket Guide to Nursing Diagnoses*. St. Louis, CV Mosby, 1984

Ziegler SM, Vaughan-Wrobel BC, Erlen JA: *Nursing Process, Nursing Diagnosis, Nursing Knowledge: Avenues to Autonomy*. Norwalk, CT, Appleton-Century-Crofts, 1986

North American Nursing Diagnosis Association
St. Louis University School of Nursing
3525 Caroline Street
St. Louis, MO 63104

Concept Media
"Nursing Diagnosis and Care Planning"
P.O. Box 19542
Irvine, CA 92713
(714) 660-0727 or 800-233-7078

Nursing Diagnosis Video Tapes
St. Clare Hospital Video Productions
515 22nd Avenue
Monroe, WI 53566
(608) 328-0167

REFERENCES

1. Shamansky SL, Yanni CR: In opposition to nursing diagnosis: A minority opinion. Image 15:47, 1983

2. Gebbie KM, Lavin MA (eds): *Classification of Nursing Diagnoses: Proceedings of the First National Conference*. St. Louis, CV Mosby, 1975

3. Fry VS: The creative approach to nursing. Am J Nurs 53:301, 1953

4. Abdellah, FG: Methods of identifying covert aspects of nursing problems. Nurs Res 6:4, 1957

5. Durand M, Prince R: Nursing diagnosis: Process and decision. Nurs Forum 5:50, 1966

6. Chambers W: Nursing diagnosis. Am J Nurs 62:639, 1962

7. Gordon M: Nursing diagnoses and the diagnostic process. Am J Nurs 76:1298, 1976

8. American Nurses' Association: *Nursing: A Social Policy Statement*. Kansas City, MO, American Nurses' Association, 1980

9. American Nurses' Association: *Standards of Nursing Practice*. Kansas City, MO, American Nurses' Association, 1973

10. Popkess-Vawter SA, Pinnell N (eds): Accentuate the positive. Am J Nurs 10, 1987

11. Carpenito LJ: *Nursing Diagnosis: Application to Clinical Practice*. Philadelphia, Lippincott, 1983

12. Griffith JW, Christensen PJ: *Nursing Process: Application of Theories, Frameworks, and Models*. St. Louis: C.V. Mosby, 1982

13. Hurley ME: *Classification of Nursing Diagnoses: Proceedings of the Sixth Conference*. St. Louis, CV Mosby, 1986

14. Kim MJ, McFarland GK, McLane AM (eds): *Classification of Nursing Diagnoses: Proceedings from the Fifth National Conference*. St. Louis, CV Mosby, 1984

15. Gordon M: *Nursing Diagnoses: Process and Application*. New York, McGraw-Hill, 1982

16. North American Nursing Diagnosis Association: *North American Nursing Diagnosis Taxonomy I*. St. Louis, North American Nursing Diagnosis Association, 1986

17. Campbell C: *Nursing Diagnoses and Intervention in Nursing Practice*. New York, Wiley, 1978

18. Doenges ME, Moorhouse MF: *Nurse's Pocket Guide: Nursing Diagnoses with Interventions*. Philadelphia, FA Davis, 1985

19. Duespohl TA: *Nursing Diagnosis Manual for the Well and Ill Client*. Philadelphia, Saunders, 1986

20. North American Nursing Diagnosis Newsletter. St. Louis: North American Nursing Diagnosis Association, 13:1, 1986

21. Kim MJ: Physiologic nursing diagnosis: Its role and place in nursing taxonomy. In Kim MJ, McFarland GK, McLane AM (eds): *Classification of Nursing Diagnoses: Proceedings of the Fifth National Conference*. St. Louis, CV Mosby, 1984, pp 60–62

22. Guzzetta CE, Dossey BM: Nursing diagnosis: Framework, process, and problems. Heart and Lung 12:281, 1983

23. Aspinall MJ, Tanner CA: *Decision Making for Patient Care: Applying the Nursing Process.* New York, Appleton-Century-Crofts, 1981

24. Carnevali DL, Mitchell PH, Woods NF, Tanner CA: *Diagnostic Reasoning in Nursing.* Philadelphia, Lippincott, 1984

25. Maslow AH: *Motivation and Personality.* New York, Harper & Row, Pub, 1970

26. Henderson V: *The Nature of Nursing.* New York, Macmillan, 1966

27. Weed LL: *Medical Records, Medical Education, and Patient Care.* Cleveland, Press of Case Western Reserve University, 1969

28. West N: The Subjective Description of Breathlessness: A Nursing Diagnosis. University of Kansas, unpublished Master's Thesis, 1986

29. Barnard K: The ANA's social policy statement on nursing. In Kim MJ, McFarland GK, McLane AJ (eds): *Classification of Nursing Diagnoses: Proceedings of the Fifth National Conference.* St. Louis, CV Mosby, 1984, p 2

30. North American Nursing Diagnosis Association: *Development/Submission Guidelines for Proposed New Nursing Diagnoses.* St. Louis, North American Nursing Diagnosis Association, 1986

31. Kim MJ, Moritz DA (eds): *Classification of Nursing Diagnoses: Proceedings of the Third and Fourth National Conferences.* New York, McGraw-Hill, 1982

32. North American Nursing Diagnosis Association: Presentations for the scientific sessions. Seventh Conference on Classification of Nursing Diagnoses. St. Louis, North American Nursing Diagnosis Association, 1986

33. Chinn PL, Jacobs MK: *Theory and Nursing: A Systematic Approach.* St. Louis, CV Mosby, 1987

34. Champagne M, Neelon V, McConnell E: Acute confusion in the hospitalized elderly: Patterns and early diagnosis, presentations for the scientific sessions. Seventh Conference on Classification of Nursing Diagnoses. St. Louis, North American Nursing Diagnosis Association, 1986

35. Fadden T, Fehring R, Kenkel-Rossi E: Clinical validation of the diagnosis anxiety, presentations for the scientific sessions. Seventh Conference on Classification of Nursing Diagnoses. St. Louis, North American Nursing Diagnosis Association, 1986

36. Cattaneo CJ, Lackey NR: Impaired skin integrity, presentations for the scientific sessions. Seventh Conference on Classification of Nursing Diagnoses. St. Louis, North American Nursing Diagnosis Association, 1986

37. Lee H, Frenn M, Jacobs C, Sanger M, Strong K: Delphi survey to gain consensus on wellness and health promotion nursing diagnoses, presentations for the scientific sessions. Seventh Conference on Classification of Nursing Diagnoses. St. Louis, North American Nursing Diagnosis Association, 1986

38. Metzger KL, Hiltunen E: Diagnostic content validation of ten frequently reported nursing diagnoses, presentations for the scientific sessions. Seventh Conference on Classification of Nursing Diagnoses. St. Louis, North American Nursing Diagnosis Association, 1986

39. Janken JK: Identifying patients with the potential for falling, presentations for the scientific sessions. Seventh Conference on Classification of Nursing Diagnoses. St. Louis, North American Nursing Diagnosis Association, 1986

40. Lazure LL, Cuddigan J: Clinical validations of decreased cardiac output: Differentiation of defining characteristics according to etiology, presentations for the scientific sessions. Seventh Conference on Classification of Nursing Diagnoses. St. Louis, North American Nursing Diagnosis Association, 1986

41. Clinton J: Nursing diagnoses research methodologies. In ME Hurley (ed) *Classification of Nursing Diagnoses: Proceedings of the Sixth Conference.* St. Louis, CV Mosby, 1986, pp 159–176

42. Dodge JS: What patients should be told: Patients' and nurses' belief. Am J Nurs 72:1852, 1972

43. Haferkorn V: Assessing individual learning needs as a basis for patient teaching. Nurs Clinics N Am 6:199, 1971

44. Miller P, Shada E: Preoperative information and recovery of open-heart surgery patients. Heart and Lung 7:486, 1978

45. Heim E, Blasser A, Waidelich E: Dyspnea: Psychophysiologic relationships. Psychosom Med 34:405, 1972

46. Kellams SE: Ideals of a profession: The case of nursing. Image 9:30, 1977

47. Bixler GK, Bixler RW: The professional status of nursing. Am J Nurs 59:1142, 1959

48. American Nurses' Association: *Code for Nurses with Interpretive Statements.* Kansas City, MO: American Nurses' Association, 1976

49. American Nurses' Association: First position on education for nursing. Am J Nurs 66:515, 1966

50. Toth RM: Reimbursement mechanism based on nursing diagnosis. Kim MJ, Moritz DA (eds): *Classification of Nursing Diagnoses: Proceedings of the Third and Fourth National Conferences.* New York: McGraw-Hill, 1982, p 90

51. New Jersey State Department of Health: A prospective reimbursement system based on patient case-mix for New Jersey hospitals 1976-1978 (SSA Contract No. 600-77-0022). Trenton, NJ, Annual Report, 1, 1977

52. Halloran EJ, Kiley M, Nosek L: Nursing complexity, the DRG, and length of stay, presentations for the scientific sessions. Seventh Conference on Classification of Nursing Diagnoses. St. Louis: North American Nursing Diagnosis Association, 1986

53. Gebbie KM: Fee based reimbursement using nursing diagnoses, paper delivered

at the Seventh Conference on Classification of Nursing Diagnoses. St. Louis, North American Nursing Diagnosis Association, 1986

54. Smalley BH: Nursing diagnosis. Kennedy & Pfeifer (eds): *Current Practice in Nursing Care of Adults.* St. Louis, CV Mosby, 1979, pp 240–251

55. Ratilff CV: Computerized nursing diagnoses: A survey. Paper presented at the University of Kansas Nursing Alumni Association Fall Business Meeting. Kansas City, KS, 1986

56. Grier MR: Health information systems: Toward computerization of nursing diagnosis. In Hurley ME (ed): *Classification of Nursing Diagnoses: Proceedings of the Sixth Conference.* St. Louis, CV Mosby, 1986, pp 168–176

JAMES D. VAIL, RN, DNSc

CHAPTER 8 *Patient Classification Systems*

Background and Overview

Determining staffing requirements and costing out nursing are two of the most challenging, and perplexing, problems currently facing nurse managers. Traditionally, staffing of nursing personnel was planned based on the number of beds occupied in a given clinical area, and the cost of nursing was usually billed on the board-and-breakfast side of the ledger. Within the past two decades, however, the nature and volume of the nursing workload have been significantly altered by: increasingly complex technology, the trend toward specialization, emphasis on health teaching, personalization of service to patients, and ongoing evaluation of personnel performance and patient care. These very factors are some of the same factors that must be considered when trying to determine the monetary worth of nursing. Consequently, realistic staffing and costing out nursing can no longer be considered a function of patient census alone. In fact, departments of nursing have been mandated by the Joint Commission on Accreditation of Hospitals (JCAH) to define, implement, and maintain a system by which the quantity and quality of available nurse staffing is based on identified requirements for nursing. Specifically, the JCAH requires that nursing departments maintain a system for determining patient requirements for nursing care on the basis of demonstrated patient needs, appropriate nursing intervention, and priority of care, and that specific nursing personnel for each nursing unit should be commensurate with patient care requirements and staff expertise.[1] The use of a well-developed, reliable, and valid patient classification system can assist nursing departments in carrying out this mandate.

Traditionally, nursing staffing needs were decided based on the daily inpatient census coupled with a predetermined number of care hours per patient day.[2] Such an outdated methodology falsely assumed that nursing care requirements were the same for all patients; hence, it became necessary to develop a more accurate procedure for determining staffing requirements.

In 1947 the National League for Nursing Education (now the NLN) examined the nursing care requirements of pediatric patients and suggested staffing be based on four factors graded on a three-point scale of intensity: degree of illness, activity, adjustment, and procedures.[3] In the early 1950s the US Army Nurse Corps developed a patient classification system according to nursing care needs. This system initially contained nine categories, later reduced to four categories based on four critical factors that were believed to influence nursing care requirements the most. Those four factors were: nursing procedural requirements, physical restoration, instructional needs, and emotional needs.[4] This prototype system was used by the Army Nurse Corps until about 1985, at which time a new factor evaluation system was implemented following a number of years of development and testing.

R.J. Conner of Johns Hopkins Hospital used work measurement techniques to identify components of direct patient care.[5] Patients were categorized as self-care, partial care, or total care and, for each group an average number of nursing care hours per patient was determined. Although this method quantified workload, Conner's system failed to address indirect nursing care and overlooked such professional activities as instruction, observation, assessment, and emotional support.

Aydelotte and Tener studied patient workload in relation to staffing and concluded that when staff numbers were increased without a corresponding increase in workload, the staff still did not deliver more direct care.[6]

PURPOSE AND NEED

Simply stated, the purpose of a patient classification system is to determine the intensity of nursing care for a patient or a group of patients, including both direct and indirect nursing care requirements.[7] However, this process alone has no inherent use. For a patient classification system to be useful, the data generated from classifying patients must be linked to a staffing methodology for the purpose of determining staffing requirements based on the identified intensity of nursing care.[8] Throughout the text of this chapter, the concept **intensity of nursing care,** as opposed to the concept **acuity of patient care,** will be used. Acuity of patient care is a misnomer, since it relates to the "degree" of patient illness and not necessarily to the amount of nursing care required. In other words, staffing should be allocated according to the intensity of nursing care and not necessarily to the "degree" of illness, as the "acuity of patient care" concept implies. For example, there may be a number of surgical patients who are scheduled to undergo elective surgery such as hernia repair, cataract extraction, tubal ligation, or reconstructive surgery. These patients are far from being "ill"; however, each patient individually, and all the patients as a group, will generate several "intense" nursing care hours based on their identified preoperative nursing care needs. Therefore the concept "intensity of nursing care" better characterizes the overall nursing workload situation than does the notion of "acuity of patient care."

The actual **classification of patients** alone, that is, the placement of patients into distinct nursing care requirement groups, has limited use.[9] At its very best it tells you only how much *direct* nursing care time is needed over any specified period of time. How useful is this information? Not very useful unless the classification data can then be linked to a mechanism that embodies an *indirect* nursing care factor that, in turn, is linked to a staffing methodology that will allow a manager to determine the current number of staff necessary to provide the care required, or to *predict* the number of staff necessary to provide care across all work shifts.[10] **Direct nursing care time** is defined as that time required for those activities that take place in the presence of the patient and/or family. These activities are behavioral and observable. **Indirect nursing care time** is defined as that time required for those activities and tasks performed away from the patient and/or family and include such tasks as: communication, planning care, assessing needs, preparation of medications and equipment, and team conferences. **Unavailable for patient care time** (nonproductive time) includes those activities of personnel not directed toward patient care or unit management that detract from time available for patient care.[11] The majority of these tasks are performed off the nursing unit. Some systems allow for as much as 22 percent nonproductive time,[12] while others[13–15] allow for as little as 15 percent. For a patient classification system to be useful for both predicting staffing requirements and assisting in measuring productivity, it must include all three measures of time: direct care time, indirect care time, and unavailable for care time. The concept "unavailable for care" time instead of "nonproductive" time has been used throughout this chapter because there can be unaccounted for nonproductivity in both direct and indirect care times.

The data acquired through the use of a valid and reliable patient classification system can be useful at several levels of management. At the patient care unit level, it may be used as a basis for prioritizing care and for qualifying the levels of care needed by each patient so that nursing personnel may be assigned appropriately in terms of their expertise. At this level it can also provide a mechanism for quality audits. Sampling can be done to measure whether care indicated as necessary on the patient classification instrument is being given and documented.

At the middle management level, data generated from a patient classification system can be used to estimate staffing requirements for nursing units based on workload so that adequate personnel may be provided to meet patient needs. It also provides an objective method for assigning temporary personnel where they will be used most effectively. Information generated from a patient classification system may be used on a daily basis as an objective means for directing admissions to various patient care units. For example, units with heavier workloads could receive the less acute admissions in an effort to balance workloads among units.

At the hospital level aggregate data from all the patient care units may be used to establish manpower plans for various categories of nursing personnel, and is one of the primary justifications for nursing budgets. The information may also be useful in justifying interim requests for additional personnel in various categories as staffing needs change caused by mission changes.

At the corporate level, where several hospitals make up the corporate structure, aggregate data from the various hospitals within the corporation may be used to generate monthly, quarterly, and annual summary management reports. These reports are useful in studying productivity and workload to staffing ratios between and among hospitals.

Giovannetti[9] believes that almost all patient classification systems are used in conjunction with some quantification—an estimation of the nursing care resources associated with each category of care. The need for patient classification is to respond to the variable nature of the demand for nursing care. It has been frequently demonstrated in hospitals that there may be wide swings in the demand for nursing care from day to day and from shift to shift, and that these fluctuations are independent of the number of patients in the patient care unit. Only in patient care units where requirements for nursing care are largely homogeneous, such as in self-care units or in some highly specialized care units, is this not likely to be true. The impact of this variability is such that the number of patients in a nursing unit may not be an adequate indicator of the demand for care. Thus the traditional methods for determining nursing personnel resources based on average care-hours per patient-day have been found to yield insensitive measures of demand.

A patient classification system that incorporates a staffing methodology can become a strong management tool at every level of management. For nursing managers to make sound administrative decisions about staffing needs and requirements as well as manage the quality, quantity, and utilization of personnel in a productive, cost-effective manner, they must make use of well-established measurement tools. Only by employing instruments of impeccable validity and reliability can accurate, acceptable data be produced for justifying all levels of managerial decision-making.

Figure 8-1 delineates the dynamics of a patient classification. The process begins with the classification of patients into categories of care. This determines the number of direct nursing care hours required. The total hours of nursing care required and the recommended number and mix of personnel needed to meet these requirements are then calculated based on

FIGURE 8-1

Dynamics of the Workload Management System

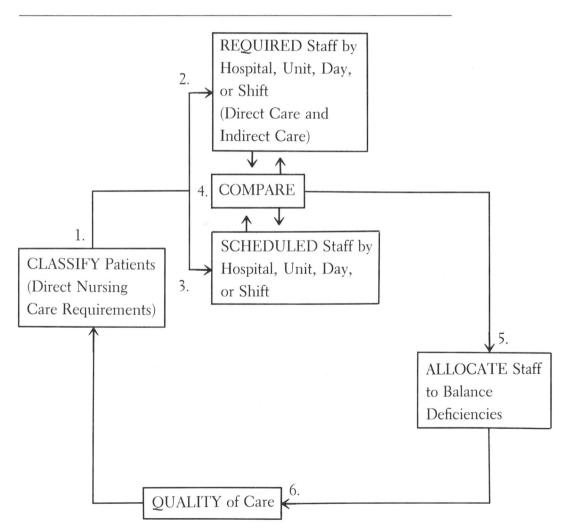

the number of patients in each category. The *actual* number and mix of personnel assigned is then compared with the *recommended* staffing to determine if staffing levels are above, below, or within the recommendations. If staffing levels for the workload to be accomplished differ from recommended levels, staffing can be adjusted to balance the variation. The number and mix of nursing personnel available to provide patient care may significantly impact on the quality of care actually delivered.

TYPES OF CLASSIFICATION SYSTEMS

Basically, there are two types of patient classification systems: the prototype system and the factor-evaluation system. In the prototype system patients are rated on a number of characteristics simultaneously, while in the factor-evaluation system the characteristics are evaluated one by one. Abdella and Levine[4] define the two types of systems as follows:

In the **prototype evaluation system,** several mutually exclusive and exhaustive patient classification categories are established. Each category is fully described in terms of the characteristics of the typical patient in that category. The patient is classified into that category in which his or her characteristics match the prototype characteristics most closely.

In the **factor-evaluation system,** specific elements of care (sometimes referred to as critical indicators of care) are delineated and the patient is rated on each of the elements. Each element may be weighted to represent a specific amount of time. Each element may then be measured to yield a subscore. All subscores are then totaled to yield an overall score that places the patient into a specific category based on nursing care requirements.

The two types are also commonly referred to as "subjective" (prototype evaluation) and "objective" (factor-evaluation) patient classification instruments. In the early stages of development, it was believed that the prototype evaluation, with its broad descriptions, could too readily be interpreted differently by different nurse raters. A great deal of subjectivity appeared to be involved in the selection of the patient category. On the other hand, the factor-evaluation type, by enumerating specific condition states or descriptors, was thought to result in total objectivity on the part of the rater. It is now recognized that the labels *subjective* and *objective* are misleading and, indeed, some measure of subjectivity on the part of the rater is and should be involved in both types. No system should disregard the element of "professional judgment," yet, professional judgment is quite "subjective" in terms of not being quantifiable, but is quite necessary in the day-to-day practice of giving or managing patient care.

Table 8-1 and Figure 8-2 provide examples of the prototype and factor-evaluation instruments respectively. A comparison of the two examples will readily reflect the limitations of the prototype system because of its

TABLE 8-1

Prototype Patient Classification System

Category I	-	A patient who requires neither nursing care nor professional nurse supervision and where daily living and health needs can be met in an ambulatory care setting.
Category II	-	A patient who requires a minimal amount of nursing care and supervision, displays mild symptoms, a need for little treatment and/or observation, some assistance in meeting ADL requirements, and a need for only slightly controlled activities.
Category III	-	A patient who requires moderate nursing care and is usually termed moderately ill. He/she displays: • a need for frequent treatment and/or observation and/or instructions. • a need for partially controlled activities. • a moderate deviation from acceptable behavior.
Category IV	-	A patient whose nursing care is so complex or time-consuming that he requires the equivalent of a full-time nurse at all times. Exhibits: • extreme symptoms—usually termed acutely ill. • a need for life-sustaining measures and/or continuous treatment and/or observation and/or information and/or instructions. • a need for full assistance with ADL. • a need for rigidly controlled activities. • a pronounced deviation from acceptable behavior patterns.

insensitivity in quantifying nursing care activities. For example, the prototype system uses such terms as "minimal," "moderate," "frequent," "complex," and "extreme" to describe patient needs, all of which are unquantifiable concepts.

ISSUES TO CONSIDER WHEN SELECTING OR DESIGNING A CLASSIFICATION SYSTEM

Although there are literally hundreds of patient classification systems (PCS) available today, they all have a singular purpose, even though their methods and instruments may vary. Sixteen years ago Aydelotte[2] reported some 40 pieces of patient classification literature, and it is likely that this number has since quadrupled. It is probably safe to say, even though there is no official

FIGURE 8-2
Factor-evaluation Patient Classification System

PATIENT ACUITY WORKSHEET				NAME OF PATIENT								
For use of this form, see HQDA LTR 40-85-6; the proponent agency is the OTGS.												
NAME OF HOSPITAL		UNIT										
SIGNATURE		DATE & TIME										
Point Values	CRITICAL INDICATORS		Acuity Code									
	VITAL SIGNS (MANUAL TPR, BP)		A1-A3									
(1)	Vital signs qid or less		1									
(2)	Vital signs q4h or x 6		2									
(4)	Vital signs q2h or x 12		3									
(8)	Vital signs qid or x 24		4									
(2)	Rectal or axillary temp or apical pulse qid or more		5									
(2)	Femoral or pedal pulses or FHT q4h or more		6									
(2)	Tilt tests q4h or more		7									
(6)	Post-op, post-partum, post-delivery (infants)		8									
(3)	Vital signs q3h or x 8		9									

	MONITORING	A3-A7																		
(2)	Intake and output q8h	20																		20
(8)	Intake and output q2h	21																		21
(2)	Circulation or fundus checks q2h or x 12	22																		22
(3)	Neuro checks q4h or x 6	23																		23
(6)	Neuro checks q2h or x 12	24																		24
(2)	CVP or ICP (manual) q2h or x 12	25																		25
(6)	Cardiac/apnea/temp/pressure monitors (not cumulative)	26																		26
(6)	Transcutaneous monitor	27																		27
(4)	A-line or ICP (monitor) or Swan Ganz set-up	28																		28
(2)	A-line or ICP (monitor) reading q2h or x 12	29																		29
(2)	PAP/PA wedge reading q4h or x 6	30																		30
(4)	PAP/PA wedge reading q2h or x 12	31																		31
(2)	Cardiac output tid	32																		32

DA Form 5445-R, Jul 85

count, that just about every hospital across the nation uses some type or form of a patient classification system. A patient classification system may be defined as a method of identification and classification of patients into mutually exclusive, homogeneous care groups or categories, and the quantification of these categories as a measure of nursing effort required.

The space limitations of this chapter preclude the listing and discussion of all the systems, whether commercial or self-developed, that are available for use; however, in the information sources section, a few of the more commonly known systems have been listed and briefly discussed.

Whether a hospital is planning to develop its own patient classification system or purchase one of the commercial systems, there are some important criteria that should be considered prior to the initial investment of both time and finances. First, several questions such as the following must be answered:

- How much will it cost to develop and test a PCS?
- How much will it cost to purchase a commercial system?
- What do you want a PCS to do?
- How is it to be used?
- Can it be used as a measure of productivity?
- Can it be used to profile staffing requirements in all patient care units?
- Can it be used to predict staffing requirements?
- How much time will be involved in both implementing and monitoring the system?
- How much of the staff's time will be required to classify patients?
- Can reliability and validity be maintained?
- Who will carry out the system?

These are but a few of the questions that should be addressed *before* a department of nursing decides to develop or purchase a system. It is recommended that since there are a variety of systems already available, the department of nursing choose one that would provide the desired information and adapt that system to the individual institution. There could be some problems with this process unless there is appropriate administrative support and personnel resources to make the proper evaluation and adaptation. This method could, however, save an institution both time and money. If the department of nursing decides to develop and test its own system, they may run the risk of sacrificing validity and reliability. Most of the commercial systems have been well tested over time and part of their legitimacy is claiming the system to have high validity and reliability.

Outlined in Table 8-2 are some of the criteria believed to be important when *selecting* a commercial patient classification system. Listed in Table 8-3 are criteria that should be considered when planning to develop a PCS.

TABLE 8-2

Criteria for the Selection of a PCS

- Accuracy
- Ease of use
- Representativeness
- Objectivity
- Discriminating
- Predictive capacity
- Ease of monitoring
- Ease of teaching, understanding, and maintaining
- Direct nursing care
- Indirect nursing care
- Established reliability, and validity
- Affordable
- Quantification
- Staffing ratios
- Provider mix

If the criteria in Table 8-3 are met, then the product resulting from the efforts of developing and testing a PCS must also meet the criteria listed in Table 8-2.

Health Management Systems Associates[16] identified a number of system performance criteria that should also be considered when either selecting a commercial system or designing a hospital specific system. Those criteria are:

TABLE 8-3

Criteria to Consider When Designing a PCS

- Available, qualified research personnel
- Full administrative support
- Support personnel (data collectors, clerical, statistical)
- Designated funds
- Adequate time allocation
- Computer support

- *Comprehensive*—The system should classify all patients according to levels of required nursing care and determine the amount of nursing time required to care for those patients. The system should apply to all inpatients, should be easily adaptable to outpatients, and should account for both direct and indirect care.
- *Data Output*—The system should produce in each hospital a series of daily and monthly reports that are useful both in the operation of the hospital and in the corporate planning and budgeting of resources. The reports should be timely and provide information on actual patient days, actual nurse staffing, and nursing workload by patient category, by shift, by ward, and by personnel category.
- *Data Input*—The same definition of patient classes should be used throughout the hospital, and in the case of hospital corporations the same system and definitions should be used throughout all hospitals within the corporation. The definitions should be simple to understand and the procedures for using it speedy and reliable. The basic data on each patient should be created at each nursing station each day.
- *Validity*—The system should measure what it purports to measure initially and on an ongoing basis. The appearance of validity should also be maintained. The validity of the patient categories and the time for direct care can be assessed on a hospital-wide basis, using expert opinions and objective data.
- *Reliability*—The hospital must assure that unsystematic variation between raters, between wards, and between hospitals in the case of hospital corporations, over time, is maintained at a reasonable level. The reliability of the PCS should be assessed fairly frequently (monthly, initially, and then at least quarterly thereafter).
- *Implementation*—The system must be capable of being operated both manually and as part of an automated system. An implementation plan should be developed that includes a training and orientation program and assignment of coordination responsibility within the hospital, and in the case of hospital corporations, throughout the corporation.
- *Cost*—System costs, both in terms of investment costs and funds, and nursing time to operate the system, should be considered in relation to benefits. These costs should be predicted.
- *Objectivity*—Objectivity is closely related to the reliability of the method. A classification instrument that uses precise and well-defined measures will produce high levels of interrater reliability.
- *Compatibility*—The system should be compatible with the existing automated systems within the institution, and with future automation plans.

To address the question "Who will carry out the system?" requires a look at the entire department of nursing, and how much administrative support and guidance the department is willing to provide. Experts believe that the system should be "carried out" by the entire department. The roles and responsibilities of nurses at each level of practice, from the Chief Nurse Executive (Director of Nursing) to the staff nurse, can be and should be clearly delineated if the patient classification system is to work effectively as a management tool. This includes the nursing education and staff development staff, and the nursing quality assurance nurse. The basic roles and responsibilities are:

- *Chief Nurse Executive*—The Chief Nurse Executive (CNE) makes the final decision about which system the department will use. He/she establishes policy that will govern the implementation, monitoring, and use of the system. The CNE will use the data generated from the patient classification system to assist in managing the department and to address the needs of the department to higher management. The CNE must know the system, how it operates, and what kind of data it can generate for management purposes. The CNE has no day-to-day operational responsibility for the system at this level.
- *Assistant to the Chief Nurse Executive*—The assistant to the chief is the "operations" officer. The responsibility of this position is to see that the policies are carried out and that reports are submitted in a timely fashion and are available for the CNE. The assistant meets with the middle managers (supervisors) and informs them of policy, instructs them as to their role in the implementation and monitoring of the system, and establishes suspense dates, based on policy, for receiving management reports.
- *Middle Managers (Supervisors)*—The role of the middle manager is crucial to the success of the patient classification system as a management tool. The middle manager must not only know *how* to use the data generated by the system, he/she must also know how to *use* the classification instrument and must become an "expert classifier." It is the responsibility of the middle manager to 1) see that the system is operational on a daily basis; 2) ensure that the data generated by the system are accurate; 3) conduct interrater reliability tests to ensure that the system continues to provide reliable data; 4) use the data on a day-to-day basis to manage staff in a specific nursing division; 5) communicate both problems and successes of the system to the assistant director and to the head nurses; and 6) provide guidance to head nurses on the use of the system. The role of the middle manager cannot be overemphasized. Whether the system works or fails will depend largely upon

how astute middle managers are at managing. The middle manager prepares monthly summary reports for the assistant director.

- *Head Nurse*—The responsibility of the head nurse is to see that patients are accurately classified according to policy. It may be every shift, once every 24 hours, or once weekly. The head nurse ensures that staff nurses are classifying patients accurately and conducts interrater reliability tests as necessary to identify any problems that may exist. The head nurse must also become an expert classifier. Daily summary reports are prepared by the head nurse and provided to the middle manager. The head nurse may conduct unit specific in-service programs on the system for new personnel. The head nurse uses the classification data on a day-to-day basis for assigning staff to patient care situations according to their expertise and the needs of the patient, and to prepare staffing schedules. If head nurses are responsible for their budgets, the information generated from a valid and reliable PCS will assist them in establishing and predicting their budgetary needs, and will help to justify their FTEs. The data from the PCS may also assist the head nurse in conducting nursing care audits.
- *Staff Nurse*—This is the place, as they say in industry, "where the rubber hits the road." The responsibility of the staff nurse is to *classify* patients as accurately as possible. The staff nurse should have thorough instructions on the classification instrument and how to use it. It is not the responsibility of the staff nurse to prepare daily or monthly summary reports, or to conduct the required monthly or quarterly interrater reliability tests. If the classification information generated by the staff nurse is incorrect, then all the data subsequently generated from the classification information will also be incorrect, and therefore, useless. In order to have as accurate data as possible, it is strongly recommended that the nurse who is providing care to the patient be the one who classifies that patient.
- *Nurse Education and Staff Development Staff*—The responsibility of the education and staff development personnel is to ensure that there is an ongoing orientation and training program for the staff who will be using the system at all levels. If a commercial classification system is purchased, the education staff should make inquiry as to the availability of existing education programs for that system. If a system is designed and developed by the institution, it is the responsibility of the education staff to develop instructional media appropriate for the system. A crucial component to ensure that a patient classification system is properly utilized, and achieves and maintains reliability, is a well-designed and implemented educational program. Experience has demonstrated that it may

take several months to achieve and maintain an acceptable reliability coefficient.

- *Quality Assurance Nurse*—The responsibility of the QA nurse is to assist in the identification and resolution of problems in nursing care as they relate to the classification system. Recommendations are made to the assistant director of nursing for the purpose of ensuring adequate quality control mechanisms. The QA nurse must know the system, how it works, and for what purposes the data are used. The QA nurse has no day-to-day operational responsibility for the system.

Impacts on the Nurse, the Consumer, and Society

THE NURSE

When the decision is made to implement a patient classification system, the impact will be felt by all nurses across all department lines. The process of implementation should be done in such a way that acceptance of the system will be maximized and the stresses brought on by the major changes will be minimized. The use of the change model developed by Donnelly and Associates[17] may be helpful to nursing administrators when the decision is made to implement a patient classification system. They describe change as consisting of eight subsystems: 1) forces for change, 2) recognition of need for change, 3) diagnosis of underlying problem, 4) identification of possible change techniques, 5) recognition of limiting condition, 6) selection of change techniques, 7) implementation of change, and 8) monitoring process and result. Huckabay[18] suggests that the implementation of a classification system should follow a planned, logical sequence that includes directing, controlling, and evaluating. She suggests that personnel first be informed about the system and the rationale and purposes for selecting and implementing a patient classification system. A working committee is then selected and should consist of nurses from a variety of practice areas, including administrative nursing personnel. The nursing education and staff development division must select and train in-service instructors who will actually teach the staff. The instructional process will include hands-on practice in actual patient care situations. Interrater reliability testing should be conducted and the predetermined level of agreement should be attained before staff are allowed to use the system for actual data analysis. It has been suggested that two nurses classifying the same patient or group of patients should agree 90 to 95 percent of the time. Also, in the directing phase there needs to be continual positive reinforcement.

In the controlling phase, a feedback system needs to be put into place to make sure that things are progressing as planned, that target dates are being met, and that the preestablished level of reliability is being maintained. The middle managers, the in-service instructors, and the QA nurse can each play an important role in this feedback system.

The evaluation phase is the final step before any major changes are implemented. In this phase it is determined whether the objectives have been met for implementing the system. Major problems are identified and any changes to improve the system are discussed and evaluated.

During the implementation of a classification system, scheduling of personnel and staffing patterns may need to change, at least temporarily, to accommodate training schedules. Once in-service programs begin, it is most important that personnel on all three shifts be taught simultaneously. Depending on the size of the department, it may take from 30 to 60 days to instruct all the nurses properly on how to classify patients and how to prepare the management reports that result from the classification data. Managers must recognize that changes in scheduling and staffing patterns may result in additional personnel problems. Huckabay and Skonieczny[19] have identified a range of problems, including complaints of staff, difficulty in motivating staff, cheating, resistance to change, and stress experienced by staff, that can be relieved by proper planning of the implementation. Therefore, a well-planned and consistent approach to the initial implementation of the system and the installment of monitoring mechanisms become of primary importance to assure that the system maintains continuity, reliability, validity, and user acceptance.

THE CONSUMER

We would all like to believe that additional staffing equates to quality of care. However, we have all seen "understaffed" units that provide "quality" care as measured by all the common indicators of care, ie, no medication errors, no falls, positive patient care satisfaction reports, comprehensive nursing care documentation, etc. It must be remembered that a patient classification system, at its very best, is a management tool and while it serves to help determine the number and mix of personnel required, it still has the weakness of not being able to clone additional staff. Probably the greatest impact a patient classification system has on the consumer is one that is largely unknown to the consumer—it identifies nursing care needs and pinpoints the number and mix of personnel and thus gives nurse managers data for negotiating additional permanent staff or on a shift-by-shift basis. It is an objective way of utilizing float personnel, or, if float personnel are not available, it can provide support for moving a patient to a unit that can provide the care required. In this way, if in no other, the patient classification system serves to improve the quality of care for the consumer.

SOCIETY

As health care costs continue to spiral upward, society will continue to apply pressure at various levels of government to identify mechanisms through which quality health care needs can be obtained economically. The federal government has been cognizant of the need to address problems of quality, and in the passage of the Tax Equity and Fiscal Responsibility Act of 1982 has made an attempt at safeguarding the quality of care by incorporating peer review organizations (PRO) into the act. The federal government has also recently contracted with 48 PROs and one super PRO to monitor quality of care, and most recently moved into the area of monitoring HMOs.[20] The problem that confronts nursing is that the PRO does not monitor the quality of care rendered according to nursing standards. Since the admission of patients to hospitals is a referral for nursing care, the focus of monitoring care needs to shift toward nursing's role in providing cost-effective care. A PCS can perform a definite role in relating determination of severity of illnesses and intensity of nursing care to the cost of nursing resources. Joel[21] makes the case that the nurse executive today needs a patient classification system to assist him or her in internal management decision making and in detailing nursing's contribution to the fiscal integrity of the facility. She writes, "the ultimate goal of any patient classification system is to provide care for those who need it the most."[21]

Giovannetti suggests that perhaps one of the least credited advantages of a well-developed and operational patient classification system is its ability to lessen the monumental problems associated with the determination and allocation of nursing personnel. She writes, "freed from some of the daily struggles associated with staffing, nurses may transfer their energies to other current and critical problems such as implementing standards of care and developing outcome measures."[9] If there is no other benefit to society than this alone, then society should demand the use of a PCS in every hospital, nursing home, and every other major institution in which nursing care is provided on an ongoing basis.

Future Considerations

Health care across the nation is one of the most inflationary components of the American economy. Over the past two decades, health care costs have skyrocketed to the point where routine health care by the average American living on an average or below average income is sometimes difficult to obtain. These spiraling costs can be attributed to many factors; however, two of the major reasons that can be attributed to increased costs are 1) tremendous growth within the health care system secondary to increased technological advances and research and 2) the passage of medicare and medicaid legislation in 1965—amendments to the Social Security Act. Medicare and medicaid provided health insurance coverage to two groups who were vulnerable to illness and its associated costs—the elderly and the poor. So, the very thing Congress tried to do to help the disadvantaged and stem the cost of health care, was the thing that opened the way to further increase the cost of health care delivery.

After the enactment of medicare and medicaid, the number of hospital admissions and physician visits greatly increased, since most insurance policies paid predominantly for inpatient services. Acute-care facilities grew in size and technological sophistication at an uncontrolled and unregulated rate. Their growth financed by the insurance carriers, both governmental and nongovernmental, guaranteed payment for inpatient services to both the hospital and the physician.

As a consequence of this growth, there was a need for personnel to care for the increased numbers of patients in the hospital and to operate the technology. Increases in the number of patients and in technological complexity tended to increase the price of health care services. The higher price did not affect the demand for services by individuals, however, because the out-of-pocket costs to patients were negligible. Hospital administrators were not overly concerned with the costs of operating the system because they were being reimbursed based upon reasonable costs. Because of the way the system was financed, there were no economic incentives to be fiscally responsible.[22] Fifteen years later, the government, finally realizing that it could no longer afford to pay for health care on a cost or reasonable-cost basis, sought to create a competitive environment to reduce health care costs.

In 1982 the passage of the Tax Equity and Fiscal Responsibility Act (TEFRA) significantly influenced the health care market by creating an incentive to reduce costs. TEFRA changed the amount of reimbursement hospitals receive for inpatient services and required the development of legislation for the Prospective Payment System (PPS).[23]

The PPS became effective in October 1982 in all states except those granted waivers by the Health Care Financing Administration (HCFA). HCFA, a division of the Department of Health and Human Resources, administers the PPS. The PPS reimburses hospitals based upon their case mix of diagnosis related groups (DRGs). Each of the 470 DRGs has a weight and rate assigned to it. The **DRG rate** is the amount of money the hospital will receive for a given DRG. The environment created by the prospective payment system, based on DRGs, limits the amount of money coming into the system, thereby forcing hospitals and physicians to operate differently and assume a business orientation with emphasis on the costs associated with providing care per DRG. This process of cost reduction has had a profound effect upon nursing as a profession and upon its product, nursing care—the first and foremost reason why patients are admitted to hospitals.

Changes in reimbursement have resulted in more acutely ill hospitalized patients who require more extensive nursing intervention and, yet, spend less time in the hospital. Since these patients are discharged earlier than they were before the institution of the PPS, it has produced a drain on the nursing resources to meet the increased demand for nursing care. While hospital costs may have decreased, not only have home health care costs increased, but the need for a greater number of qualified home health care personnel has increased also, thus increasing the overall costs of operating a nursing service.

Sovie et al[24] believe the most effective management of patient care resources under prospective payment systems requires new knowledge and a comprehensive and integrated patient care and financial information system. One data element that is essential to both components of such a management information system is the identification of the nursing care hours associated with the DRGs that constitute a hopsital's case-mix. One way to do this is to study the severity of illness within DRGs, using a nursing patient classification system. The literature describes several studies that have attempted this approach, and their results are promising.[24–26]

The basic problem with the DRG system as it impacts nursing is the assumption that within a DRG patients do not differ in their nursing care requirements. This obviously is a false assumption, thus leading to early hospital discharges before adequate nursing care can be completed.

It is obvious that prospective payment systems based on fixed prices for patients with similar medical problems encourage physicians and hospitals to deliver *medical* care as efficiently as possible so that they can retain costs savings. The problem with this is that the "nursing factor" has been largely overlooked.

How will nursing plan for the inevitable changes inherent in future health care needs, increased incidence of chronic illness, changes in health care settings, and prospective payment mandates? The answer lies in the use of collaboration and consultation in research, clinical practice, and education. Conway-Welch writes:

> Well-prepared clinicians will hold the key to decreasing the length of stay in the hospital, decreasing the number and severity of complications, and decreasing the need for and use of diagnostic and therapeutic services. The need for early discharge will call for increased collaboration between nursing service and nursing education, and between nurses and physicians, on both the staff and faculty level. Nursing's secret to survival in this DRG world is the creation and

management of information, innovative use of human resources and assertive action to establish the autonomy of nursing practice.[27]

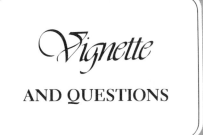

AND QUESTIONS

The Nursing Corporation of America (NCA) has long been convinced that patient census is an inadequate basis for planning nursing budgets and staff levels within its nursing departments in the group of corporate hospitals it serves.

The trend toward shorter stays and increased nursing intensity has led to understaffing in the nursing area. In addition, the Chief Nurse Executives managing the nursing departments desire a more precise measurement of patient needs and subsequently required nursing personnel to operate their departments on a day-to-day basis.

The president of NCA appointed a task force to review the various systems being used and asked for recommendations about which *one* of the systems could be used in all of the hospitals served by the NCA.

The task force found that five different patient classification systems were being used in the corporation's seven hospitals. There was a clear need for a patient classification system, but the purposes for which they were being used were not consistent with the mission of the NCA. Both prototype and factor evaluation systems were being used, thereby making it difficult to assess budgetary and staffing needs across all hospitals. Some of the systems took as little as one minute or less to classify a patient, while others took up to 25 minutes per patient. In some of the hospitals the head nurses were classifying all the patients, while in others staff nurses and nursing assistants were classifying patients. Staffing patterns on like units between hospitals varied widely and there was no mechanism to determine nursing costs or quality of care.

The preliminary evaluation of the five systems found none of the systems adequate for NCA-wide implementation, and concluded that none of the five systems was clearly superior to the others.

1. Based on the findings of the task force, what might be the next step for the Nursing Corporation of America?

2. Why would it be important for the NCA to use the same patient classification system in *all* of the hospitals?

3. What criteria would be important to consider when trying to identify a specific system for the corporation?

4. How might the implementation of a single system be approached for multiple hospitals?

5. Do you think a quality assurance mechanism could be built into a patient classification? If so, how?

6. Do you think a patient classification system can be used to determine the cost of nursing care? If so, how?

INFORMATION SOURCES

CASH Patient Classification System

CASH is the acronym for Commission for Administrative Services in Hospitals. This system categorizes patients according to types of illness, emotional status, medication and treatments ordered, and general health. The number of care hours needed are then calculated from the number of patients in each category. This system is a prototype system and is based on four categories of care requirements. Janet Georgette describes this system in more detail in Staffing by patient classification, *Nursing Clinics of North America*, June 1970, 329–331.

Holloran System

Holloran, Edward: *Holloran Systems: A Computerized Nursing Information System.* University Hospitals of Cleveland, Cleveland, Ohio, 1982.
This system is a computerized nursing information system (NIS), which uses a factor evaluation classification instrument as one of its components. The goal of the NIS is to accurately and validly describe resource requirements and allocation of nursing personnel. The classification instrument uses nursing diagnoses as its conceptual frame of reference.

GRASP System

Meyer, Diane: *GRASP: A Patient Information and Workload Management System.* Morgenton, NC, MCS, Inc, 1978.
This is a patient information and workload management system. The patient classification instrument is a factor evaluation system based on critical indicators of care. The GRASP system provides a basis for determining and analyzing the cost of nursing care. The workload measurement instrument permits analysis of data by individual patient, as well as by DRG and cost center. GRASP is a trademark of MCS, Inc, exclusive agents.

Time Spent in Indirect Nursing Care

Misener TR, Frelin AJ: Time Spent in Indirect Nursing Care. Final Report, 83-004, Defense Technical Information Center (DTIC), Alexandria, VA, 1983.

The overall purpose of this study was to objectively measure the percentage of time spent by nursing personnel on inpatient clinical services providing direct and indirect care. Nursing service staff were monitored every ten minutes on each selected shift for a total of 107,700 data points. Vail and Associates have used these data along with the data from the Sherrod Nursing Care Hours Standard Study to develop, test, and implement the Workload Management System for Nursing (WMSN).

San Joaquin System

Murphy LN, Dunley MS, Williams MA, et al: Methods for Studying Nurse Staffing in a Patient Unit, DHEW Publication No. (HRA) 78-3. Washington, DC, US Government Printing Office, 1978.

The San Joaquin instrument uses four patient care categories in a factor evaluation form. Nine critical indicators are listed on the instrument with a set of definitions available for user reference. The classifier checks each activity describing the patient's care requirements. The number of checks are then added by column and columns are totaled to derive a category of care. A weighted factor is included to handle tie scores.

Saskatchewan System

Saskatchewan System. Hospital Systems Study Group (HSSG), University of Saskatchewan, Saskatchewan, Canada.

This system involves a four-category factor-evaluation instrument. Five major groupings of nursing care are further subdivided for a total of 13 critical indicators. A set of indicators, specific definitions, and a decision tree are available to assist the user with accurately classifying patients.

Nursing Care Hour Standards Study

Sherrod SM, Rauch TM, Twist PA: Nursing Care Hours Standards Study, Parts I - VIII, Health Care Studies Division, Academy of Health Science, Fort Sam Houston, TX, 1981.

This study proposed an improved patient classification system for the following inpatient areas: coronary care, medical/surgical, obstetrics, psychiatry, neonatal and pediatrics and their concomitant intensive care units. This PCS is based on the results of over 37,000 time measurements where the mean times for 357 direct nursing care activities were established. This system addressed direct nursing care time only. It has been cited as the most comprehensive and best documented task list in the nursing literature (Giovannetti, 1982).

Workload Management System for Nursing
Vail JD, Norton DA, Rimm EA: Workload Management System for Nursing. Nursing Research Service, Walter Reed Army Medical Center, Washington, DC, 1984.
The Workload Management System for Nursing (WMSN) is a two-part system: 1) a factor-evaluation classification system that places patients into one of six discrete categories, and 2) a system linked to a staffing methodology that determines the number and mix of personnel recommended to provide nursing care. The system measures both direct and indirect nursing care requirements and is based on concurrent and prospective classification. The WMSN incorporates the findings and recommendations of both Sherrod's Nursing Care Hour Standards Study and Misener's Indirect Nursing Care Study. Research results demonstrated a valid, reliable, quantifiable classification system that can be used to predict staffing requirements at unit, hospital, and corporate levels.

REFERENCES

1. Joint Commission on Accreditation of Hospitals: *Accreditation Manual for Hospitals.* Chicago, Joint Commission on Accreditation of Hospitals, 1984

2. Aydelotte MK: *A Review and Critique of Selected Literature, Nursing Staffing Methodology.* US Department of HEW, PHS, DHEW Publication No. 73-4333, 1973

3. Grant LM: *A Study of Nursing Services in One Children's and Twenty-one General Hospitals.* New York, National League for Nursing Education, 1948

4. Abdella FG, Levine E: *Better Patient Care Through Nursing Research.* New York, Macmillan, 1965

5. Conner RJ, Flagle C, et al: Effective use of nursing resources; A research report. Hospitals 35, 1961

6. Aydelotte MK, Tener ME: *An Investigation of the Relation Between Nursing Activity and Patient Welfare.* Iowa City, Iowa State University, 1960

7. Jelinek R: Patient classification systems. In Gilles DA (ed): *Nursing Management: A Systems Approach.* Philadelphia, Saunders, 1982

8. Meyer D: *GRASP: A Patient Information and Workload Management System.* Morganton, NC, MCS, 1978

9. Giovannetti PJ: Understanding patient classification systems. J Nurs Adm, February, 1979

10. Montgomery JS, Kelly M: *A Comparative Analysis of Patient Classification Systems for Nursing Personnel Staffing Naval Hospitals.* Bethesda, MD: Research Department, Naval School of Health Sciences, National Naval Medical Center, 1981

11. Williams MA, Murphy LN: Subjective and Objective Measures of Staffing Adequacy. J Nurs Adm 9:21, November, 1979

12. CASH, Nursing Service Staff Utilization. Huckabay LM: In *Patient Classification: A Basis for Staffing.* New York, NLN, Publ. No. 20-1864, League Exchange No. 131, 1981

13. Williams GN: Workload measurement: How many on the job? How long? Mod Hosp, Sept 1969, 133

14. Sauer JE: Cost containment and quality assurance, too. Hospitals 46:78, November 1, 1972

15. Misener TR, Frelin AJ: *Time Spent in Indirect Nursing Care, Technical Report.* Alexandria, VA, Defense Technical Information Center, Defense Logistics Agency, 1983

16. Health Management Systems Associates. *A Review and Analysis of Two Patient Classification Systems,* Vol. 1, Final Report, Department of the Army, Office of the Surgeon General, (OTSG:CN), December, 1982

17. Donnelly J, Gibson J, Ivancevich J: *Fundamentals of Management: Function, Behavior, Models.* Austin, Business Publication, 1971

18. Huckabay LM: *Patient Classification: A Basis for Staffing.* New York, National League for Nursing, 1981

19. Huckabay LM, Skonieczny R: Patient classification systems: The problems faced, Nurs Health Care, February, 1981

20. Shaffer FA, (ed): *Costing Out Nursing: Pricing Our Product.* New York, National League for Nursing, 1985

21. Joel LA: Costing out nursing in nursing homes. In Shaffer FA (ed): *Costing Out Nursing: Pricing Our Product,* NY, National League for Nursing, 1985

22. DiVestea N: The changing health care system: An overview. In Shaffer FA (ed): *Costing Out Nursing: Pricing Our Product.* NY, National League for Nursing, 1985

23. Bertram D: DRG Reimbursement—A Comprehensive Review. NYSCPA Newsletter, October 1984

24. Sovie MD, Tarcinale MA, et al: Amalgam of nursing acuity, DRGs and costs. Nurs Manag 16:3, 1985

25. Rieder KA, Kay TL: Severity of illness within DRGs using a nursing patient

classification system. In Shaffer FA (ed): *Costing Out Nursing: Pricing Our Product*. NY, National League for Nursing, 1985

26. Dhalen AL, Gregor JR: Nursing costs by DRG with an all-RN staff. In Shaffer FA (ed): *Costing Out Nursing: Pricing Our Product*. NY, National League for Nursing, 1985

27. Conway-Welch C: DRGs, nursing education, and nursing service: A collaborative effort for survival. In Shaffer FA (ed): *Costing Out Nursing: Pricing Our Product*. NY, National League for Nursing, 1985

MARLENE R. VENTURA, RN, EdD, FAAN

FRANCES CROSBY, RN, EdD

Quality Assurance: The Appraisal of Health Care Delivery

CHAPTER 9

Background and Overview

Increased emphasis is being placed on quality assurance activities by federal and state governments, third party reimbursers, accrediting agencies, health care professionals, and consumers themselves. There are many definitions and interpretations of quality and each has merit for consideration in selected instances and contexts. To more fully understand the multi-dimensionality and complexity of quality, one needs to think about the definitions, assessment approaches, and assurance activities and their relationships with nursing practice.

Zimmer, as early as 1974, reported that **quality assurance** involves identifying standards for excellence, evaluating care against those standards, and then taking action to correct deficiencies and achieve the standards. It is accounted for by "implementing systematic evaluation to make sure that delivered care is at the optimum achievable degree of excellence and by continuously taking action to secure improvements."[1]

Quality of health care has been defined as the "goodness" and "badness" of health care. Donabedian[2] reported that the "balance of health benefits and harm is the essential core of a definition of quality." He describes it as "the evaluative dimension of the elements and interactions in the medical care process."[3] More specifically, it entails the identification of the impact of services delivered upon the health of the people served and a comparison of actual impact with desired impact according to established goals.[4]

Appraisal of quality in the delivery of health care has evolved in response to the interaction of a number of factors affecting health care at the time. Most efforts in the appraisal of quality of care have been related to correcting abuses, setting minimum standards, and stimulating improvements.[5] Recent interest in scientifically evaluating programs and in professionals monitoring their own practice has offered additional impetus for appraising quality of care.

Historically, nurses have demonstrated a commitment to quality assessment and assurance. Florence Nightingale, in the mid-1850s, urged that nursing care be evaluated, and compiled hospital sickness statistics (morbidity and mortality) to bring about reform in the British military health care system.[6] Schroeder and Maibusch have identified Nightingale's work as the "initiation of quality assurance or quality control process," ie, standard setting, comparison of care to that standard, and the initiation of action to bring about desired change.[7]

Demands for a systematic evaluation of medical care later appeared around 1910 as a result of an expose of poorly educated physicians and inadequate facility conditions.[8] In response, the American College of Surgeons was formed to serve as an accrediting mechanism to improve standards of medical education, and facility conditions were evaluated through a nationwide survey of hospitals.

In the 1950s a system to evaluate quality of care was designed in Michigan. A panel of physicians participated in consensus rounds to identify criteria, related to 18 different diagnoses, used for medical record review to determine appropriateness of length of stay by diagnosis.[9]

Concern for assessment of quality in health care reached a peak in the 1970s and has been referred to as the issue of the 70s, with nurses taking a leading role.[10] Emphasis in quality assurance became even more pronounced with the enactment in 1972 of PSRO legislation, Public Law 92-603.

A review of literature on quality of care in nursing reveals many approaches and tools designed to measure nurse performance and patient care. Names associated with quality assurance, such as Marie Zimmer, Norma Lang, Carol Lindeman, Marie Phaneuf, Mabel Wandelt, Doris Slater Stewart, Doris Bloch, Robert Brook, and Avedis Donabedian, became familiar.

APPROACHES TO QUALITY ASSESSMENT

A number of approaches have evolved over the years to assess quality, and the one most frequently referred to is that of Donabedian.[11] This approach divides components of health care to be evaluated into structure of health care, the process of providing health care, and outcomes.

When quality of care is assessed by means of a **structure evaluation,** the environment in which the care is delivered is assessed. The instruments for delivering care and their organization are appraised, with the assumption that when specific conditions are met, good care will occur.[12]

Process evaluations measure the components of care that have been delivered and are provider-focused. They may be retrospective, as when audits or chart reviews are conducted, or they may be concurrent, as when the delivery of care is directly observed and judged.

Outcome evaluations measure the quality of care received as reflected in specific anticipated end results. Zimmer[13] describes these as the "alteration in health status of the patient caused by goal directed nursing care activities." Outcome assessments are usually patient-focused.

In addition to those described above, attempts have been made to assess patient satisfaction, continuity of care, accessibility, efficiency, and provider satisfaction, just to name a few, as other parameters of quality.

SPECIFIC ASSESSMENT METHODOLOGIES

From the 1950s to the 1970s a focus was on the development of specific instruments to measure quality of nursing care. The development of the Nursing Audit began in 1952, but was not published until 1972,[14] and revised in 1976.[15] It was the belief at that time that nurses "responsible for the provision of care were accountable for its quality and that given an audit method . . . were capable of passing judgment on the quality."[16] This was, in essence, the evolution of peer review. The Nursing Audit evaluated the quality of nursing care through the appraisal of the nursing process as reflected in the clinical record of discharged patients. The framework for the Phaneuf Audit, as it was also called, was the delineation of seven functions of professional nursing as developed by Lesnick and Anderson.[17] A record was reviewed, each item was rated, and a score was computed. Care provided was then described as excellent, good, incomplete, poor, or unsafe.

The Slater Nursing Competencies Rating Scale[18] was created to evaluate competencies of a nurse in the performance of care to patients. The scale yielded both a descriptive and a numeric score and could be used in any setting where nurses provided care. Eighty-four items were rated, with the performance of the nurse judged as best nurse, between, average nurse, between, poorest nurse, or not applicable or not observed. The numerical values for performance ranged from 5 to 1, with a value of 5 being best nurse. An overall score was obtained by tabulating an average of item scores.

The Quality Patient Care Scale (QualPacs)[19] was developed using the Slater Nursing Performance Rating Scale as a basis. QualPacs measured the quality of nursing care received by patients in any setting where nurse-patient interactions occurred. The standard used for rating the item was the care delivered by a first-level staff nurse, and each of 68 items was also rated on a 5-point scale. It differed from the Slater Scale in that the observation was of the patient, and ratings were made of the care received from all nursing providers, as opposed to the nurse, who is rated using the Slater Scale.

In 1972 a contract was initiated from the Division of Nursing, United States Department of Health, Education, and Welfare (now Health and Human Services) to the Rush-Presbyterian-St. Luke's Medical Center and Medicus Systems Corporation of Chicago to develop a method to monitor quality of nursing care in hospitals. The development of this methodology was based on the review of existing process measures. The resulting approach,[20-22] referred to as the HEW–Rush–Medicus Methodology for Monitoring Quality of Nursing Care, combined chart review, patient and staff interviews, and direct care observation for data collection of quality of care on a nursing unit. The instrument, with 257 criteria, had its own patient classification system.

Horn and Swain[23] were funded by the National Center for Health Services Research to develop a series of criterion measures of nursing care that measured health status from an outcome standpoint. The instrument contained 539 outcome criteria by utilizing the eight universal and ten health deviation self-care demand categories of Orem.

Other instruments to measure quality of care also appeared during the 1970s. Around that same time, work had begun in developing generic models or frameworks for conducting quality assurance activities. The model approach was an alternative from the standardized methodologies previously described and was directed at a process to address quality assessment with the uniqueness of the given agency and patient population. It allowed for the opportunity to focus on a specific issue.

The American Nurses' Association formed nursing practice divisions to develop practice standards and developed prototypes of criteria for specific patient groups. In 1974 Norma Lang developed a model for quality assurance[24] that the American Nurses' Association integrated into its quality assurance activities.[25] Emphasis at this time was placed on developing criteria, establishing standards, and refining models.[26-28]

At the same time, the Joint Commission on Accreditation of Hospitals added quality assurance to its evaluation criteria, requiring departments to implement an ongoing quality assurance program to identify problems and initiate and evaluate corrective actions. In 1984 the Joint Commission made significant changes in the quality assurance chapter in its accreditation manual. The previous problem-focused approach was replaced with an emphasis on an organization-wide program focusing on the planned, systematic, ongoing monitoring and evaluation of important aspects of patient care and services.[29] The Joint Commission developed a model[30] in 1985 to provide a framework in monitoring and evaluating processes. This model consisted of nine steps and was intended to assist health care facilities in demonstrating compliance to the standards put forth by the Joint Commission. Additional changes are predicted, with increased emphasis being placed on assessment of outcomes of care.

In 1987 the Joint Commission on Accreditation of Hospitals was renamed the Joint Commission on Accreditation of Health Care Organizations. Their role on accrediting facilities and providing educational programs for health care professionals has been expanded to include ambulatory health care organizations, home care programs, hospice programs, hospitals, long-term care organizations, and psychiatric and substance abuse organizations.

State health departments, to a greater extent, and some federal agencies, too, have become increasingly concerned about quality of health care in hospitals, nursing homes, home health care agencies, and related institutions. They, too, in many instances have specific criteria that have to be met and conduct on-site reviews. If deficiencies are noted, specific actions need to be taken to correct them. In some cases the criteria developed are very specific and stringent.

Nursing today is integrating many facets of quality assurance in its practice areas. It includes, but is not limited to, developing quality assurance activities at the unit level,[31] developing standards,[32] and developing frameworks that integrate standards into practice and quality assurance activities.[33]

For a more thorough review of specific studies addressing the assessment of quality of nursing care, the reader is referred to the work of Lang and Clinton.[34] For additional resources on quality assurance approaches, standards, and criteria, the reader is referred to the information sources at the end of this chapter.

DEVELOPING A QUALITY ASSURANCE PROGRAM

Quality assurance includes both measuring the level of care provided and improving it when necessary. As previously described, there are a number of ways of setting up a quality assurance program and these vary in their steps. Programs can be centralized or decentralized, or have a combination of both. However, any approach should have as a goal the improvement of the delivery of health care to clients and the development of strategies to maintain a desirable level of care once it is achieved. Excellence in care is based on the most recent and best knowledge derived from the sciences and humanities, and that knowledge, when translated into practice, has the least unfavorable outcomes.

One of the first steps in the development of a quality assurance program is a written description of 1) the scope of services provided to clients within a setting; 2) quality assurance committee structure and its relationship to other committees; 3) the delineation of lines of responsibility for quality assurance activities; 4) the nature and extent of interface with other programs or individuals also conducting quality assurance activities within an organization; 5) procedures to be followed; 6) methods by which the program will be evaluated; and 7) type of documentation required. This description can be a written document or one of the policy statements developed by the institution.

The second step is the determination of the relevant areas to be reviewed and, if needed, some prioritization. Factors such as incidence and prevalence, likelihood of placing clients at risk, known problem areas, and lack of compliance with established guidelines or standards of care can enter into the decision to select an area for review. Emphasis should be placed on clinical areas, but consideration can be given to administration, research, and education issues. Input regarding the importance of areas for quality assurance review should be obtained from relevant individuals and groups.

After the areas of interest have been identified, specific statements are written that describe the expectation or desirable aspect of care to be delivered and evaluated. Specific measurable criteria are then delineated to represent the desirable aspect of care. These criteria define what data are to be collected and allow for a comparison of "what actually is" with what was predetermined as "ought to be." These criteria statements can focus on structure, process, or outcomes of care. They are derived from the health care literature, from policies and procedures of a local institution, and from the knowledge and experience of nursing experts.

These criteria, which operationalize the standard of quality, need to be written so that the individuals using them have a clear delineation of what is being observed. They should assess a single entry and should be measurable, clear, and concise. It is preferable to try the criteria out in a pilot phase so that any changes in wording or time frame can be made before widespread data collection is initiated. Considerations at this time should also be given to who will collect the data, what is the data source, what is the time frame, and what type of instructions or orientation will be needed to collect accurate data. Once the procedure is established, data collection can occur.

The third step is the analysis of data. Analysis is dependent on the type of data that have been collected; how the data have been reported by unit, by clinical area, and by Nursing Service; and what type of statistics are important. For example, should numbers be reported or should percentages be used? If the latter is selected, what is the nature and size of the sample from which percentages will be derived? This is especially important when describing the data to other individuals and attempting to make any comparisons with other institutions or data found in the literature.

Analyzing data by groups of patients, by areas, by unit, by shift, or time of day is also helpful. This approach allows one to look for any patterns that may exist. Several rounds of data analysis may be necessary. The staff may review existing results and suggest further analysis.

Appropriate individuals need to be included in the review of the data, the identification of areas that can be improved, and actions to achieve that improvement. If the data are determined to reflect that a satisfactory level of care is identified, then several options are available. These include continuing to monitor the area at the previously designated intervals, altering the interval schedule, or reexamining the criteria to make sure that they are measuring the aspect of care identified. If the level of care assessed is less than satisfactory, then the areas requiring improvement need to be identified and an action plan developed to reduce the incidence of occurrence and to improve care.

Action plans may take many forms, but they should include the nature of the desired change, the individual responsible for the change or coordinating the change, a time frame for the change to occur, and some indications of when the aspect of care will be reevaluated. Proposed changes can include changes in policies and procedures within an institution, changes in the use of equipment, and changes in the knowledge, attitude, and behavior of providers.

After the action plans have been initiated, a follow-up review is conducted at a selected interval. The time frame should be significant enough to have allowed for the appropriate changes to have taken place. The follow-up assessment can be done using the same criteria as before, especially if some comparisons are to be made. However, if there are serious problems with the criteria that will threaten the validity of the data collection, appropriate changes should be made.

The fourth step is to document and communicate the results of the data collected to selected individuals. Documentation should be a formal written report. Format may vary from institution to institution. It should be available for the annual review of the program. Some reports generated may be monthly, quarterly, semiannual, or yearly. These reports may be sent to selected individuals or to committees as designated by the institution.

Impacts on the Nurse, the Consumer, and Society

THE NURSE

An effective quality assurance program has an impact throughout the health care system. The nurse delivering care, the patient receiving care, and the institution and society in which the system operates are all influenced. It is difficult to identify all the areas where benefits may be realized, since they are numerous and their impact may influence various sectors of society simultaneously. Quality assurance activities have a direct impact upon the nurse. They identify areas where high quality of nursing care is delivered. They also evaluate provider performance. Deficits in patient care demonstrate the need for additional or altered nursing actions. Quality assurance activities also identify where changes may need to occur that impact other health care disciplines or the institution as a whole. Nurses need to understand the nature of quality assurance in institutions and what specifically is their role in the process. They need to know how quality assurance fosters good health care, how activities are initiated, how best to develop criteria, how to bring about desired change, and what types of reports may need to be generated. Nursing personnel can benefit from quality assurance if they develop a positive attitude toward quality assurance, as opposed to viewing it as something that is imposed upon them by the institution or by outside agencies. The accountability implied in quality assurance fosters professional autonomy. Inherent in nursing, as a profession, are internal evaluation and self-monitoring procedures. Identification of problem areas either in the delivery of nursing care or in patient outcomes leads to a problem-solving process of exploring alternative nursing care actions. This allows for creativity within practice as well as the opportunity to apply research findings to practice or to conduct research. The latter will assist in validating findings in current practice or in answering important clinical questions. The ability to confirm the effectiveness of nursing actions contributes to quality of care and to job satisfaction. Systematic evaluation of the effects of alternative approaches to patient care demonstrates to the nurse that care components need to be assessed and modified as indicated, and that change is an acceptable occurrence. When desired results are found, the quality assurance process provides positive feedback to the individual nurse for his/her efforts and performance.

Quality assurance activities have increased nurses' adherence to standards of practice, involvement in patient education and health counseling, documentation of care provided, and documentation of patients' and families' responses to care. Such activities more fully help describe the scope of practice and the effectiveness of nursing interventions on improving and maintaining health. The development of the *Journal of Nursing Quality Assurance* and other journals, such as the *Journal of Health Promotion*, provides additional vehicles for nurses to communicate the results of quality assurance activities.

When less than desirable results are obtained, the opportunity for staff development and performance appraisal exists. The quality assurance process maintains accountability and responsibility for the care delivered by individuals, by nursing units, and by an overall organization. The care delivered and its appraisal can be traced to identify patterns and/or issues that need to be addressed. While identification of problem areas may be perceived as threatening, scrutiny, or censure, a positive view of it as growth promoting and assuring high quality care better serves its purpose. Ultimately, the way the quality assurance staff conduct quality assurance programs and the feedback they provide, along with the nurses' perception of the activities, determine whether quality assurance is a valuable or fearful experience.

THE CONSUMER AND SOCIETY

Consumers benefit directly from quality assurance activities because of the positive outcomes of care and because of the interaction process between patient and provider. Measurements of patient outcomes are the ultimate validators of quality of care and provide the means to determine the effect of care upon the patient. The purpose of quality assurance is to assure positive health care for patients. While various approaches may be used, all quality assurance programs strive for the improvement of care for groups of patients. An ongoing process of self-monitoring is most effective. When patient needs are identified via quality assurance assessments, deficits in patient care can be remedied. Quality assurance programs that observe the patient's environment and assess the patient's needs for selected nursing interventions, the appropriate use of siderails, number of medication incidents, and patient satisfaction levels, for example, all foster the individual patient's safety and well-being. This ultimately promotes the therapeutic value of the patient's experience by taking ongoing steps to monitor his experience. Those actions that relate to the appropriate assessment to be made for the patient and enhance the implementation of the most effective nursing interventions also enhance therapeutic nursing care.

Patients have benefited from having their health education needs assessed and specific programs developed to address those needs. Just to cite some examples, the incidences of pressure ulcers and patient falls have been identified and decreased by quality assurance activities. Infection control and medication incident assessment and tracking are other concrete examples of the benefit of quality assurance activities upon the patient. Discharge planning has been facilitated by documentation of outcome criteria and nursing interventions.

Quality assurance provides a channel for input from patients as consumers of health care services. Some health care agencies invite consumers to participate in planning of care and may identify committees where consumer input would be most beneficial. Quality assurance activities help define the consumer's expectations of nursing care. Increasing evidence is being obtained to support the notion that consumers are being informed to a greater extent regarding health care and quality assurance.

Quality assurance activities seek to afford public accountability for the care that health care providers make available. The program monitors the accessibility to care, which affects the consumer dimension of the community. Ongoing quality assurance monitors the currency of health care procedures and cost of care provided in the community.

Self-monitoring of the quality of care is an essential ingredient in the profession of nursing. It stresses the "social contract between society and professions, whereby society grants the professions authority over functions . . . and permits them considerable autonomy. . . . In return, the professions are expected to act responsibly, always mindful of the public trust."[35]

Future Considerations

A number of considerations are germaine to the issue of quality assurance activities for the future. These are not necessarily identified in any order. The first consideration deals with increasing the involvement in the quality assurance process of those nurses directly involved in patient care. This could be accomplished by decentralizing quality assurance activities, identifying quality assurance liaison representatives at the unit level, and increasing staff membership on quality assurance committees. The second issue is increasing the involvement of various disciplines, when appropriate, in quality assurance activities and identifying strategies to integrate nursing service quality assurance activities with those of others in the institution. Efforts need to be directed to focus on clinical issues of importance for nursing from a concurrent and prospective data collection basis. Better strategies need to be developed to track quality assurance activities, assure that the corrective action has occurred, and reassess the impact of these actions in a timely fashion. The use of computers and software for quality assurance will be of benefit and have an impact on the data collection procedures, analyses, and the generation of information collected.

Emphasis should be placed on determining outcomes of nursing care and methods to assess those outcomes. Increased consideration should be given to prospectively identifying standards of care and standards of nursing practice as an integral part of quality assurance activities.

Quality assurance will play a key role in monitoring an acceptable balance between quality and cost. There will be a need to evaluate and intervene in the appropriate use of resources in health care delivery and increase access to health care. Quality assurance will need to be extended to outpatient, extended, and home care services. These activities will need to be interfaced with inpatient monitoring efforts.

Strategies to enhance documentation of nursing care and to integrate the nursing care plan with ongoing documentation in the medical record is an issue. The balance between confidentiality and freedom of information will need to be addressed.

Quality assurance needs to be given a prominent place in nursing education and practice. The quality assurance concepts currently taught in schools of nursing at various levels and in continuing education programs should be examined. Further, a model curriculum to incorporate quality assurance content into undergraduate, graduate, and continuing nursing education programs should be designed and evaluated.

Service agencies need to review the expectations they have for nursing staff and the type of orientation and support resources that are provided for quality assurance. The interrelationships of problem solving, quality assurance, evaluation, and research activities need to be clarified and encouraged.

The nature and scope of quality assurance is evolving and as such has created a state of influx as organizations have attempted to meet internal and external requests. In addition, the external agencies that incorporate quality assurance into their credentialing criteria vary, creating an ambiguous and sometimes conflicting expectation of quality assurance programs. The health care agencies and external agencies need to coordinate efforts so expectations are complementary and can be fulfilled.

Changes will continue to occur in quality assurance as advancements in technology, prospective payment systems, and nursing profession and practice also evolve as professional nurses and consumers assume greater leadership roles in health care. We should accept the fact that changes in quality assurance are inevitable and welcome them, since these refinements demonstrate growth and concern for the quality of care that is provided and the cost for that care.

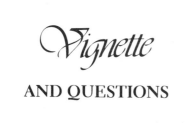

Vignette

AND QUESTIONS

The numbers of patient falls are increasing in a health care institution and the director of nursing has brought this to the attention of the quality assurance nurse and the members of the quality assurance committee. The director of nursing has asked that this problem be addressed and that a plan of action be developed.

The committee needs to review the format currently used to report patient falls to determine what types of information have been collected retrospectively and how complete was the information collected. At the same time, the committee members would want to designate a few individuals to conduct manual searches and a computer search of the literature, and others may want to contact other institutions to determine their experience regarding patient falls. This would enable the committee to have some background on previous studies, identified factors that place a patient at risk, and intervention programs that have been established. Several members of the committee would review the completed incident forms for patient falls for a predefined period of time, most likely the last 12 months. This would allow for an analysis of any monthly cyclical trends. The committee members should identify what types of information that have already been collected would be important to review as part of this quality assurance activity. These may include, but not be limited to, unit, sex, age, number of days hospitalized, when fall occurred, mobility status, mentation, elimination needs, number of previous falls, medications taken within 48 hours, day of week, time of day, location of fall, general description of what patient was doing at the time of the fall, outcome of the fall, and treatment required.

The members of the committee may want to develop a data sheet that would be used to compile the data. The incident forms would be sorted by month and a member of the committee would extrapolate the information from the incident forms onto the data collection sheet. A short orientation program would be initiated to insure that the members of the committee are interpreting the items consistently. Only incident forms involving a patient who has fallen should be used. If these cases are to be summarized by month, the number of patients treated for the month should also be obtained, so that the number of incidents can be interpreted in light of the numbers of patients treated. Other statistics might also be used.

Data would be summarized by month for a 12-month period and any observed trends reported. Specific information as to type of fall, location, nursing unit, and outcome of fall should also be described. After the data have been reviewed, the committee would identify the major findings and any recommendations. If the data available from the incident forms are not sufficient to identify trends or factors that impact on falls, a recommendation can be made to conduct a prospective study of patient falls. This would include having the nurse who reports a patient fall complete a data collection sheet that would include some of the information described earlier.

The committee would also want to discuss such issues as what is the current expectation or policy on patient safety; to what extent is it being carried out; what elements described in the literature or obtained from others may be applicable, ie, fall risk assessment tool, fall prevention program, or better reporting on the incident form. One recommendation for the action plan might be to develop a fall prevention program to reduce the occurrence of patient falls.

The following are questions for further discussion:

1. What items might be included on a data collection instrument?

2. What steps should be taken to insure that the data collection sheet for patient falls is completed accurately and in a timely fashion?

3. What trends may be observed that would have clinical significance?

4. What might be some key elements in a policy statement on patient safety?

5. What might be included in a fall prevention program?

6. How would one evaluate the effectiveness of a program?

7. What would be the role of the staff nurses, head nurse, nursing instructor, and nursing supervisors in reducing the numbers of patient falls in an institution?

INFORMATION SOURCES

American Nurses' Association and Sutherland Learning Associates, Inc: *Nursing Quality Assurance Management/Learning System: Guide for Nursing Quality Assurance Coordinators and Administrators.* Northridge, CA, Sutherland Learning Associates, Inc, 1982

Cantor M: *Achieving Nursing Care Standards: Internal and External.* Wakefield, MA, Nursing Resources, Inc, 1978

Carter J, Hilliard M, Castles M, et al: *Standards of Nursing Care: A Guide for Evaluation.* 2nd edition, NY, Springer, 1976

Davidson S: *Nursing Care Evaluation: Concurrent and Retrospective Review Criteria.* St. Louis, CV Mosby, 1977

Donabedian A: *Explorations in Quality Assessment and Monitoring, Volume II: The Criteria and Standards of Quality.* Ann Arbor, MI, Health Administration Press, 1982

Duke University Hospital Nursing Service: *Guidelines for Nursing Care: Process and Outcome.* Philadelphia, Lippincott, 1983

Joint Commission on Accreditation of Hospitals: *The QA Guide: A Resource for Hospital Quality Assurance.* Chicago, Joint Commission on Accreditation of Hospitals, 1980

Joint Commission on Accreditation of Hospitals: *Monitoring and Evaluation in Nursing Services.* Chicago, Joint Committee on Accreditation of Hospitals, 1986

Karch A: *Concurrent Nursing Audit: Quality Assurance in Action.* Thorofare, NJ, Charles B Slack, Inc, 1980

Mayers M, Norby R, Watson A: *Quality Assurance for Patient Care: Nursing Perspectives.* New York, Appleton-Century-Crofts, 1977

Tucker S, Breeding M, Canobbio M, Jacquet G, Paquette E, Wells M, Willmann M: *Patient Care Standards.* St. Louis, CV Mosby, 1975

Williamson J, Hudson J, Nevins M: *Principles of Quality Assurance and Cost Containment in Health Care.* San Francisco, Jossey-Bass, 1982

Williamson J, Ostrow P, Braswell H: *Health Accounting for Quality Assurance: A Manual for Assessing and Improving Outcomes of Care.* Rockville, MD, American Occupational Therapy Association, 1981

REFERENCES

1. Zimmer M: Quality assurance for outcomes of patient care. Nurs Clin North Am 9(2):307, 1974

2. Donabedian A: *Explorations in Quality Assessment and Monitoring; Vol. I, The Definition of Quality and Approaches to its Assessment.* Ann Arbor, MI, Health Administration Press, 1980, p 27

3. Donabedian A: Promoting quality through evaluating the process of patient care. Med Care 6(3):182, 1968

4. Kerr M, Trantow D: Defining, measuring and assessing the quality of health services. Public Health Rep 84(5):415, 1969

5. Sheps M: Approaches to the quality of hospital care. Public Health Rep 70(9):884, 1955

6. Kopf E: Florence Nightingale as statistician. Res Nurs Health 1(3):93, 1978

7. Schroeder P, Maibusch R: *Nursing Quality Assurance—A Unit-Based Approach.* Rockville: Aspen Systems Corporation, 1984, p 4

8. Lembcke P: Evolution of the medical adult. JAMA 199(8):111, 1967

9. Payne B: Continued evolution of a system of medical care appraisal. JAMA 201(7):127, 1967

10. Hegyvary S: Prospective payment: Focus on quality of care. *Nursing Research and Policy Formation: The Case of Prospective Payment.* Missouri, American Nurses' Association: 1984, p 51

11. Donabedian A: *Explorations in Quality Assessment and Monitoring; Vol.* I, p 90

12. Donabedian A: Part II. Some issues in evaluating the quality of nursing care. Am J Public Health 59(10):1833, 1969

13. Zimmer M: A model for evaluating nursing care. Hospitals, JAHA 48:91, 131, 1974

14. Phaneuf M: *The Nursing Audit, Profile in Excellence*. New York, Appleton-Century-Crofts, 1972

15. Phaneuf M: *The Nursing Audit, Self-Regulation in Nursing Practice*. New York, Appleton-Century-Crofts, 1976

16. Phaneuf M: *The Nursing Audit, Self-Regulation in Nursing Practice*, p 2

17. Lesnick M, Anderson B: Nursing Practice and the Law, ed 2. Philadelphia: Lippincott, 1955

18. Wandelt M, Slater D: *Slater Nursing Competencies Rating Scale*. New York: Appleton-Century-Crofts, 1975

19. Wandelt M, Ager J: *Quality Patient Care Scale*. New York: Appleton-Century-Crofts, 1974

20. Jelinek R, Haussmann R, Hegyvary S, Newman J: A *Methodology for Monitoring Quality of Nursing Care, Part I*. Washington DC: US Government Printing Office, DHEW Publication No. 76-25, 1975

21. Haussmann R, Hegyvary S, Newman J: *Monitoring Quality of Nursing Care, Part II*. Washington DC: US Government Printing Office, DHEW Publication No. 76–7, 1976

22. Haussmann R, Hegyvary S: *Monitoring Quality of Nursing Care, Part III*. Washington DC: US Government Printing Office, DHEW Publication No. 77–70, 1977

23. Horn B, Swain M: *Development of Criterion Measures of Nursing Care, Volume I and II*. Springfield, VA: National Technical Information Services (NTIS Nos. PB267004 and 267005), 1977

24. Lang N: A Model for Quality Assurance in Nursing. (unpublished doctoral dissertation), Marquette University, Milwaukee, 1974

25. American Nurses' Association, A *Plan for Implementation of the Standards of Nursing Practice*. Kansas City, MO: American Nurses' Association, 1975

26. Zimmer M: Quality assurance for outcomes of patient care, p 217

27. Hover J, Zimmer M: Nursing quality assurance: The Wisconsin system. Nurs Outlook April:242, 1978

28. Bloch D: Evaluation of nursing care in terms of process and outcome: Issues in research and quality assurance. Nurs Res 24(4):256, 1975

29. Joint Commission on Accreditation of Hospitals, *Monitoring and Evaluation in Nursing Service*. Chicago: Joint Commission on Accreditation of Hospitals, 1986

30. Joint Commission on Accreditation of Hospitals, *Monitoring and Evaluation in Nursing Service*, p 11

31. Schroeder P, Maibusch R: *Nursing Quality Assurance.*

32. Mason E: *How to Write Meaningful Nursing Standards.* New York: Wiley, 1984

33. Marker C: The Marker umbrella model for quality assurance: Monitoring and evaluating professional practice. J Nurs Qual Assur 1(3):52, 1987

34. Lang N, Clinton J: Assessment of quality of nursing care. In Werley H, Fitzpatrick J (eds): *Annual Review of Nursing Research*, Vol. 2. New York, Springer Publishing Company, 1984, p 135

35. Phaneuf M: *The Nursing Audit: Self Regulation.* p xiii

SARA T. FRY, RN, PhD

Ethical Dimensions of Technology and Consumer Care

CHAPTER 10

Background and Overview

New developments in technology have created unprecedented opportunities in health care. Yet the uses of technology often pose distressing value conflicts for nurses, consumers, and society. The conflicts may be as minor as discussing a pregnant woman's general fears before undergoing a prenatal diagnostic technology or as complex as deciding whether to engage in experimental efforts to manipulate the genetic endowment of an embryo conceived in the laboratory.

Prior to the 1970s, the limited use of technology in health care did not cause value conflicts for the majority of individuals. The question of whether or not a patient ought to be kept alive by artificial life support was not morally imperative when there was no technology to maintain life support of the patient. The question of whether or not one ought to tell prospective parents that their unborn child had a serious genetic abnormality was not an issue when there was no technology available to diagnose genetic abnormalities with demonstrated accuracy during the first trimester of pregnancy. Beginning in the 1970s, however, the explosive development of technology steadily created pressing moral conflicts as new technological advances provided opportunities to alter life and death. Focusing on the "edges of life," these advances gave health professionals the opportunity to intervene in procreation and birth while, at the same time, the opportunity to prolong life or delay the time of death. Prenatal diagnostic technologies, genetic screening, and genetic engineering have been associated with many value conflicts surrounding procreation and birth. Artificial life support mechanisms, the artificial heart, and innovative cardiovascular surgery have been associated with value conflicts surrounding the prolongation of life.

This chapter will examine the impacts of new technological advances in health care on the nurse, the consumer, and society. Case situations will demonstrate the types of value conflicts experienced in the use of technology to intervene in procreation and birth or to prolong life. Additional questions will encourage the reader to consider the significance of important human values in health care and the role of the nurse in protecting and promoting these values.

Impacts on the Nurse, the Consumer, and Society

THE NURSE

Technologies that alter procreation have enabled millions of infertile couples throughout the world to conceive and bear children. Other technologies to combat otherwise untreatable disorders are enabling individuals to develop the capacity to produce needed bodily defenses. The nurse participating in the use of these technologies often faces ethical problems. The nurse might face the question of whether or not altering the process of procreation is an immoral tampering with nature. The nurse might also face more specific questions concerning the use of leftover embryos for research or the use of altered human genetic material. The following two cases demonstrate the value conflicts experienced by nurses when confronted by these questions.

CASE 10.1—THE NURSE AND IN VITRO FERTILIZATION

Pamela Sorrenson has heard about an impending opening of an in vitro fertilization clinic in her community and the availability of several nursing positions on the clinic staff. Curious about the clinic and in vitro fertilization, Mrs. Sorrenson applies for a position. On interview, her responsibilities are explained and she is given a tour of the almost completed laboratories and the unit. She is impressed, but has some nagging questions about the moral issues involved with in vitro fertilization and the process itself. When she tries to discuss these questions with the medical director, he seems to brush away her concerns and focus on the novelty of the technology, the benefit of its use to childless couples, and the social demand for the service. Mrs. Sorrenson, however, is concerned about some very basic questions about fertilization of human ova, conception, and the values she has usually associated with these human events. She wonders whether she can work effectively in an environment that treats the traditional "mysteries of life" as simply scientific events that can be manipulated by human intervention. She also wonders what guidelines the clinic will have for the treatment of fertilized ova that are not implanted in the prospective pregnant woman. Will they be used for other purposes? Or will they be discarded in the sink drain? If they are stored for any period of time, what policies will the clinic have for discarding them at a later date? These are issues of fundamental importance to Mrs. Sorrenson and impact on both her professional and personal values.

The questions facing Mrs. Sorrenson are ones that have been widely discussed by theologians and ethicists.[1-3] Many people question the demystification of the birth process. Those who favor a "natural law" position urge that certain biological processes are the natural way of procreating. Thus, anything that artificially manipulates the procreation process or that alters human germ cells violates the natural order of things.

Others have questioned whether or not in vitro fertilization is a form of experimentation. If it is experimentation, the subject of the experimentation would be nonconsenting, since the subject is the embryo. In what sense could the experimentation of in vitro fertilization be said to be beneficial for the embryo created by the process? Some would argue that in vitro fertilization is only beneficial to the adults who seek it. They perceive a child as beneficial to *them*, but the child is not benefited in any moral sense. Yet the growing number of babies born as a result of in vitro fertilization demonstrates that these babies are not at any greater risk than those conceived naturally. Despite the absence of risk, the underlying question of benefit is still an important moral issue where the technology of in vitro fertilization is concerned. This seems to be one of the fundamental questions troubling Mrs. Sorrenson in this case situation.

Another fundamental question concerns the morality of disposing of leftover embryos. Some experts in the field have argued that extra embryos are essentially the property of the man and woman who produced them. Since couples have the right to abort fetuses, they should also have the right to destroy any embryos produced by in vitro fertilization. Does this right also mean that couples have the right to do other things with the embryos they have produced? Do they have the right to sell them to laboratories, for example, to be maintained until more mature or to be the subjects of research? Do couples have the right to dispose of their embryos in any way that they want? Should society create norms of proper disposal? Should couples receive financial compensation for sharing their extra embryos? Or should the embryos become the property of the state and be available to other couples who want to conceive but are unable (or uninterested) in supplying their own ova? Before Mrs. Sorrenson or any nurse agrees to work in a clinic offering a birth technology such as in vitro fertilization, these questions must inevitably be faced.

CASE 10.2—PARTICIPATING IN GENETIC ENGINEERING

Tricia Holmes is a staff nurse at a major clinical research center. She is part of a nursing care team that provides services to bone marrow transplant patients. The research team is attempting some innovative techniques that involve removal of bone marrow tissue from individuals affected with an untreatable metabolic disorder, exposure of the human tissue to gene splicing techniques in laboratory, and reimplantation of the bone marrow tissue into the patient. It is anticipated that the patient would then have a capacity to produce the needed metabolic substance and overcome the disorder.

Ms. Holmes and the other nurses on the team would provide the same nursing care services for these patients as they currently do for all bone marrow transplant patients. The use of this technology, however, promises to initiate new and potentially controversial technologies. For example, the same technology could be used to make other changes in the basic genetic structure in human beings. Eventually, efforts would be made to modify germ cells which make it possible to transmit new genetic material from one generation to the next. The result would be an introduction of new genetic material into the human species.

Ms. Holmes is being asked to participate in this new research effort. She recognizes that the research will probably meet local and national standards of the institutional IRB (Institutional Research Board) and that the investigators on the research team are acting in good conscience. She must decide, however, whether it is ethical for *her* to participate in this type of research.

In assessing this type of research, Ms. Holmes will need to consider all the standard questions involving research involving human subjects.[4,5] She will need to evaluate 1) the objectives and rationale of the proposed research; 2) research design; 3) the risks and benefits; 4) selection of patients; 5) informed consent; and 6) privacy and confidentiality afforded the prospective subjects of research. Additional questions will also need to address the potential risks of altering DNA material, disrupting other genes, and any untoward side effects of gene alteration.[6] The technology is so new that not all of its side effects and risks are known at the present time.

The most fundamental question to be faced is whether there is something morally wrong about human efforts to manipulate genetic material and reintroduce new genetic material into the cells of human beings.[7] Most medical interventions prior to this decade have left the genetic nature of the human species undisturbed. Now, however, there is potential to make dramatic changes in the genetic composition of the human species. Ms. Holmes and other nurses must decide whether or not to participate in procedures where this change may take place. Of particular importance is whether increased use of this type of technology with somatic cells will be extended to germ cells, with all the potential of introducing genetic material into the next generation that may eventually prove harmful to the human species. These are just a few of the ways by which birth technologies and genetic engineering may impact on the nurse.

THE CONSUMER

The consumer is directly concerned with many uses of technology. Opportunities to combat otherwise fatal diseases and to prevent chronic and often debilitating disorders are being afforded any patient in a well-equipped hospital or medical center today. Some of the more dramatic technologies are being used to combat cancer with limited success.[8] Other technologies are commonly used in the treatment of heart disease, one of the most common diseases of the twentieth century.[9] Individuals who, in the past, might have died from coronary artery disease and fatal coronary artery occlusion, can now be kept alive by modern technologies that enable medical teams to replace blood vessels, remove obstructions from major arteries, and prevent serious damage of the heart muscle before it occurs. Yet patients are not always fully informed about the nature of their treatment and are not aware of alternative treatments available.[10,11] Since many patients are in critical condition when the use of these technologies is proposed, there is also reason to believe that informed consent is an unattainable ideal where the majority of technological advances are concerned. The following two cases demonstrate the impact of technology use on the lives of two consumers who were not fully informed about the consequences of technology where they were concerned.

CASE 10.3—THE CANDIDATE FOR THE FIRST ARTIFICIAL HEART IN HUMANS

The Institutional Review Board (IRB) that approved Barney Clark as the first artificial heart recipient had a very difficult job. The research protocol selected subjects from a group of patients whose cardiac condition could not be ameliorated by any other treatment. The subjects would be in the New

York Heart Association Class 4 stage of cardiac dysfunction (significant cardiac symptoms at bed rest) for a minimum of eight weeks. The life expectancy of such a subject was estimated at several weeks to several months.

Once a candidate was selected, however, the really difficult questions became obvious. The IRB had to determine how informed consent would be obtained for the first artificial heart implantation in a human. Of special concern were the means and adequacy of informed consent. Would severely debilitated subjects falsely perceive the impending implantation as the key to survival? How could any patient, aware of his impending death, accurately assess the research project for risks and benefits? Since this was a procedure involving the use of a new technology in humans, how could anyone accurately assess the life-style changes that would inevitably occur? Most of all, how could the limitations of the procedure be assessed when the subject to be selected had no options but death in the near future?

The 11-page consent form that Barney Clark signed supposedly was designed to address all of these concerns. But no one was really certain what "informed consent" meant in this procedure and where Mr. Clark was concerned. The use of the artificial heart transplantation is a new technology that poses significant moral concern for consumers. Should the IRB have approved the protocol?

As with all new technology, it can be questioned whether the first artificial heart transplant was therapy or research and whether this made a difference in the moral consideration of the technology's use. If Mr. Clark volunteered for the surgery because it was in his interest to do so, given the alternatives, then he was volunteering for innovative therapy. It is not certain that informed consent would be required for innovative therapy. However, since data would be gathered throughout the procedure and Mr. Clark's recovery, the use of the technology could also be considered research. Interventions and tests would be given and publications would be made based on interpretations of the data obtained. If a research component was involved in the use of the technology, then the research protocol would have to be reviewed by the IRB and must meet informed consent requirements. Regardless, the fact that the proposed procedure was ethically problematic would suggest that it should have been reviewed by some committee. There was always the danger that Mr. Clark, by virtue of his condition and limited alternatives, was coerced into consenting to the transplant surgery. Informed consent to treatment is a pressing moral problem in the use of any life-extending technology.

The fact that Mr. Clark did not live long after implantation of the artificial heart raises additional questions. During his recovery, Mr. Clark was never free from the equipment used to maintain his heart function, nor did he ever leave the hospital environment for an extended period of time. Whether there was ever any real benefit to him from participating in the research and therapy involving these types of constraints is questionable. Certainly, he lived longer than he would have lived without the implantation. Yet the losses of freedom, privacy, and confidentiality from the procedure were significant. Did the benefits outweigh these harms from participating in innovative therapy using a new and untested technology in health care?

CASE 10.4—IS CONSENT REQUIRED TO CLONE CONSUMER BLOOD PRODUCTS?

John L. Moore was diagnosed as having hairy-cell leukemia, a rare and potentially fatal form of leukemia in 1980.[12] He underwent a splenectomy to slow down his form of leukemia and subsequently enjoyed an extraordinary recovery from his leukemic disorder. Four years later, he was still visiting his physician's clinic twice a year for blood tests and an examination. His physician told him that his blood had some unique characteristics that were of interest to him and his research staff.

On one visit, Mr. Moore questioned the consent form that he was asked to sign prior to having his blood drawn for testing. He asked exactly what research was being conducted on his blood and whether there were any commercial products or potential financial interests involved in the research being performed on his blood. When his questions were not answered to his satisfaction, he refused to sign the form. He later retained an attorney to investigate the use of his blood for research. To his surprise, he found that his physician, recognizing the unique properties in his blood, had sold it for commercial biomedical production. As a result, a for-profit biogenetic firm had been granted exclusive access to Mr. Moore's blood cells and their products in exchange for payment to the physician of approximately half a million dollars and other advantages, accruing to both the physician and his employer. The biogenetic firm had cloned the unique genetic sequence of Mr. Moore's white blood cells responsible for producing useful substances in the treatment of leukemias. This had all been done without Mr. Moore's knowledge and consent. He sued the physician, the research institution, and the biogenetic firm. In 1985 he testified before the Subcommittee on Investigations and Oversights, House Committee on Science and Technology, in Hearings on the Use of Human Patient Materials in the Development of Commercial Biomedical Products. His case has raised many questions about the use of technology to reproduce body materials without the consent and knowledge of the individual. Should individuals share in the financial gain resulting from the cloning of their unique body cells? Or should all such profit be used to mass produce the technology for the use of all citizens who can benefit from the product?

The use of one's blood for the production of commercial products is a modern miracle and a pressing moral concern for the consumer. Mr. Moore gave consent to the withdrawing of his blood and to the use of his blood for research. But he had presumably not been told that his blood would be used to develop a cell line that would have potentially significant financial implications. Without this type of information, how could he have given an adequately informed consent? Can he withdraw his consent and prevent the future production of commercial biomedical products from his blood cells? Or should all consumers be expected to contribute to the welfare of society by voluntarily contributing their body products once it is known that they have unique capabilities from which others may benefit?

One of the arguments currently being advanced to increase the supply of donor organs hinges on mandatory contribution of organs from some types of patients and a national listing of available organs for the availability of all.[13] Given the potential use of donor organs and unique blood products to combat disease, it can be argued that all citizens should be required to donate organs and body products in order to enhance the overall health of the state. Is this morally obligatory for the consumer or merely morally praiseworthy when consumers do contribute organs and body products? Can consumers be required to do this? Or is contribution a voluntary act on the part of the consumer? More important, what criteria will be used to determine who receives a modern technological advance and who does not? What role will individual citizens have in establishing the criteria that will be used to choose recipients of the technology and who will apply the criteria to real life cases? Obviously, the use of technology to enhance the health of citizenry poses some interesting questions about the ultimate liberty and freedom of individuals where their personal bodies are concerned.

SOCIETY

While the growing use of technology promises to enhance the health of citizens in unprecedented numbers, our society is experiencing tremendous costs for essential as well as for the more exotic technological services.[14] The care of a severely ill, low birth weight infant in a neonatal intensive care unit may well cost over $1200 per day. The long-term care of an adult patient on kidney dialysis may cost even more. Because many technological advances in health care are costly, they require judgment as to whether they should be used on selected patients. Their use also requires careful assessment of their anticipated benefits and harms to the individual patient.

At issue in many decisions involving the use of costly technological advances is a fundamental conflict between the patient's welfare and the welfare of society as a whole. Often the net benefits of a technology use to an individual patient are obvious, yet when the cost of the procedure is viewed from the societal perspective, the benefits do not seem to be as great.

At other times, the use of the technology for the individual patient does not seem to be that beneficial. Yet the benefits, according to society, seem to mandate the technology's use in patient care. The following two cases demonstrate some types of conflicts involving societal values that arise from technology use in health care.

CASE 10.5—WHEN THE COST OF CARE IS PROHIBITIVE

Four-year-old Bobby Monroe has acute leukemia. While on chemotherapy, he has suffered several relapses and is very sick. His physicians have suggested a bone marrow transplant to improve his condition. At this point in his disease, this is the only procedure that offers him a reasonable hope of survival. Yet no one expects the treatment to offer a total cure for Bobby's condition. Although Bobby receives Medicaid assistance, the bone marrow transplant will be a costly procedure and involves months of treatment for which his family must travel to a distant medical center. In conference, the social worker informs Bobby's parents that the estimated cost of the treatment would use more than two-thirds of the annual Medicaid budget allotted for Bobby's entire state. Should Bobby's parents be urged to seek out this treatment because it is available?

Is it fair for one citizen, even someone as ill as Bobby, to receive a major share of the state's Medicaid budget? If technological services are dispersed solely on the basis of need, then Bobby, like anyone else, has a claim to the services. However, if services are disbursed in equal shares to those eligible, then surely Bobby would be receiving more than his share. The question of fairness is a major consideration where the distribution of crucial technological advances in health care is concerned.[15]

Yet the cost of treatment, in relation to the expected benefits of the treatment, also needs to be considered. The treatment will not cure Bobby's disease process. At best, it will allow him time to combat the disease and put him in remission. Is this a benefit of such moral significance that two-thirds of the Medicaid budget for Bobby's state should be used to pay for the technology? Could other individuals benefit equally or even more significantly than Bobby from the use of the funds in other ways? Should the most recent technological advances always be used for treatment, as opposed to more traditional means of treating health problems?

Certainly, deciding benefit of treatment depends, in part, on the "track record" of the treatment, its potential, and expected benefits to the identified patient. But even if benefit of this treatment for Bobby could be ascertained or even quantified, does this mean that benefits from other uses of the money would automatically be inferior to the benefits of Bobby's treatment? Surely, the nature of "benefits" is a subjective evaluation and should not be entirely based on objective facts—the results of lab tests, numerical values, etc. Who is to say how morally significant one set of benefits is in comparison with another set of benefits? Technology use, therefore, cannot be decided entirely on the basis of individual benefits, and cannot be based entirely on the basis of costs. Both individual benefits and costs are important to the decision, but no decision can be adequately made solely on the basis of individual benefits and costs. If that is the case, what other alternatives does a society have when considering the use of a technological advance in health care? The following case suggests another criterion that might be selected by a society for deciding to use a technological advance in health care.

CASE 10.6—SHOULD ALPHA-FETOPROTEIN SCREENING BE REQUIRED OF ALL PREGNANT WOMEN?

Staff nurses of a community-based prenatal care program have been informed that all patients admitted to the program will undergo maternal serum alpha-fetoprotein (MSAFP) screening at six to seven weeks of pregnancy. The test, drawn by fingerstick, will indicate whether or not a pregnant woman is at risk for bearing an infant with a neural tube defect (NTD). No informed consent will be required for the test; admittance to the prenatal care program automatically implies consent to perform standard tests throughout pregnancy.

When the nurses question why the test is being performed on all patients without additional consent, they are told that the test is being performed as a community service to help reduce the public cost of supporting infants born with NTDs. It is assumed that if the pregnant woman knows that she is bearing a NTD-affected infant, she will want to abort the pregnancy. Since the initial cost of the MSAFP test is negligible and the continued cost of caring for a child with a NTD is great, the potential cost-saving to the community is considerable, even if only one or two affected pregnancies per 1000 births are aborted as a result of the testing. The community health agency believes the screening of all pregnant women admitted to the program to be of considerable value to the community in terms of costs averted that would otherwise be needed to support disabled children.

Prenatal diagnostic technologies have dramatically increased the number of fetal abnormalities that can be detected during the prenatal period.[16] MSAFP testing is one test performed early in pregnancy that provides the opportunity for a noninvasive approach to diagnose abnormality in the fetus. An important goal in prenatal diagnosis is to develop techniques that can be employed as early as possible in pregnancy and that are as noninvasive as possible to the fetus and to the pregnant woman. Since fetal cells normally pass in small numbers into the maternal circulation, the development of techniques that can be performed early in pregnancy and that allow fetal abnormalities to be detected by examination of fetal cells obtained from maternal blood is very desirable. Hence, MSAFP testing is widely accepted as a prenatal diagnostic technology in early pregnancy. It is not expensive, it is noninvasive, and it indicates risk of bearing a NTD-affected infant. Additional testing provides final evidence of the type, character, and extent of the structural defect within the fetus.

Participation in diagnostic testing for prenatal abnormalities has largely been viewed as a voluntary act on the part of the pregnant woman. However, there is reason to believe that because of the low risk and cost of the initial screening test and the potential benefits to parents in the form of knowledge that can result from the test, MSAFP testing should be mandatory for all pregnant women in the United States.[17] Mandatory testing, however, raises some important moral questions.

First, we need to ask whether some disorders are so costly that society can mandate testing for their presence in the pregnant woman. Is the care of a NTD-affected child in the community so costly that a positive result on the initial screening test means that the pregnant woman must submit to additional testing involving different benefits and risks to the fetus and the woman? At least one study has suggested that NTDs pose a substantial financial burden on society that could be effectively averted through the abortion of NTD-affected fetuses.[18] Is the cost of caring for disabled children a significant factor in deciding whether or not to have mandatory prenatal diagnostic testing, using new and available technologies?

Second, we need to ask whether the degree of invasiveness of the testing is important to the use of the prenatal diagnostic technology. Since additional testing may be more invasive to the woman and may limit her personal liberty in significant ways, does this have any bearing on whether additional testing can be mandated or not? It has been argued that tests that are more invasive to the pregnant woman and that pose risk to the woman or her fetus can only be undergone voluntarily.[19,20] Even then, constraints on the voluntary choices of the pregnant woman for testing increase with the duration of the pregnancy and the viability of the fetus. Obviously, the rights of the fetus increase throughout pregnancy. At what point in pregnancy can the rights of the fetus outweigh society's right to impose mandatory testing on the pregnant woman? These are questions that must be faced by society before mandatory testing for fetal abnormalities can be initiated, even at the initial testing level for MSAFP.

Future Considerations

As the availability of technological advances makes it possible to alter procreation and birth and delay the time of death, the moral justification for technology use becomes an important endeavor. Nurses must justify their choices to participate in projects when the use of technology to benefit individual patients is proposed. Knowledge of the technology, its benefits and risks, its costs, and moral implications will necessarily influence the nature of the nurse's justification for technology use. Consumers must justify their expectations and rights claims to technological advances, especially when the availability of the technology is limited and the cost of the technology is great. The issue of informed consent where technological advances are concerned is a pressing issue as the use of technology borders on research activity. Is informed consent merely an ideal that can never be realized where treatment with new technologies is concerned? The consumer needs to be realistic about the limitations of informed consent in forms of treatment using new and marginally tested technologies. This does not mean, however, that informed consent to treatment should not be morally required for the protection of consumer rights and liberties.

Society must also justify decisions related to the funding of technological advances, the availability and use of the technology, and the reporting of the technology's risks and expected benefits. The use of technology in health care with the potential to alter the genetic endowments of the next generation needs to be discussed in the public arena and moral considerations of this technology must be addressed. The uses of computer technologies and their effects on confidentiality of health record data and the privacy of individuals will also require public discussion in the future. Quality of life, impacts on future generations, and the basic liberties of individuals are all relevant issues that must be considered by society before final adoption of any new technological advance. Finally, questions of fairness and justice will need to be considered and consumer access to new technologies will need to be shaped by policy initiatives. All of these factors will enter into societal justifications for technology use.

Nadia Rinke is a community health nurse who has been asked to participate in a new screening program. Based on genetic screening techniques developed in the early 1980s, the screening program will draw blood samples from preteenage children to detect genetic conditions having an impact on intelligence. The tests will also be used as a reasonably accurate predictor of significant mental function deficits of future offspring

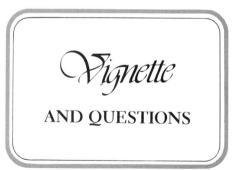

Vignette

AND QUESTIONS

of community residents. Although the screening test is not 100% accurate, the test is reliable enough that the test results can be used to make procreation decisions. Since the deficits detected are clearly linked to genetic anomalies of offspring, pressures are being generated to make the diagnostic tests mandatory for all preteenage children. Those individuals who do bear children later on in spite of unfavorable test results will not be eligible for public education of the child or public funds for the care of the child. The goal of the program is to prevent the suffering and expense generated by the birth of mentally defective children and to decrease the frequency in the gene pool of genes responsible for mental deficiency.

Mrs. Rinke is not sure that it is morally permissible for a nurse to participate in this type of screening program. She must give her supervisor an answer tomorrow. She does not know if her present employment status will be affected if she decides not to participate. What should she do?

Mrs. Rinke must decide whether or not it is permissible for a community health nurse to participate in mandatory genetic screening of preteenage children. She must weigh her responsibilities as a nurse, as a citizen, and as an individual where the detection of genetic abnormalities is concerned. The risks and benefits of the screening test and its results must be discussed, the issue of mandatory versus voluntary screening needs to be addressed, and the informed consent of individuals, especially minor children, must be considered. Mrs. Rinke must also consider whether the use of this technology is research or treatment. If those children with unfavorable test results are expected to refrain from bearing children, then the screening test is a "treatment" of sorts. Yet, since data will be collected and compared with incidence of birth defects in the community, over time, then it seems that the screening program is also research. Certainly, the impacts of this genetic screening technology on the nurse (as a professional), the consumer (as a target of the technological advance), and society (as the means by which standards for the use of the technology are decided), must be considered.

1. What value conflicts are in this case situation? for the nurse? for the individual consumer? for society?

2. Who will benefit from the use of this technology? Do the benefits outweigh the risks?

3. What potential harms might result from participating in the screening program? from not participating in the screening program?

4. Will the test results be used for other purposes? at the present time? in the future?

5. Should testing of this type be voluntary or mandatory? What arguments could you offer for your choice?

6. What are the moral justifications for making the technology

available? Does moral justifiability have any bearing on whether or not the test is mandatory?

7. Who should decide to offer screening programs of this type? the state? the laboratory developing the test? the health professions?

8. How will the test results be communicated?

9. Who will have access to test results?

10. Should individuals be prevented from bearing children once it is known that they have a significant possibility of bearing genetically defective and mentally deficient children? Whose decision is this?

INFORMATION SOURCES

American Nurses' Association: *Code for Nurses with Interpretive Statements*. Kansas City, The Association, 1985

Beauchamp TL, Childress JF (eds): *Principles of Biomedical Ethics*, ed 2. New York, Oxford, 1983

Fletcher J: *The Ethics of Genetic Control: Ending Reproductive Roulette*. Garden City, NY, Anchor Books, 1974

Fletcher JC: The morality and ethics of prenatal diagnosis, in Milunsky A (ed): *Genetic Disorders and the Fetus*. New York, Plenum Press, 1979, p 621

Gastel B, Haddow JE, Fletcher JC, Neale A (eds): *Maternal Serum Alpha-fetoprotein: Issues in the Prenatal Screening and Diagnosis of Neural Tube Defects*. US Government Printing Office, 1980

Reich WT (ed): *The Encyclopedia of Bioethics*. New York, Free Press, 1978

President's Commission for the Study of Ethical Problems in Medicine and Biomedical and Behavioral Research: *Making Health Care Decisions: A Report on the Ethical and Legal Implications of Informed Consent in the Patient-Practitioner Relationship*, vol I. US Government Printing Office, 1982

President's Commission for the Study of Ethical Problems in Medicine and Biomedical and Behavioral Research: *Deciding to Forego Life-Sustaining Treatment: Ethical, Medical, and Legal Issues in Treatment Decisions.* US Government Printing Office, 1983

President's Commission for the Study of Ethical Problems in Medicine and Biomedical and Behavioral Research: *Screening and Counseling for Genetic Conditions: The Ethical, Social, and Legal Implications of Genetic Screening, Counseling, and Education Programs.* US Government Printing Office, 1983

The Totally Implantable Artificial Heart: A Report of the Artificial Heart Assessment Panel of the National Heart and Lung Institute (June 1973). DHEW Publication No. (NIH), 74

Veatch RM, Fry ST: *Case Studies in Nursing Ethics.* Philadelphia, Lippincott, 1987

REFERENCES

1. Kass KR: Making babies—The new biology and the "old" morality. The Public Interest Winter:18, 1972

2. Ramsey P: Shall we "reproduce"? JAMA 220 (June 5 and June 12):1346, 1480, 1972

3. Kass LR: "Making babies" revisited. The Public Interest Winter:32, 1979

4. National Commission for the Protection of Human Subjects of Biomedical and Behavioral Research: *The Belmont Report: Ethical Principles and Guidelines for the Protection of Human Subjects of Research.* US Government Printing Office, 1978

5. US Department of Health and Human Services: *Final Regulations Amending Basic HHS Policy for the Protection of Human Research Subjects: Final Rule: 45 CFR 46.* Federal Register: Rules and Regulations 46 No. 16: 8366, January 26, 1981

6. Working Group on Human Gene Therapy: Points to consider in the design and submission of human somatic-cell gene therapy protocols. Recombinant DNA Technical Bulletin 8:116, 1985

7. Walters L: The ethics of human gene therapy. Nature 320:225, 1986

8. Vadhan-Rha S, et al: Phase one trial of recombinant interferon gamma in cancer patients. J of Clinical Oncology 4(2):137, 1986

9. Christopherson LK: Heart transplants. Hastings Cent Rep 12 (February 1982):19

10. Faden R, Beauchamp TL (in collaboration with King NNP): *A History and Theory of Informed Consent.* New York, Oxford, 1986

11. Levine RJ: *Ethics and Regulation of Clinical Research.* Baltimore, Urban & Schwarzenberg, 1981

12. Statement of John L. Moore Before the Subcommittee on Investigations and Oversights, House Committee on Science and Technology, Hearings on the Use of Human Patient Materials in the Development of Commercial Biomedical Products, October 29, 1985

13. *Organ Transplantation: Issues and Recommendations: Report of the Task Force on Organ Transplantation.* US Government Printing Office, 1986

14. Roberts SD, Maxwell DR, Gross TL: Cost-effective care of end-stage renal disease. Ann Internal Medicine 92:243, 1980

15. Beauchamp TL: Morality and the social control of biomedical technology. In Bondeson WB, et al (eds): *New Knowledge in the Biomedical Sciences.* Dordrecht, Holland, D. Reidel, 1982

16. Kolata G: First trimester prenatal diagnosis. Science 221:1031, 1983

17. Fry ST: The ethical dimensions of policy for prenatal diagnostic technologies: The case of maternal serum alpha-fetoprotein screening. Adv Nurs Sci 9(3):44, 1987

18. Layde PM, Von Allmen SD, Oakley GP: Maternal serum alpha-fetoprotein screening: A cost-benefit analysis. Am J Public Health 69:566, 1979

19. Kolata GB: Mass screening for neural tube defects. Hastings Cent Rep 106:8, 1980

20. Walters L: Ethical perspectives on maternal serum alpha-fetoprotein screening. In Gastel B, Haddow JE, Fletcher JC, et al (eds): *Maternal Serum Alpha-Fetoprotein: Issues in the Prenatal Screening and Diagnosis of Neural Tube Defects.* US Government Printing Office, 1980

DOROTHY JEAN WALKER, RN, PhD, JD

Health Care Litigation: A Case for Professional Liability Coverage

CHAPTER 11

Background and Overview

For health care providers, "It [is] the best of times, it [is] the worst of times, . . ."[1] It is a time when health care technology has reached its acme; it is a time when health care providers are torn between a desire to serve and fear of being sued by the very persons they serve. It is a time when the mechanism of professional protection (professional liability insurance) is being strained beyond the financial reach of many health care providers. It is a time of great debate when at least one proposed solution (a cap on overall recovery) could leave some victims of health care malpractice undercompensated and unable to provide for their own care in the future. It is a time of rumor and fear among health care providers. Most of all, it is a time to take a serious, comprehensive, and scientific look at what, in fact, is occurring.

Although isolated instances of "provider-before-patient" attitudes may be found, the general disposition of most health care professionals is that of "patient-before-provider." This has been the case historically and continues to hold true today, even in the face of rising financial risk to health care providers themselves.

The recent patient's rights movement is generally thought to be an outgrowth of the consumer movement of the 1960s. Actually, its roots predate the 1960s by more than 2000 years. Hippocrates (?460–?366 BC), whose principles of medical science formed the basis for medical theory developed in the 1800s, required his students to take an oath regarding rules of conduct between a doctor and his patients. Even today, many graduating medical students take this oath. Although its ethical precepts have been reinterpreted and expanded to accommodate modern society and advances in health care technology, they have never been abandoned by the health care professions. It, therefore, is not surprising that the Oath of Hippocrates

THE OATH OF HIPPOCRATES

I SWEAR BY APOLLO, THE PHYSICIAN, AND AESCULAPIUS AND HEALTH AND ALL-HEAL AND ALL THE GODS AND GODDESSES THAT, ACCORDING TO MY ABILITY AND JUDGMENT, I WILL KEEP THIS OATH AND STIPULATION:

TO RECKON him who taught me this art equally dear to me as my parents, to share my substance with him and relieve his necessities if required; to regard his offspring as on the same footing with my own brothers, and to teach them this art if they should wish to learn it, without fee or stipulation, and that by precept, lecture, and every other mode of instruction, I will inpart a knowledge of the art to my own sons and to those of my teachers, and to disciples bound by a stipulation and oath, according to the law of medicine, but to none others.

I WILL FOLLOW that method of treatment which, according to my ability and judgment, I consider for the benefit of my patients, and abstain from whatever is deleterious and mischievous, I will give no deadly medicine to anyone if asked, nor suggest any such counsel; furthermore, I will not give to a woman an instrument to produce abortion.

WITH PURITY AND WITH HOLINESS I will pass my life and practice my art, I will not cut a person who is suffering with a stone, but will leave this to be done by practitioners of this work. Into whatever houses I enter I will go into them for the benefit of the sick and will abstain from every voluntary art of mischief and corruption: and further from the seduction of females or males, bond or free.

WHATEVER, in connection with my professional practice, or not in connection with it, I may see or hear in the lives of men which ought not to be spoken abroad I will not divulge, as reckoning that all such should be kept secret.

WHILE I CONTINUE to keep this oath unviolated may it be granted to me to enjoy life and the practice of the art, respected by all men at all times but should I trespass and violate this oath, may the reverse be my lot.

frequently is referred to in current literature on confidentiality and disclosure of patient information.[2]

In modern times, nursing has been seen to flex its muscles on behalf of patients. In 1959 the National League for Nursing (NLN) issued the first patient's bill of rights—a listing of 15 rights of patients that the NLN believed nurses were responsible for upholding. More than a decade later (1972), the American Hospital Association (AHA) developed the "AHA Patient's Bill of Rights."[3] Although not itself legally binding, the AHA statement served as a model for many hospitals that chose to develop their own patient's bill of rights. By 1973 states had begun enacting patient's rights laws. The hospital patient was no longer being denied access to even such basic information about him/herself as temperature and blood pressure readings. Today these patient's rights laws run the entire gamut from their right to care to the right to refuse care.

The rise in American public consciousness of human rights generally and of patient's rights specifically lends credence to the frequently identified need of nurses to better understand the legal implications of their nursing actions so that they may better ensure the rights of their patients and, incidentally, protect themselves. Unless health care providers, as a group, can determine what they, as individuals, are doing wrongfully that harms patients, they cannot rationally move their educational and practice systems in directions that will obliterate that harm.

Furthermore, unless health care providers are able to and, in fact, do bring about such movement, the financial cost to themselves for professional liability protection can be expected to continue to escalate—if not indefinitely, at least for some time in the future. Current efforts to cap money awards, should they be successful, are unlikely to bring about a rollback in the cost of professional liability premiums. Furthermore, even if such rollback should occur, it would in no way diminish the continuing responsibility of health care providers to move toward safer practice. That goal can be approached only by the efforts of health care providers themselves. It follows in a logical pattern that entry into the process toward safer care requires a clear picture of what is occurring in the broad field of health care litigation, particularly in the area of professional malpractice.

LEGAL CONCEPTS OF INTEREST TO HEALTH CARE PROVIDERS

The dark cloud of "lawsuits" appears to hang increasingly heavy over the health care industry. The industry needs to determine whether the magnitude of the threat is illusionary or real. In either event, the *best self-protection* available to the health care provider is the continuous updating of professional knowledge and skills. Of course, the responsible health care

NLN PATIENT'S BILL OF RIGHTS

The National League for Nursing believes nurses are responsible for upholding these rights of patients:
- People have the right to health care that is accessible and that meets professional standards, regardless of the setting.
- Patients have the right to courteous and individualized health care that is equitable, humane, and given without discrimination as to race, color, creed, sex, national origin, source of payment, or ethical or political beliefs.
- Patients have the right to information about their diagnosis, prognosis, and treatment—including alternatives to care and risks involved—in terms they and their families can readily understand, so that they can give their informed consent.
- Patients have the legal right to informed participation in all decisions concerning their health care.
- Patients have the right to information about the qualifications, names, and titles of personnel responsible for providing their health care.
- Patients have the right to refuse observation by those not directly involved in their care.
- Patients have the right to privacy during interview, examination, and treatment.
- Patients have the right to privacy in communicating and visiting with persons of their choice.

- Patients have the right to refuse treatments, medications, or participation in research and experimentation, without punitive action being taken against them.
- Patients have the right to coordination and continuity of health care.
- Patients have the right to appropriate instruction or education from health care personnel so that they can achieve an optimal level of wellness and an understanding of their basic health needs.
- Patients have the right to confidentiality of all records (except as otherwise provided for by law or third-party payer contracts) and all communications, written or oral, between patients and health care providers.
- Patients have the right of access to all health records pertaining to them, the right to challenge and to have their records corrected for accuracy, and the right to transfer of all such records in the case of continuing care.
- Patients have the right to information on the charges for services, including the right to challenge these.
- Above all, patients have the right to be fully informed as to all their rights in all health care settings.

The National League for Nursing urges its membership, through action and example, to demonstrate that the profession of nursing is committed to the concepts of patient's rights.

provider will wish to supplement the protection of quality and current practice by procuring adequate professional liability coverage. The nurse may ask: "If I am a good nurse, one who keeps current, do I need liability coverage? Wouldn't the fact that I carry insurance serve to invite a lawsuit?" The answer to the first question is "yes." The answer to the second question is "no."

The need for self-protection is better comprehended if one gains an understanding of the legal milieu in which controversies arise between patient and health care provider. This requires that the health care provider grasp the meaning of a number of legal concepts. First, a legal entanglement will not arise unless the patient feels that he/she has suffered some injury wrongfully at the hands of the health care provider. When this occurs, the patient becomes a **plaintiff** or **complainant,** meaning a person who has initiated a legal action against another person, who, in turn, becomes a **defendant** or **respondent.** There may be more than one person on either or both sides of a dispute.

It is interesting to note that, at law, a person may be a **natural person** (such as a physician, nurse, dentist, etc.) or an **artificial person** (such as a hospital, nursing home, insurer, etc.). The plaintiff(s) and the defendant(s) are the **parties** to the legal action, even though any number of other *persons* may have been involved in the actual situation that gave rise to the "suit."

Suit is a generic term that is often applied to any proceeding by one person(s) against another or others in a court of justice. "Suits" against health care providers by patients generally are more accurately called **legal actions** or **actions at law.** An action at law is a judicial proceeding whereby a party(ies) prosecutes one or more others for a wrong done. In order to bring an action, the plaintiff must have a **cause of action** (a claim in law and facts that is sufficient to demand judicial attention to the enforcement of a right or the redressing of a wrong). Of course, if the plaintiff is to be successful he/she must prove the allegations made.

Actions between patients and health care providers fall primarily in the area of law known as **torts.** A tort by definition is a legal wrong, independent of contract, committed upon the person or property of another. A tort is not a crime, per se. However, the same act may be both tortious and criminal. A tort gives rise to liability (an obligation to pay money) based upon fault. Essential elements of a tort are the existence of a legal duty owed by the defendant to the plaintiff, a breach of that duty, and a causal relation between the defendant's behavior and the resulting damages to the plaintiff. **Damages** are monetary compensation awarded to an injured party in recompense for a legal wrong suffered at the hands of another.

The causal connection between the breach of duty and damages must be shown to be both **actual** (real) and **proximate** (legal). **Proximate cause** is that which, in a natural and continuous sequence, is unbroken by any efficient intervening cause and without which the injury would not have occurred. Proximate cause encompasses the concept of **foreseeability**—that which was foreseen or with due diligence ought to have been foreseen by the offending party. It functions as a legal mechanism to cut off at an identifiable point the liability of the **tort-feasor** (wrong-doer; one who commits a tort) for injuries that actually flow from the tortious act.

A tort may be either intentional or negligent, but, except in the very limited circumstances of strict liability, liability is not found in the absence of fault on the part of the defendant. This does not mean that the defendant is a bad person, an evil-doer. For the most part, insofar as the fault concept relates to health care providers, it simply means that the defendant, by whatever quirk of judgment motivated, has caused harm by an act or omission that failed to meet the applicable **standard of care,** ie, has failed to exercise the degree of care and skill that a reasonably prudent person with the same education and experience practicing in the same community would exercise under the same or similar circumstances.

Regardless of the extent of the injury sustained by the patient, the health care provider will not be found liable for mere maloccurrence—there *must be* some fault basis for liability. Furthermore, the *allegation* that an act or omission was tortious is not sufficient to make it so. The allegation must be admitted by the defendant *or* proven by the plaintiff. The burden of proof always rests upon the party making the allegation (the plaintiff) and must be borne by a **preponderance of the evidence.** Evidence preponderates whenever it is more convincing to the trier of fact (usually a jury) than is the opposing evidence.

Not only is the burden of proof cast upon the plaintiff, but there also exists another set of laws, called **statutes of limitation,** which act in favor of the defendant. The purpose of a statute of limitation is to fix the time within which the aggrieved party *must* take judicial action or else be barred forever from pursuing his/her rights. Statutes of limitation exist in every state. However, their lengths vary from state to state and according to the cause of action to which they apply. Furthermore, the length of time allowed may be modified by certain circumstances, such as the age or competency of the injured party.

Of major importance in any malpractice case are the holdings of cases already decided. Such cases may be looked to as precedent setting. A **precedent setting** case is a previously decided case that is recognized as an authority for the disposition of future cases. The authority of a precedent setting case is exerted on subsequent cases through the legal doctrine of **stare decisis.** This doctrine holds that once a court has laid down a principle of law as applicable to a certain set of facts, it will adhere to that principle, and apply it to all future cases, where the facts are substantially the same. The doctrine, although not inviolable, permits the prior rule to be repudiated only on a showing of good cause. Such rules of court are binding (to the extent that *stare decisis* binds a court) in the same court and in other courts of equal or lower rank in subsequent cases where the very point is again in controversy.

A feature of stare decisis that frequently is misunderstood is its lack of legal effect as between jurisdictions. **Jurisdiction** is a fairly complex legal concept, one aspect of which is territorial in a geographic sense. *Stare decisis* means that a rule of law handed down by a court in one jurisdiction (New York, for example) would have no legal effect in another jurisdiction (Kentucky, for example). However, since a court confronted with deciding a case of **first impression** (one that presents an entirely novel question of law within the jurisdiction) has no binding rule(s) of law to guide it, it may take judicial notice of the rules of law in other jurisdictions and apply them to the case at bar. Thus, the influence of a rule of law may extend beyond the territorial boundaries of its binding authority.

For the very reasons set forth in the preceding paragraph, literature on health care law invariably touches upon cases decided in a number of states. If this were not done, the cases discussed would fail to address a number of important legal issues simply because a health care case of first impression regarding each possible cause of action will not have arisen in each jurisdiction.

LEGAL ACTIONS OF INTEREST TO HEALTH CARE PROVIDERS

Actions in Negligence.   **Negligence** is the most frequently litigated health care tort. It is the failure of the health care provider to exercise that degree of care which a prudent provider of similar education and experience would exercise under the same circumstances. Negligent errors are of many types. Errors in medication,[4] mistaken identification,[5] burns from misused or faulty equipment,[6] faulty positioning,[7] and patient falls[8] are but a few.

A question often asked by staff nurses is: Can I be held liable for the mistakes made by another nurse (or student or aide) with whom I work? The answer is "No." Only an employer may be held liable for the negligent act of an employee.[9] A staff nurse is not an employer. Neither is a nurse supervisor, nor a nurse educator. These nurses are subject to liability only for their own negligent acts—which may include, eg, the negligent failure to adequately supervise an aide or student. Employer liability of this type occurs under the legal doctrine of **respondeat superior** (let the superior reply). It comes as a surprise to many that the "superior" (employing hospital, physician, nursing home, etc.) has the legal right to recover from the tort-feasor employee the amount of the award granted under the respondeat superior doctrine.

A second doctrine of institutional liability, **corporate liability,** is totally different in its premise. Corporate liability is not based on the transference of an employee's wrongful conduct to the institution, but on *the wrongful conduct of the institution itself*.[10] The tort is committed by the institution in its corporate capacity—often in the form of failure to provide adequate staff, safe procedures, or a safe environment.

It should be clearly understood that, regardless of the doctrinal underpinning of a cause of action which is in reference to negligence, no liability may be found *unless an injury resulted* from the negligent act. This literally means that a nurse may carelessly administer a wrong drug to the wrong patient, via a wrong route, and not be liable for the negligent nursing action *if* the patient fortuitously is unharmed by the chain of medication errors.

Intentional Torts.   The eight **intentional torts** that are of greatest interest to the nurse—battery, assault, libel, slander, invasion of privacy, disclosure of confidential information, false imprisonment, and the infliction of mental distress—are discussed below. An intentional tort, unlike negligence, may cause liability to attach to the tort-feasor, even though the victim suffers no injury. An intentional tort is one that involves a willful act that violates some right of the patient (plaintiff). Such tort requires that the *result* be *intended* by the actor or be *reasonably certain* to follow the act. An intentional tort does *not* require that the tort-feasor intend to do evil.

Assault and battery, although frequently thought of as a single entity, are separate and distinct torts. A **battery**[11] is an unauthorized touching that either is injurious or would be offensive to the reasonable person in the situation of the plaintiff. In the context of the health care industry, charges of battery may arise whenever a treatment is performed 1) without the patient's consent, 2) after patient consent has been withdrawn, or 3) by a health care provider other than the person regarding whom the consent was given.

The tort-feasor may be held liable in battery even though the plaintiff actually benefited from the unauthorized touching—as from the administration of much needed blood or medication. The unauthorized touching that may give rise to a legal action of battery (an intentional tort) is a different specie of absence of consent than absence of *informed consent*. The latter action is in reference to negligence. This distinction is very important inasmuch as the plaintiff must prove injury in a negligence case, but need not show injury in order to establish an alleged battery.

Once the concept of battery is grasped, an understanding of **assault** easily follows. An assault is merely a threatened battery. It is complete when, by action or words, the health care provider puts the plaintiff in apprehension of being touched without authorization and in a manner that would be harmful or offensive to the reasonable person in the same or similar situation. An actual touching need not occur. Indeed, if it does occur the assault becomes a battery.

Defamation is the publication (communication to a third person) of something that is injurious to the good name or reputation of another. There generally is no legal cause of action called defamation. However, libel and slander are two causes of action that are founded on defamation. Truth[12] and (in some cases) privilege[13] are defenses against charges of libel or slander.

Libel traditionally has been thought of as written or printed defamation (the form of defamation that impacts upon the eye). **Slander** traditionally has been described as spoken defamation (defamation in a form that impacts upon the ear). However, more recent years have seen a redefinition of these legal actions to accommodate advances in technology. Today, libel generally is defined as a defamatory publication in the form of some fixed media (including, eg, audio recordings); slander as a defamatory publication in the form of transient media (including, eg, broadcast defamation, even if it is made from a written script).

Invasion of privacy is the legal cause of action that is available when the plaintiff's right to privacy (the right to be left alone or the right to be free from unwanted publicity) is violated. In invasion of privacy actions, truth is *not* a defense; privilege is. If the defendant is to prevail, it must be shown that there existed a legal right to publish the matter at issue.

The right to privacy is not absolute. Each state has a fundamental right and duty to enact and enforce laws promoting the public health, safety, and welfare, even if such laws conflict with the right of privacy of some of its citizens.[14]

Unauthorized disclosure of confidential information, like invasion of privacy and unlike libel and slander, may be based on the publication of material that is entirely true. Unlike invasion of privacy, which is the violation of a right accorded to all citizens, disclosure of confidential information,[15] in the health care context, is based on a duty owed by the health care provider to the patient. It also differs from invasion of privacy inasmuch as less extensive publication may be necessary to render a disclosure actionable.

False imprisonment is the unlawful restriction of a person's liberty. In the health care context it includes physical restraint and unlawful detention.[16] Even when a patient poses a threat to himself or others, no more force than is reasonably necessary to restrain him may be used. Furthermore, the duration of the restraint or detention may not exceed reasonable time to ensure the safety of the patient or of those threatened by him.

Infliction of mental distress is less well developed as an independent cause of action. Actually, liability for this tort may be based on either negligent or intentional misconduct. The plaintiff most often prevails where the mental anguish was the result of a direct physical injury or the plaintiff can prove some resultant physical manifestation of injury (eg, ulcers, a diagnosed phobia or mental breakdown, etc.). Liability will not be found against the defendant for mere insults, indignities, threats, annoyances, or petty oppressions that are not otherwise tortious. However, liability will be found for conduct that an average member of the community would characterize as "outrageous."[17]

Impacts on the Nurse, the Consumer, and Society

In recent days there has been within the health care industry, echoed and fostered by insurers of health care providers, an outcry against accelerating activity in malpractice litigation accompanied by spiraling costs to health care providers and consumer alike. If it is true that legal actions brought against health care providers are increasing in numbers disproportionate to population growth, or that the sizes of jury awards and out-of-court settlements are overreaching the capacity of the health care industry to pay, there is a pressing need for health care providers collectively to take action to stem the tide.

The key word is *if.* If the foregoing assertions are true, on the assumption that damages are paid only where fault is admitted or proved, it follows that either 1) health care malpractice (to be distinguished from mere allegations of malpractice) is on the rise, 2) injuries sustained by patients are increasing in severity, or 3) patients, after a long period of quiescence, are beginning to assert their legal rights of redress for wrongfully inflicted injuries. If these are indeed the facts, there seems little room to question that the burden of correction lies squarely with the health care providers themselves.

However, if the assertions are not true, it seems that the escalation in cost for adequate protection against liability must be the result of some financial phenomenon that is unrelated to the quality of care given. If this is the case, the problem is not, in the strict sense, one for health care providers alone. The burden of getting at the root of the trouble, therefore, would more fairly be shared by the industry, the consumers, and society as a whole.

A beginning place might well be a carefully conducted scientific study of what is actually occurring. To this end, the Virginia study of health care litigation between the years 1970 and 1986, inclusive, recently conducted by the author might serve as an example.

The Virginia study produced some surprising results. However, findings of the study can be put into proper perspective only by a clear understanding of the study's limitations. For data accessibility reasons the study was limited to cases decided by the Virginia Supreme Court (the highest court in the state) during the relevant years. Because of this limitation, many controversies among health care providers or between health care consumers and health care providers no doubt went unnoted.

Since the Virginia Supreme Court is an appellate court, the excluded (though highly important) disputes included all cases that 1) went to judgment but were not appealed beyond the trial court level, 2) were settled by the parties during trial, 3) were dismissed by the trial court, 4) were settled by the parties before trial, or 5) were not prosecuted beyond the initial filing. Furthermore, the study did not include injuries for which no health care provider was ever proceeded against, either because the injured party 1) elected not to pursue his/her legal rights for such reasons as general respect or affection for the tort-feasor or fear of having a future need of the services of the tort-feasor or the tort-feasor's colleagues, 2) did not have the emotional or physical stamina to pursue his/her legal remedy, or 3) was unaware that the injury sustained at the hands of the health care provider(s) was legally compensable.

A comprehensive review of the syllabi of all cases decided by the Supreme Court of Virginia between 1970 and 1986, inclusive, led to the identification of 100 cases that conformed to the study's constraints. Given the implications of current popular debates on likely causes of increased malpractice premiums, these cases revealed startling results.

Approximately the same number of cases were decided over the first ten years of the study period as were decided over the last seven. Thus, the cases might be viewed as showing only a modest increase in numbers over time, with the sharpest increase having occurred during 1979-1980.

If one keeps in mind that the study involved only 100 health-related cases over a 17-year period, an even greater surprise is in store when these cases are separated into business-related and practice-related categories. **Business-related** cases are those that deal solely with the business and financial rights and growth of the various health care providers. These include such things as disputes over the selling and buying of stocks or property, legal actions to recover outstanding bills, determination of whether an employee's injury is compensable under workman's compensation, establishing responsibility for inadequate performance on construction contracts, and the acquisition of certificates of need. **Practice-related** cases are those growing out of behaviors of the health care provider in the role of health care provider, ie, professional behaviors of a health care provider toward a health care consumer.

When the 100 observed cases are separated into business-related and practice-related groups, they are seen to be equally divided. Fifty are business-related and 50 are practice-related. The 50 practice-related cases may be divided further into two groups—malpractice and other.

For the Virginia study, the term **malpractice** was used in its comprehensive sense, ie, to include not only negligence, but also to encompass all potential sources of liability in connection with professional health care services. Thus, malpractice was defined as actions or omissions on the part of the health care provider for which a patient or patient's next-of-kin (if the patient is incompetent or has failed to survive the health care received) may seek to recover damages. The malpractice cases studied grew out of a range of negligence actions, among which were counts of failure to diagnose and treat, negligent treatment, wrongful death, wrongful birth, and failure to warn.

Other practice-related cases addressed concerns of vital interest to the health care provider, but did not involve professional activities for which a health care provider was sued by a health care recipient. These cases dealt with such things as revocation of license, libelous statements by the press, assisting the police to secure evidence when the criminal suspect is a patient, criminal charges against a health care provider, and failure to maintain sidewalks in a safe condition.

When the practice-related cases were thus divided, the malpractice cases were found to number only 43. Table 11-1 shows the professional-identity profile of the health care providers who were defendants in the 43 malpractice cases. Since some cases had multiple defendants, the total number of defendants by classification exceeds the total number of cases. As might have been expected, the leading class of defendants was shown to be physicians. In 31 of the 43 cases, the defendant or one of the defendants was an MD. These data are identified by legend numbers 1, 2, 3, and 4 in Table 11-1. The second greatest number of defendants of a single class were the 14 hospitals, hospital associations, and clinics that are shown by legend numbers 2, 3, 6, and 7. It also is of interest to note that there were five cases of dental malpractice.

In only three malpractice cases were nursing activities traceable. One of the 1979 cases named an unidentified nurse as a defendant to the action.[18] In a 1980 case,[19] a nurse defendant had been either nonsuited or found not liable at the trial level. In the 1980 case brought against a drug company,[20] a nurse had administered the medication that caused the injury, although she was not named a defendant in the legal action.

Further analysis showed that in 22 of the malpractice cases the plaintiffs prevailed. This is approximately half of the malpractice cases decided. It means, of course, that defendant health care providers also won half of the cases appealed to the Supreme Court. However, unless interpreted with great care, these data are misleading. Cases "won" on appeal by the patient-plaintiff may ultimately be lost to the defendant on issues that are of greater concern to health care providers.

Cases won by the plaintiff are indicated on Table 11-2. The double-p (pp) indicates that the case was **remanded** (sent back to the trial court for further proceedings, usually for trial or retrial on some point). When this occurs either party may win; ie, there is no guarantee that the plaintiff will continue to prevail in the remanded case.

That a plaintiff may win before the Supreme Court and yet lose may seem a contradiction in terms. However, it can and does occur. The sole

TABLE 11-1

Professional Identities of Health Care Providing Defendants in Malpractice Cases Reported by the Supreme Court of Virginia between 1970 and 1986, Inclusive. n = 43.

1 = One or more MDs and/or MD, PC
2 = MD(s) and hospital, hospital assoc, clinic, radiological assoc., or other HCP*
3 = MD and hospital and nurse
4 = MD and attorney
5 = Attorney
6 = Hospital, or hospital assoc., or hospital and HCP
7 = Clinic and HCP
8 = Dentist or dentist's insurer
9 = Chiropracter
10 = Patient's committee
11 = Drug company

Number of cases	1970	71	72	73	74	75	76	77	78	79	80	81	82	83	84	85	86
10																	
9																	
8										01	01						
7										01	01						
6										01	01						
5										02	02						01
4										03	02						01
3								01		07	03		02	01		01	01
2				02	01		01	02		08	05		06	01		01	06
1	01	01		08	08		01	02	04	09	11	08	10	02		02	08

Year in Which Case Was Decided

* HCP = Health care provider

TABLE 11-2

Malpractice Cases Reported by the Supreme Court of Virginia between 1970 and 1986, Inclusive, in Which Plaintiff (Patient) Prevailed. n = 22.

jf = Plaintiff prevailed and judgment final
pp = Plaintiff prevailed but case remanded for further proceedings
— = Case decided but plaintiff did *not* prevail

Number of cases	1970	71	72	73	74	75	76	77	78	79	80	81	82	83	84	85	86
5										pp	—						
4										pp	pp						
3								pp		jf	pp		jf	pp		pp	jf
2				—	pp		—	pp		pp	pp		pp	pp		pp	pp
1	—	—		—	—		—	—		—	jf	—	—	pp	pp	—	—

Year in Which Case Was Decided

issue decided by the Supreme Court may be, for example, whether the statute of limitations has run out, thus leaving the plaintiff time-barred from pursuing the action. The Court may find that the plaintiff's action is *not* time-barred. Yet, when the plaintiff pursues his/her case before the lower court, the jury may find for the defendant health care provider(s).

If the data in Table 11-2 are read as if superimposed over Table 11-1, the "losing" health care providers can easily be identified. On these two graphs, the cases are placed in the same order from top to bottom within the bar that is representative of each given year.

THE NURSE

Even as the escalating cost of liability coverage persists in arousing dread among health care providers generally, it continues to appear that the medical profession, followed closely by health care institutions, still bears the brunt of the alleged liability crunch. Certainly this has been the case traditionally.

Although nursing is moving toward full recognition as a profession, many nurses continue to operate on the assumption that they are sheltered from liability by doctors and employing institutions. This belief often is erroneous and may lead to a lack of adequate concern on the part of nurses for their own protection. (Ask yourself: How well do I understand the extent to which I am protected by my employer's or my own liability insurance policy?)

Nurses were involved (or at least appeared to be involved) in only seven percent of the 43 malpractice cases decided by the Supreme Court of Virginia over a period of 17 years. In one case[21] the defendant health care providers prevailed. In a second case[22] the nurse was found not liable at the trial level. In the third case[23] the nurse was not made a party to the legal action, although it was nursing behavior that, at least in part, caused the injury to the patient. Are these cases indications that nurses practice their profession from a sheltered position? Not necessarily. It is important that studies, such as the Virginia study, neither create nor foster a milieu of erroneous security for nurses.

For their own protection, nurses should 1) keep themselves appraised of changes in nursing, 2) develop technical and judgmental skills that are commensurate with the advances in their respective fields of nursing, and 3) assume responsibility for securing adequate professional liability coverage, whether through their employers or independent of them. If these things are done, the nurse will have taken reasonable precautions to secure protection against the financial impact of health care accountability. In addition, patients will benefit directly by reason of generally receiving better and safer care, from which should follow a diminution in patient need for financial compensation.

THE CONSUMER

The **health care consumer** may be defined as a person in need of *and* receiving health care services. Under this definition it is highly likely that each member of the (US) population shall at some time during his/her life be cast in the role of consumer. This, of course, includes persons who, in their career roles, are health care providers.

Consumers collectively will benefit to the extent that awareness of the propensity of the consumer to exercise his/her legal rights presses health care providers to improve the quality of care given. To the extent that patients (or relatives of patients who do not survive the health care received) are successful in righting their legal wrongs, they retain the financial ability to care for themselves.

The cost of financial protection to the individual health care provider, particularly to the physician and the hospital, is at the root of the present concern. Blame sometimes is laid at the door of the poor unfortunate consumer who has the temerity to seek legal redress for physical injuries that were wrongfully inflicted—to seek nothing more than to exercise his/her legal rights. It becomes easy to overlook the fact that health care providers when in the role of consumer enjoy comparable protection under the legal system. In fact, most attorneys who practice in the health care field would attest to the difficulty with which a plaintiff's case arising in the health care area can be won.

Even when the plaintiff wins, the award may be reduced by reason of being deemed excessive.[24] Furthermore, if a malpractice action is brought without probable cause, the health care provider may file a motion for judgment against opposing counsel for malicious prosecution or wrongful use of civil proceedings.[25]

SOCIETY

Society may be defined as the organized pattern of relationships among institutions and individuals interacting in a variety of roles toward a common end. When society is viewed thus, the common end, as it refers to the health care area, must be optimal health care for all residents (not limited to citizens) under conditions that are affordable to individuals and/or institutions.

One would be hard-pressed to mount an argument that the cost of health care to the consumer (or to the consumer's health care underwriter) is not closely linked to the health care provider's cost of doing business. The two will continue to rise (or fall) together, since cost to the consumer is driven by expenses of the provider. Expenses of the provider include the premium that must be paid for professional liability protection.

Recently, some health care providers have claimed that they are being put out of business by the prohibitive cost of malpractice coverage, since they cannot afford adequate protection and dare not practice without it. If an exodus of health care providers from the field should occur, health care services, which already are strained beyond capacity (in some locales), may become virtually unavailable to many.

On the other hand, the situation of the individual victim of health care malpractice may be likened to that of the injured innocent victim of an automobile accident. The ordinary citizen is horrified when confronted with a report of highway carnage, doubly so if the account includes a tale of gross irresponsibility or hit-and-run. The expectation is that each driver will assume responsibility for his/her actions, even to the extent of assuming financial responsibility for injuries unfortuitously inflicted upon another. How much greater is the responsibility of the health care provider who, by definition, assumes the role of fiduciary to each health care recipient for whom he/she/it cares?

Future Considerations

Members of legal, financial, and health care institutions find a variety of explanations for the malpractice coverage dilemma. Positions argued run the gamut from ungrateful patients through greedy lawyers and incompetent doctors to unwise investments by insurance underwriters. The strength of each argument fluctuates with the articulateness of the contender. Various solutions with varying degrees of acceptability are also proposed. All of these things are discussed in the popular media[26] with varying degrees of balance.

That there is a malpractice liability crisis cannot be denied. That it must be attended to also is indisputable. But it must be addressed rationally, giving weight to fact rather than emotion. This requires, as a beginning point, that facts be identified and separated from innuendo. It is important to determine whether the rate of malpractice claims is on the rise and, if so, whether the increase is nationwide or isolated to identifiable geographic pockets. It is equally important to ascertain the size of awards and the extent of the injuries for which large awards are being made. Finally, it is of utmost importance that health care providers identify health care activities that are most likely to lead to verdicts of liability. It is only when such data are carefully gathered and analyzed that the health care industry will be able to move rationally and effectively toward cost containment with quality care for all.

Staff nurse Smith was assigned to care for Mrs. Brown, who was admitted to the hospital with abdominal pain and fever. Her physician, Dr. Green, made the diagnosis of cholecystitis. He ordered bed rest, intravenous fluids, antibiotics, and a series of four injections, to be given over four days, of a combination of demerol and Vistaril IM.

Vignette

AND QUESTIONS

Nurse Smith gave all four injections into the gluteal area, alternating sides. Mrs. Brown was a large woman who was grossly overweight. The first two and the fourth intramuscular injections were given without incident. However, immediately following the third injection into the right buttock, Mrs. Brown complained of "very bad pain in her hip." Ice packs were prescribed and immediately applied.

Examination of the area the next morning revealed a reddish discoloration and hardening under the skin with blisters forming. Over a period of seven days, the inflammation spread to a very large area with raised blisters, a dark discoloration, and insensitivity to touch indicating that necrosis of the tissue had occurred.

Four debridements were performed over a period of three weeks. The wound was irrigated and packed with gauze four times each day by the nursing staff. Dr. Green is certain that the third injection was not given deep enough, ie, that it entered the subcutaneous tissue rather than the muscle.

During the sixth week, a skin graft to the area was performed. Skin was removed from Mrs. Brown's thigh for this purpose. When released from the hospital during the eighth week, Mrs. Brown had a large concave hole in her right hip and hospital and medical bills far in excess of her health insurance coverage. Her family are urging her to consult an attorney.*

1. What might the nurse have done to avoid litigation?

2. What can the nurse do to prepare for litigation?

3. What is likely to be the advice of the nurse's attorney?

4. If an action is filed, who are likely to be named as defendants?

5. What defense is each defendant likely to try to mount?

6. What is likely to be the outcome of a trial?

* Facts taken from Pfizer v. Jones, 221 Va. 681, 272 S.E.2d 43.

7. Do you think the outcome that you expect would be fair? If not, to which party(ies) do you think the expected outcome of the trial would be unfair?

You might wish to review the *Pfizer* case to see how the actual case was decided. Why do you think the defendant who was actually named was the one to be named? Do you think the decision was fair? If not, to whom was it unfair? Why?

INFORMATION SOURCES

Bernzweig EP: *The Nurse's Liability for Malpractice: A Programmed Course*. 4th ed. New York: McGraw-Hill, 1987

Creighton H: *Law Every Nurse Should Know*. 5th ed. Philadelphia, Saunders, 1986

Rhodes AM, Miller RD: *Nursing and the Law*. 4th ed. Rockville, MD, Aspen Systems Corporation, 1984

REFERENCES

1. Dickens C: *A Tale of Two Cities*. Chicago, The Fountain Press, 1949, p 1

2. See, eg, Annas GJ: *The Rights of Hospital Patients*. New York, Avon Books, 1975, p 125. Also see, eg, Rhodes AM, Miller, RD: *Nursing and the Law*, 4th ed. Rockville, MD, Aspen Systems Corporation, 1984, p 259

3. *Nurse's Legal Handbook*. Springhouse, PA, Springhouse Corporation, 1984, p 65

4. Mahoney v. Wake Hosp. Sys., Inc., 262 S.E.2d 680 (N.C. Ct. App. 1980)

5. Southeastern Ky. Baptist Hosp., Inc. v. Bruce, 539 S.W.2d 285 (Ky. 1976)

6. Porter v. Patterson, 107 Ca. App. 64, 129 S.E.2d 70 (1962)

7. Porter v. Patterson, 107 Ca. App. 64, 129 S.E.2d 70

8. Leavitt v. St. Tammany Parish Hosp., 396 So.2d 406 (La. Ct. App. 1981)

9. Crowe v. Provost, 52 Tenn. App. 397, 374 S.W.2d 645 (1963)

10. Darling v. Charseston Community Memorial Hospital, 33 Ill.2d 326, 211 N.E.2d 253 (1965). See also Sanchez v. Bay General Hospital, 172 Cal. Rptr. 342 (Cal. Ct. App. 1981) and Story v. McCurtain Memorial Management, Inc., 634 p.2d 778 (Okla. Ct. App. 1981)

11. Schloendorff v. New York Hospital, 211 N.Y. 127, 105 N.E. 92 (1914)

12. Farrelh v. Kramer, 159 Maine 387, 35 A.2d 218, 193 A.2d 560 (1963)

13. Wynn v. Cole, 91 Mich. App. 517, 204 N.W.2d 144 (1979)

14. Kathleen K. v. Roberts B., 198 Cal. Rptr. 273 (Cal. Ct. of App. 1984)

15. Alexander v. Knight, 177 A. 2d 142 (Pa., 1962)

16. Big Town Nursing Home v. Newman, 461 S.W.2d 195 (Tex., 1970)

17. Johnson v. Women's Hosp., 527 S.W.2d 133 (Tenn. Ct. App. 1975); McCormick v. Haley, 37 Ohio App. 2d 73, 307 N.E.2d 34 (1973)

18. Prohm v. Anderson, 220 Va. 74, 255 S.E.2d 491 (1979)

19. Pugsley v. Privette, 220 Va. 892, 263 S.E.2d 69 (1980)

20. Pfizer v. Jones, 221 Va. 681, 272 S.E.2d 43 (1980)

21. Prohm v. Anderson

22. Pugsley v. Privette

23. Pfizer v. Jones

24. Rutherford v. Zearfoss, 221 Va. 685, 272 S.E.2d 225 (1980)

25. Ayyildiz v. Kidd, 220 Va.1080, 266 S.E.2d 108 (1980)

26. See, eg, Shuchman M, Wilkes M: Malpractice. *Washington Post Magazine*, p 6, 16, March 2, 1986

UNIT II   *Educational and Research Perspectives in Nursing*

This unit addresses aspects of education and research that influence the entire profession of nursing. The chapters in this section discuss the types and benefits of continuing education; the types and purposes of graduate education; the influence of nursing research; the structure and function of the National Center for Nursing Research; and the historical aspects of the relationship between nursing education and nursing service. It must be kept in mind that each chapter is written by a different author(s), so the styles of writing will vary. The reader may find it helpful to read the two chapters on nursing research as a set, since the content in each chapter compliments the other. After reading each chapter in this unit, the student should have a better understanding of some of the aspects of education and research that impact upon the profession of nursing.

VIRGINIA LAYNG MILLONIG, RN, PhD

CHAPTER 12　　　　　　　　　　*Continuing Education*

Background and Overview

For us who Nurse, our Nursing is a thing, which, unless in it we are
making *progress* every year, every month, every week, take my word for
it we are going *back*.
　The more experience we gain, the more progress we can make. The
progress you make in your year's training with us is as nothing to what
you must make every year *after* your year's training is over.
　A woman who thinks in herself: "Now I am a 'full' Nurse, a 'skilled'
Nurse, I have learned all that there is to be learned": take my word for
it, she does not know *what a Nurse is*, and she never *will* know; she is
gone back already.[1]

Many nurses follow this advice given by Florence Nightingale and
continue to be involved in learning activities throughout their professional
lives. Cyril Houle refers to these people as having "inquiring minds."[2]
　Nurses who are conscientious, effective practitioners continue to learn
on the job, but too often this is incidental, rather than planned, learning.
From the beginning of organized nursing, many nurses have participated in
available continuing education (CE) activities, due to interest and a general
desire for self-improvement.
　These CE activities have included a diversity of learning opportunities
and have been described in different ways, depending upon the provider,
length of time involved, setting, type of offering, and subject matter.
Definitions have been broad and many times terms with different meanings

have been used for interchangeably, ie, inservice education, staff development, continuing education. Originally CE was defined to include only noncredit learning activities. The definition has since been expanded to those learning activities that include credit offerings.

Perhaps the definition that is generally accepted by most is that of the American Nurses' Association (ANA), which defines **continuing education** as

> Those learning activities intended to build upon the educational and experiential bases of the professional nurse for the enhancement of practice, education, administration, research or theory development to the end of improving the health of the public.[3]

Postgraduate courses in nursing represent the first organized efforts in CE. Before the turn of the century, a number of postgraduate courses were offered in areas of clinical practice such as obstetric and/or psychiatric nursing.[4] Among the first were those offered by the University of Wisconsin, the University of Kansas, and the Western Interstate Commission for Higher Education. The content of classes in those early days included such topics as refresher courses for inactive nurses and the use of audio-visual aids for teaching. Elda Popiel, who along with Signe Cooper is considered the "mother of continuing education," directed her early efforts to school nurse workshops. Jo Eleanor Elliott, another pioneer in the field of nursing continuing education, developed programs for nurses in leadership positions. Her population consisted of faculty and special nursing groups such as industrial, coronary care, and school nurses.[5-7]

However, motivating some nurses to continue to learn and stay technically current is difficult. Kuramoto's study found a "failure to accept personal responsibility for continued learning."[8] Studies conducted by Puetz demonstrated that the nurses most in need of continuing education were the least likely to participate in continuing education activities.[9] Simms asserted that even though many practitioners maintain a high degree of professional competence and knowledge, most nurses participate in educational activities only when required to do so.[10]

Adult education literature suggests that habits established during a prior education experience are important factors in subsequent adult learning patterns.[11] Millonig examined nurses' educational backgrounds and participation in continuing education activities and found that educational background was a factor.[12] Those nurses with the highest level of education (master's prepared) were the most frequent participants in continuing education programs. Dolphin examined variations and intensities of attendance of registered nurses in continuing education programs and found that multiple factors influenced attendance, including job competence, job requirements, sociability, and peer pressure.[13]

The limited participation of some nurses in continuing education is not surprising, since the concept of the professional nurse as a lifelong learner is not promoted in either the practice or educational settings, as it should be, given the complex care nurses are required to provide.[14]

Schools of nursing are so intent upon providing theory and technologies that will enable the graduate to function in the practice settings, that little time is available to stress the importance of the professional nurse as a continuous learner. Decisions about what should be learned, how students are to learn, and how students should be tested for competence are made entirely by the faculty rather than by the learners. Consequently, nurses later practice unaware of their own creative resources and capabilities for planning their further learning.[15] Thus, many career nurses do not engage in ongoing educational activities. Instead, they base their nursing judgments and actions on obsolete or insufficient knowledge.[14]

MANDATORY VS VOLUNTARY CONTINUING EDUCATION

Many legislators, as well as the professional nursing community, are aware of the problem of motivating nurses to continue their learning. Hence, 11 states require documented continuing education for relicensure as a registered nurse (See Table 12-1).[16] In 1973 the National League for Nursing (NLN) passed a resolution supporting mandatory continuing education.

TABLE 12-1

State Continuing Education Requirements for Relicensure as a Registered Nurse

State	Contact Hours	Time
California	30 hours	every two years
Colorado	20 hours	every two years
Florida	24 hours	every two years
Iowa	45 hours	every three years
Kansas	30 hours	every two years
Kentucky	30 hours	every two years
Massachusetts	15 hours	every two years
Minnesota	30 hours	every two years
Nebraska	75 hours	every five years
Nevada	30 hours	every two years
New Mexico	30 hours	every two years

National Council of State Boards of Nursing, Chicago, IL, Continued Competence Survey, 1987

The 1974 ANA House of Delegates adopted a policy expressing "strong support for establishing participation in continuing education approved by state nurses' associations (SNAs) as one prerequisite for continuing registration of the license to practice the profession of nursing, that ANA assist SNAs in developing systems for implementing this requirement which will ensure interstate mobility of licensed practitioners of nursing."[17]

One major problem with this statement as it stands is that it seems to indicate that the ANA is the only body that can approve continuing education programs. This would subsequently destroy the value and/or credibility of other approval bodies.

California was the first state to require continuing education for relicensure. Legislation was passed in 1971. Eight years later, the state of Colorado was the first to reverse its decision on mandatory CE, which it then reinstated.[18]

Although thought to be the solution to lifetime licensure, mandatory CE was not without its problems. The passage of the California law marked the beginning of much debate on the topic. Originally the passage of nurse practice acts in the 1900s established requirements for entry into practice and the concept of a lifetime license remained unchallenged for many years. The pros and cons of mandatory CE have created not only a heightened awareness of the problem associated with lifelong licensure, but also groups of both health professionals and nonhealth professionals have started to examine those problems associated with both sides of the debate.

In some states legislators have favored the concept of mandatory CE as the profession attempts to serve the public better. Those who support the concept claim the mandatory requirements will force those who normally would not participate in continued learning to do so. There appears to be some truth associated with this premise. Forcing those nurses who normally would not participate may indeed motivate them to become more actively involved in the process, or better yet, create an "appetite for learning." Attendance at CE offerings not only provides continued learning activities, but also an opportunity to associate with one's colleagues and develop relationships that will, hopefully, lead to improved practice and an understanding of the importance of continued learning.

Those who oppose the mandatory concept claim that participation alone in CE will not necessarily lead to improved practice. Very few studies have been able to measure the application of learning from the classroom (seminar, workshop) to the practice setting. Other opponents claim mandatory CE will force nurses to attend any kind of offering in order to accumulate the required number of contact hours or continuing education units (CEUs) for relicensure. Still others question how to measure the appropriate learning activities for all nurses. For instance, should pediatric nurses be required to attend only those offerings with pediatric content? Will they not receive credit for attendance at any other type of offering outside of their specialty? Attendance at any kind of learning activity, though valid, does not prove that learning has occurred or been applied in the practice setting.

In addition to programmatic and content areas of controversy, other issues related to the mechanics of mandatory CE exist, such as keeping up to date with states that require CE, types of requirements, format for record keeping, and kind and amount of acceptable credits. The availability of offerings is also a major concern. The quality of offerings becomes an issue as the number of providers escalate in mandatory states. What kind of quality assurance is required for the providers of CE? Most mandatory states have limited resources for determining quality of offerings. Mandatory CE, though substantively good, is a costly enterprise, if implemented appropriately. Who is responsible for these costs—the nurse, provider, patient, or state? These are unanswered questions. At this writing the issue is far from settled. There seems to be strong agreement that some measure of continued competency is needed, but less agreement that mandatory CE is the answer. It has even been suggested that the next two decades will see the elimination of many mandatory continuing education programs and that competition will cause the survival of the fittest.[19]

TYPES OF PROGRAMS

The most common program offering continues to be the one-, two-, or three- day workshop or conference, although several long-term courses, usually focusing on complex skills and knowledge, are available. The content for these long-term courses tends to be clinically oriented, although management and education are also receiving attention. Another common design is the national conference where numerous well-known speakers present topics with an overall theme.

The self-study model, which has been in existence for some time, has recently become a more common offering. This is no doubt due to decreased attendance at workshops, seminars, courses, and conferences as a result of budget cuts for continuing education. The self-study models range from directed readings to audio and videotapes and computer programs with administration of post tests and CEUs, if an appropriate pass score is obtained.

One of the major disadvantages associated with the self-study approach is the lack of interaction with professional colleagues. The ability to develop a network of contacts that can be utilized for consultation and/or support in the practice setting is absent. Much informal learning takes place during attendence at structured, planned offerings. As a result of this dialogue exchange, nurses return to the workplace revitalized and stimulated from the social/professional interactions that take place during these programs.

Self-study approaches, though more economical and convenient, do not provide these kinds of learning opportunities.

PROVIDERS

Over the years, nursing CE has appeared in a number of settings, offered by a variety of providers. The two most visible providers have been hospitals or medical centers and, to a lesser degree, colleges and universities. The major providers today are large health care organizations, colleges and universities, professional organizations, and private entrepreneurs.

The largest providers in terms of size and number of offerings are medical centers. Their programs for nurses range from instruction regarding complex aspects of advanced technology to programs dealing with such topics as management, crisis intervention, assertiveness, and role conflict. Medical centers and hospitals have moved from providing disease-oriented programs, orientation programs, and offerings concerned with advances in technology to areas traditionally considered within the university domain.

One of the reasons for this overall programming change is the improved preparation of nurses who are directing nursing continuing education programs in hospitals and medical centers. Previously, staff development positions were held by diploma or associate degree graduates, and occasionally by baccalaureate graduates. Today, many such positions are filled by master's and even doctorally prepared nurses. In some cases even the names of the departments have changed from staff development to departments of education and research.

The second largest group of providers includes professional organizations, such as state nurses' associations and specialty nursing organizations. An informal survey of this group indicates that the larger organizations that have nurse educators responsible for planning and development usually offer the highest quality programs. Smaller organizations, with limited staff, depend upon their elected or appointed members to plan and develop their CE offerings. If the membership includes individuals who are willing to assume responsibility for these major program activities, the results may be quality CE programs. However, organizations that fail to support an experienced CE provider may find program success to be unpredictable at best. As a result, these programs may be an expensive disappointment for the nurse consumer, and they may also project a poor image of the sponsoring organization.

Colleges and universities, the third largest providers of nursing continuing education programs, were slow to enter this arena. Resources within colleges and universities for continuing education programs have not been as plentiful as those for undergraduate and graduate programs. According to most consumers and authorities in the field of CE, the quality of the programs has been good.[20]

The newest group of CE providers are the entrepreneurs, who surfaced in the 1970s. The quality of their offerings, however, is as varied as that of the providers. Many of the programs are excellent, well-planned, and academically sound. Unfortunately, others are poor, because the provider is interested in continuing education primarily as a profitable enterprise, with program development being a secondary concern. These providers are often guilty of using marketing strategies that claim that participants will gain complex skills in a matter of hours. Others advertise programs with well-known faculty and substitute faculty of lesser accomplishments. These represent just a few of the complaints heard from consumers of these programs.[21]

The entrepreneur movement grew during the last decade as a result of increased emphasis on mandatory continuing education. It also grew as specialty nurse organizations required participation in continuing education for maintenance of certification or as a condition of membership. The traditional providers did not keep pace with the demand. Entrepreneurs filled a need and took advantage of the increased market, while professional organizations and universities geared themselves to develop additional programs. The eventual effect was an oversupply of CE providers.[22] This excess resulted in universities, agencies, and entrepreneurs presenting similar programs in the same geographic area and competing for the same populations.

One positive aspect of this oversupply of providers was the healthy competition that evolved. There are definite benefits that result from competition. Each program sponsor strives to be the best and to attract the most participants.[20]

ACCREDITATION

In order to assure the quality of programs offered to the consumer, a process of review is required that can attest to their credibility. Perhaps the most familiar accreditation process known to nurses is that provided by the National League for Nursing (NLN) to schools or programs of nursing that meet certain predetermined criteria. However, the NLN does not approve continuing education offerings or programs, whether they be located in schools of nursing, professional associations, hospitals, or the private sector.

Accreditation of CE offerings is provided by the American Nurses' Association, specialty nurse associations, and other educational review boards responsible for reviewing educational programs in colleges and universities. Although the American Nurses' Association is perhaps best known for its accreditation process, many specialty associations that provide continuing education opportunities for their membership adhere to a similar type of review and approval process. These associations may also approve the offerings of other providers or develop reciprocal agreements between associations as part of their approval process. There seems to be a general agreement within the profession that the responsibility for maintenance of safe and competent practice rests with the individual practitioners, and part of that responsibility includes participation in some kind of continued learning activities.

The providers, therefore, have a responsibility to assure the consumer that continuing education offerings meet established educational standards. It is imperative that the nurse, as a consumer, is aware of the importance of programs being reviewed. The nurse should also be aware of the review process. Most programs that award continuing education units or contact hours should have been subjected to some type of review process. The nurse, as the consumer, must be aware that there are few or no states that prohibit outside providers from offering CE programs within their state. Although a central clearing house would prevent some of the "harlequin" activity that exists in CE, development of such a function has not been a possibility thus far. Again, cost is the primary factor.

Impacts on the Nurse, the Consumer, and Society

THE NURSE

If continuing education is perceived as a good thing, what effects will this have on the practicing nurse? Even within those states where mandatory CE is not an issue, the importance of continued learning is stressed. Many agencies require participation in continued learning activities of some kind for advancement.

Some agencies provide time off, as well as registration fees for their employees. Others provide a variety of compensation models, while still others provide the learning opportunity in the work setting. The major problem affecting CE programs today is the decreased monies available for participation in CE programs. With the cutbacks in funding, the educational programs have been the first to suffer. There is less money to send individuals outside of the agency to other programs and many times programs within the agencies themselves have either been cut back or even eliminated.

Perhaps the most significant concern of limited access to learning opportunities is the effect on the practice of nursing. Maintaining competency and improving standards of nursing practice have concerned nursing administrators for some time. The current half-life of nursing knowledge is five years. Half of everything the student learns in the classroom today is outdated in five years.[23] Clearly, the importance of continued learning is indisputable. Yet this same concern is not prevalent in health care agencies. More of the responsibility for ongoing education will have to be assumed by each individual nurse. If the nurse uses time off for continuing education activities, in addition to providing registration fees, will this then affect his/her participatory behavior?

A review of the literature cited earlier would tend to agree that participation would be affected. While some nurses engage in continued learning activities because they find the pursuit of learning a source of enjoyment and stimulation, others participate simply to carry out the recommendations of an authority figure or to comply with the instructions or suggestions of someone else.[14]

Although few studies are available demonstrating the relationship between participation and competency levels, few would deny the inherent problems resulting from little or no attention to continued learning. Arguments exist on both sides for providing, or not providing, access to learning opportunities. There are those who claim that if agencies are going to make CE an expectation in the work setting, they are then obliged to provide the opportunities for accessibility. There are still others who propose that if nurses are to add strength to their professional identity, then they as professionals should be responsible for their own learning. Ultimately, what has happened and will continue to happen is that the nurse is going to have to search for available programs. Decreased attendance at continuing education activities offered by universities and colleges has already affected these educational institutions, resulting in closure of many of these departments. Professional associations are also taking a close look at their current program viability. The American Nurses' Association, a long-time provider of continuing education programs, is conducting surveys among other specialty professional organizations to determine if the need exists for the association to continue to provide these services. Changing tax laws will seriously impact nurses' participation in continuing education. If the nurse will be required to participate in continuing education for job advancement, yet the employer does not provide reimbursement and the nurse cannot use this expense as a deduction for tax purposes, participatory behavior will decline further.

THE CONSUMER

Unfortunately, the consumer will be affected most seriously by this set of circumstances. Budgetary cutbacks have already altered the quality of care. Increased acuity, shortened length of stay, and a decrease in nursing resources have created a multitude of problems that have affected the entire health care system. The profession has a responsibility to provide the very best of care within prescribed periods of time. However, this can only be accomplished with an educated, well informed, competent practitioner of nursing.

Today's health care consumer is an educated consumer and the media stresses that the public has a right to be more selective in terms of their health care provider. If the public exercise this right, they also have a right to expect the best practitioner. If nurses do not assume responsibility for their own continued learning, they will lose their right to provide care. For too long nurses have relinquished many of their "nursing jobs" to others because of their claims of overwork and too much "paper work." Unfortunately, instead of retaining some of those nursing activities that were respected, nurses allowed the activities to be taken over by others, and as a result lost some of the little power they had.

If the consumer has a right to expect the best practitioner, then he also has a right to expect that "the best" is also "the safest." Licensure laws were meant to insure that those who took the licensing examination were safe to provide at least the minimal competencies expected of a nurse. How can nursing provide these competencies if the individual practitioners do not engage in continuous learning activities that contribute to their knowledge base? If nursing does not take the initiative to ensure that members of their profession are adequately prepared, the consumer may take steps to compensate for this deficit. Consumers are finding an increasing number of opportunities to become involved in consumer-protection issues, especially in environmental protection and health planning. Both the Comprehensive Health Planning and Public Health Service Amendments Act of 1966 and the National Health Planning and Resources Development Act of 1974 (PL93-641) mandated consumer involvement in the planning process.[24] Even when the consumer does not seem to be technically prepared to make judgments regarding matters of a professional nature, it has been substantiated that they usually have a clear picture of desired outcomes. Hence, most consumers are aware of inadequate care, though they may not be able to explain the rationale for its existence.

Most governing boards of institutions and health care agencies are concerned with setting standards for care and associated areas reflective of this care. However, few acknowledge the methodology in which this competency is maintained. Perhaps this is an area that deserves as much scrutiny as does an inept or incompetent practitioner.

SOCIETY

What are the implications for society at large relative to the area of continuing education in nursing? The health care area is expanding so rapidly, it is virtually impossible for even the most dedicated, self-disciplined, and motivated nurse to keep current. There are not only technological advances, but also legislative changes that affect the practice of nursing. Health care is provided in innumerable settings to diverse populations. Schools of nursing cannot begin to prepare beginning level practitioners to be competent in all areas. If society continues to be involved in the selection of care they will receive, or have some voice in the process, then nursing will have to examine the benefits of continued learning associated with practice.

Although the mandatory licensure laws are still in a state of disarray in many states, specialty nursing groups are responding to societal needs. Interestingly enough, many of these same specialty nursing groups were conceived in continuing education programs. As their credibility grew, so too did their movement out of the noncredit continuing education arena into the credit area, such as master's programs. The majority of nurse practitioner programs began in continuing education programs. Society's needs determined the future direction of these practitioners. In an attempt to enhance their credibility to the public, these same specialty nurse associations have initiated certification processes. Many of these certification programs and recertification/certification maintenance programs require some kind of continuing education. Although originally intending it to be a voluntary process within the specialty, many states now require certification as a requirement for practice.[25] For an in-depth discussion of certification, the reader is advised to refer to Chapter 3, "Credentialing: Opportunities and Responsibilities in Nursing."

Future Considerations

Many forces affect the future of continuing education. The twenty-first century is little over ten years away. It promises to be radically different from today in ways not possible to predict with any degree of certainty. Continuing nursing education has received much attention and dramatic growth within the last 15 years. Will growth continue or will it level off or even decline? We have already witnessed dramatic changes within the past five years. Is mandatory continuing education for relicensure a passing fad or a growing and permanent reality? Or will continued learning be generally accepted as part of a professional nurse's repertoire?

Many laws and regulations that have been in existence for years and new laws that are being passed each year have direct or indirect impact on continuing education. Society's expectations of the profession and the changing social climate will have their effect. Shifts in the economy have already exerted a profound influence on the rate of progress and direction of continuing education. The technological advances, seen by some as mandates for continuing education, may or may not play an important role.

Members of the profession must take steps to define the role of continuing education within the discipline of nursing.

Economics will play a major role. Who will pay the bill? Will the consumer ultimately be the one who finances continued learning by the professional nurse? If one looks at society, the health care consumer is the same individual who also shops at supermarkets and purchases drugs, clothing, and life essentials and nonessentials. They are the ones who pay for the advertising of their food, clothing, essentials, and nonessentials. They also pay for the research and marketing related to the drugs they take. The millions of dollars spent on advertising on television as well as research, whether it be scientific or marketing research, is ultimately reflected in the costs to the consumer. Health care costs are already a major problem in the industry. How can the health care industry absorb the costs of continuing education for their staff? Most health care agencies have not been socialized to the mechanics of the business world. It seems there was always someone to finance their establishment, whether it be the federal or state government, third party reimbursement, or the consumer. It was not until the prospective payment system went into effect that the "art and science" of economics was experienced as a serious deficit by those health care administrators.

These health care providers should look to the industrial model for solutions to these problems. Industry's primary concern is productivity, as it should be in the health care industry. Major industry is concerned with the productivity of their employees. The better prepared, knowledgeable employee is the more productive. Why, then, eliminate continuing education funding in a time when the more competent staff are the most productive and cost effective? Does it not behoove the employer to provide those funds that will continue to support competency levels?

The only other alternative is that individual nurses will have to bear the cost of their own continuing education. Physicians and lawyers have done so for years; however, the pay scale of physicians and lawyers is considerably greater than that of nurses. Many physicians and lawyers are self-employed and tend to see the need to "keep up." Their livelihood is dependent upon their ability to be up-to-date on the current or latest practice strategies. Nurses are not in positions to finance their own continuing learning; therefore, significant advances in salary will have to take place for this to become a reality.

Associated with cost factors is time commitment. Time and money are synonymous. If the agency is responsible for providing continued learning, the nurse may be compensated for the time away from the job while in the CE setting, and the agency will also be responsible for "covering" the job site with someone else while the nurse is pursuing this activity. If the nurses are responsible for pursuing their own continued learning, then time again becomes a factor. There are two options available. Vacation or leave time can be used, or leave without pay is the alternative. Some agencies may allow education days, but the nurse is still responsible for paying the costs. When the time factor is considered, not only is the time of the activity a concern, but associated costs may also need to be considered. Programs scheduled in the same geographic area do not present the same problems as those scheduled outside of the area requiring time and money for transportation and lodging. Not all applicable programs may be available to the nurse in his/her own community.

Perhaps the singular solution to both time and cost factors for the nurse who has either limited funds or accessibility to formal CE programs is the self-study approach. However, this approach is not without several problems. It is better than no continued learning activity, but it has limitations. It is a solitary exercise with no opportunity to question, challenge, or request clarification on pertinent areas. It requires a high level of motivation on the part of the learner. There is no opportunity to develop the nurses' "network system" and exchange ideas, concerns, successes, and failures with colleagues. Most consumers of CE would agree that as much learning occurs outside of the structured learning event as within the formal setting, when attending continuing education programs. These exchanges are not possible with the self-study approach.

The self-study approach can be cost and time effective when used in conjunction with other kinds of learning activities. It is currently being applied in a variety of innovative continuing education programs and projects. It seems to be generally accepted as a mode of learning for orientation of new employees in health care agencies. Its movement into staff development, leadership training, and specialty preparation programs seems to be a recent development. Although exciting, challenging, and rewarding, it, too, is not without potential problems and difficulties.[26]

An additional force affecting the future of continuing education is legislation in the health care system. As legislative activities are designed to change or monitor the health care system, continuing education activities for the health professions are affected. The resulting pressures toward increased productivity and cost effectiveness and quality assurance are already creating changes in the delivery of continuing education.

Less concrete than legislative forces are the social forces. There is a growing societal demand that those who perform services of any kind be competent to do so. The demands mandate the necessity of lifelong learning. The maintenance of competency traditionally delegated to the professions is increasingly being questioned by the public. The growing lack of trust is demonstrated by federal legislation creating consumer-oriented health planning agencies and in increased malpractice litigation. No longer is the learning that occurs in day-to-day practice sufficient. Continuing education is but one measure to satisfy society of the profession's commitment to strengthening competency levels.

Economic forces are perhaps the greatest force affecting the viability of CE activities. As cited earlier, decreased funding for activities is affecting not only the nurse as consumer but providers of CE located outside of the health care agency. These professional associations, colleges and universities, and entrepreneurs are seriously affected by budgetary cutbacks. Many of them have had to make dramatic changes in their CE programs and others have had to close their doors. From an economic perspective, the future is bleak.

Who will the individual practitioner of the future resemble? It seems the full responsibility for currency and competency will be assumed by the individual practitioner. Organized programs as we know them today will be but one resource available to the individual learner. Basic educational programs will have to provide the student with assessment skills to determine the need for continued learning. Independent study and self-directed learning will be an integral part of the continued learning process.

The status of mandatory continuing education is questionable and lifelong licensure is no doubt a thing of the past. A change will occur in licensure requirements and competency will be measured through some, as yet, clearly undefined process. The profession will continue to credential advanced or specialized competence through the certification process. The responsibility for relicensure and certification maintenance will be on the individual seeking continued practice privileges, while the state of the art for describing, measuring, and recording competence will be more fully developed. As a result, relicensure and certification maintenance will focus on proof of competence rather than on any one means for maintenance of that competence, and continuing education will play a role in providing a means for practitioners to maintain current knowledge and skills.

Participation in continued learning will gain the respect of society and can only help to advance the profession. The professional nurse, as a professional, is charged with a commitment to continued learning. The profession will gain the respect not only of others in the health profession, but consumers as well when this participatory behavior is translated into improved health care. To date, because of the cost and time involved, competency based studies are limited. Those that do exist usually are restricted to technological skills, for a mechanical act is relatively easy to measure. Unfortunately, most evaluations of nursing continuing education programs have been based upon subjective participant evaluations of the course content and not on objective evaluation of the skills of the participants. It seems likely that attendance at CE offerings would affect the later performance of the participants. However, a closer examination raises many questions regarding this applicability. For example, newly appointed head nurses who have completed a basic management skills course are what would appear to be an appropriate group to examine. However, to determine baseline behavior prior to the course, a pretest must be administered.

But the kind of information to be collected on the pretest needs to be determined. Secondly, an even better measurement would be an analysis of their behavior in the clinical setting prior to their taking the course. After the course is completed, how does one measure the management skills acquired by the participant? If motivation skills were part of the course, what kind of tool would be needed to measure how these nurses implemented the skills in the practice setting? Perhaps the staff were not interested in changing their behavior. Would that, then, indicate that these nurses were failures; or if there were several settings with similar staff of this kind, would this, then, indicate that the course was not appropriate? These are just a few of the variables that interfere with the measurement process. It is far easier to measure the change in participant behavior when teaching a course in the methodology of a venipuncture. Hence, in the area of continuing education and its effect on improvement in patient care research is limited.

Although the ultimate focus of evaluation in nursing continuing education should be on how changes in the quality of nursing practice affect patient outcomes, even less is found in the literature in this area. Measurement approaches and instruments are either still in their infancy stages or yet to be developed to evaluate the relationship of continuing education to improved patient care and health delivery.[27]

In summary, an examination of the history of nursing provides future direction for the profession. Social, political, and economic trends will have an influence on nursing in the next century. Nursing will be part of the "learning society." Nurses will become more adept in assessing their own learning needs and will be more selective in their learning opportunities. More continuing education will be available to larger numbers of nurses and it will be offered by a wide range of providers. Innovative teaching strategies will be used by providers; the traditional conference-workshop format will be only one of many educational approaches available. Self-directed learning will become more generally accepted by individuals, as well as licensing boards and certification and recognition programs.[28]

Remarkable strides have been made in continuing education in the last 15 to 20 years. These developments have included the establishment of voluntary and mandatory continuing education programs, creation of a mechanism for accrediting and recording participation in continuing education, an increase in publications for and about nursing continuing education, and expanded opportunities for nurses to participate in research in the area of continuing education.

These developments will continue to expand as continuing nursing education is recognized as an important component of collegiate nursing programs. Research in continuing education will grow and move from an examination of nurse learners and surveys of existing practice to extensive investigations of the impact of learning on nursing practice.

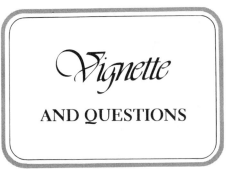

Vignette

AND QUESTIONS

Ms. Thomas graduated one year ago from a nursing program and is interested in enrolling in continuing education activities. She has "kept up" because she subscribes to a nursing journal, which she reads faithfully. However, she was recently assigned to the pediatric unit and feels she needs a course in pediatric health assessment skills. Although she completed a course in health assessment in her nursing program, the major emphasis was on the assessment of the adult. She believes a course of this kind will enhance her previously acquired skills and provide her with the necessary pediatric skills.

Having identified what her learning needs are, Ms. Thomas will now consider several other factors. She will need to determine the scope and depth of the kind of course she will need. Will a cursory overview course be sufficient, or will a several week course more appropriately meet her needs? In addition to identifying her learning needs, Ms. Thomas may also want to consider whether she is interested in pursuing a master's degree in nursing with a pediatric emphasis. If she is uncertain of her commitment and interest in pediatrics, it would probably be better if she worked in pediatrics before she made a decision. Thus the most appropriate action for her at this time is to enroll in a continuing education offering that will enhance her practice in the pediatric setting.

Since the learning needs have been identified and the kind of learning experience selected, several other questions will need to be addressed. Some of these might include the following.

1. Will the employer provide release time to take a course if the course is offered during working hours?

2. How much time will Ms. Thomas have to devote to the CE activity?

3. What contacts need to be made to determine accessibility of these courses?

4. Where are courses such as pediatric health appraisal skills offered?

5. Will the employer pay the registration fee for the course?

6. Are there rewards for taking a CE course in terms of merit pay increase or credit toward the career ladder?

7. How is the quality of the course offering determined?

8. Will contact hours or continuing education units (CEUs) be offered?

9. What additional benefits will be derived from enrollment in a CE activity, ie, will it allow one to be eligible to take a certification examination or will these contact hours or CEUs meet the licensure requirements for mandatory CE states in the event the nurse is licensed in such a state?

INFORMATION SOURCES

Universities and colleges are reliable sources for continuing education offerings if they have a department or program for continuing education. The programs can many times provide information on the quality of programs located outside of their institution.

No central clearing agency exists for continuing education offerings; therefore, responsible contacts, such as peers or other CE providers, can often provide information on program offerings.

The American Nurses' Association is a good resource for continuing education programs, including history, trends, and pertinent facts on continuing education. They also have a Council on Continuing Education. In addition, they can provide the location of the state nurses' association and contacts for programs approved by the state nurses' association.

American Nurses' Association
2420 Pershing Road
Kansas City, MO 64108
(816) 474-5720

Request placement on mailing lists of local colleges, universities, medical centers, and hospital providers of continuing education.

Specialty nurse associations are good sources for continuing education. Contact the association for placement on their mailing lists or information regarding program offerings. A list of these specialty organizations, with their addresses, follows:

American Association of Critical-Care Nurses (AACN)
One Civic Plaza
Newport Beach, CA 92660

American Association of Neuroscience Nurses (AANN)
22 South Washington Street, # 203
Park Ridge, IL 60069

American Association of Nurse Anesthetists (AANA)
216 Higgins Road
Park Ridge, IL 60068-5790

American Association of Occupational Health Nurses (AAOHN)
3500 Piedmont Road, NE, Suite 400
Atlanta, GA 30305

American College of Nurse-Midwives (ACNM)
1155 K Street NW, Suite 1120
Washington, DC 20005

American Medical Association (AMA)
535 N. Dearborn Street
Chicago, IL 60610

American Nephrology Nurses' Association (ANNA)
North Woodbury Road, P. O. Box 56
Pitman, NJ 08071

American Nurses' Association (ANA)
2420 Pershing Road
Kansas City, MO 64108

American Organization of Nurse Executives (AONE)
840 N. Lake Shore Drive
Chicago, IL 60611

American Society of Ophthalmic Registered Nurses, Inc. (ASORN)
P.O. Box 3030
San Francisco, CA 94119

American Society of Plastic and Reconstructive
    Surgical Nurses, Inc. (ASPRSN)
North Woodbury Road, P. O. Box 56
Pitman, NJ 08071

American Society of Post Anesthesia Nurses (ASPAN)
P.O. Box 11083
Richmond, VA 23230

American Urological Association Allied (AUAA)
6845 Lake Shore Drive, P.O. Box 9397
Raytown, MO 64133

Association for Practitioners in Infection Control (APIC)
505 East Hawley Street
Mundelein, IL 60060

Association of Operating Room Nurses, Inc. (AORN)
10170 East Mississippi Ave
Denver, CO 80231

Association of Pediatric Oncology Nurses, Inc. (APON)
2081 Business Center Drive # 290
Irvine, CA 92715-1117

Association of Rehabilitation Nurses (ARN)
2506 Gross Point Road
Evanston, IL 60201

American Society for Parenteral and Enteral Nutrition (ASPEN)
8606 Cameron Street, Suite 500
Silver Spring, MD 20190

Emergency Nurses Association (ENA)
666 North Lake Shore Drive, Suite 1131
Chicago, IL 60611

International Association for Enterostomal Therapy (IAET)
2081 Business Ctr. Drive # 290
Irvine, CA 92715-1117

National Association of Orthopedic Nurses, Inc. (NAON)
North Woodbury Road, P. O. Box 56
Pitman, NJ 08071

National Association of Pediatric Nurse Associates and Practitioners
(NAPNAP)
1000 Maplewood Drive, Suite 104
Maple Shade, NJ 08052–1931

National Association of School Nurses, Inc. (NASN)
P.O. Box 1300
Scarborough, ME 04074-1300

National Flight Nurses Association (NFNA)
P.O. Box 68395
Virginia Beach, VA 23455

National Intravenous Therapy Association, Inc. (NITA)
87 Blanchard Road
Cambridge, MA 02138

National League for Nursing (NLN)
10 Columbus Circle
New York, NY 10019

National Nurses Society on Addictions (NNSA)
2506 Gross Point Road
Evanston, IL 60201

National Student Nurses Association (NSNA)
555 W. 57th Street
New York, NY 10019

Nurse Consultants Association, Inc. (NCA)
P.O. Box 25875
Colorado Springs, CO 80936

The Organization for Obstetric, Gynecologic and Neonatal Nurses
    (NAACOG)
600 Maryland Avenue, SW
Washington, DC 20024

Oncology Nursing Society (ONS)
3111 Banksville Road, Suite 200
Pittsburgh, PA 15216

Society of Gastrointestinal Assistants, Inc. (SGA)
1070 Sibley Tower
Rochester, NY 14604

Society of Otorhinolaryngology and Head Neck Nurses, Inc.
    (SOHNN)
3893 East Market Street
Warren, OH 44484

REFERENCES

1. Nightingale F: *Florence Nightingale to Her Nurses.* London, Macmillan, 1914

2. Houle C: *The Inquiring Mind.* Madison, WI, University of Wisconsin Press, 1961, p 43

3. American Nurses' Association Manual for Accreditation as a Provider of Continuing Education in Nursing. Kansas City, MO, The Association, 1986, p 82

4. Cooper S: Continuing education: Yesteryear and today. *Nurse Educator* 3(1):25, 1978

5. Yoder-Wise P: Living history series: Signe S. Cooper. *J. Contin Educ Nurs* 14(5):32, 1983

6. Yoder-Wise P: Living history series: Elda S. Popiel. *J Contin Educ Nurs* 14(6):26, 1983

7. Yoder-Wise P: Living history series: Jo Eleanor Elliott. *J Contin Educ Nurs* 15(1):22, 1984

8. Kuramato A: Continuing nursing education: A necessity and opportunity. *Washington State Journal of Nursing* 50(2):38, 1978

9. Puetz B: Legislating a continuing education requirement for licensure renewal. *J Contin Educ Nurs* 14(5):5, 1983

10. Simms L: Bridging the gap between education and competent nursing practice. *The Michigan Nurse* 51(4):4, 1978

11. Cross KP: Adult learners: Characteristics, needs and interest. R. Peterson & Associates (eds): *Lifelong Learning in America.* San Francisco, Jossey-Bass, 75, 1979

12. Millonig VL: Nurses' educational backgrounds, position levels and participation in continuing education. *J Contin Educ Nurs* 16(2):70, 1985

13. Dolphin N: Why do nurses come to continuing education programs? *J Contin Educ Nurs* 14(4):8, 1983

14. Millonig VL: Motivational orientation toward learning after graduation. *Nurs Admin Q* 9(4):79, 1985

15. Allan D, Grosswald S, Means R: Facilitating self-directed learning. J. Green et al (ed): *Continuing Education for the Health Profession.* San Francisco: Jossey-Bass, p 219, 1984

16. American Nurses' Association: Facts about nursing. Kansas City, MO, The Association

17. American Nurses' Association: *Summary of ANA Policies on Internal and External Regulation of Nursing.* Kansas City, MO, The Association, December 1986

18. Yoder-Wise PS: Continuing education in nursing: Where are we today? In *Perspectives on Continuing Education in Nursing.* Cooper SJ, Neal MC (eds): Pacific Palisades, CA, NURESCO, Inc., 1980

19. Thomas C: Motivational orientations of Kansas nurses participating in continuing education in a mandatory state for relicensure. J Cont Educ Nurs 17(6):198, 1986

20. Millonig VL: University-based continuing education—what future? Nurs Econ 2(5):330, 365, 1984

21. Calderon J: The purpose of continuing education for nurses: Growth or "big bucks?" Virginia Nurse L(2):14, 1982

22. Arbruzzese R, Chodil J, Puetz B, Strauss M, Wise P: The scope of continuing nursing education as a field of practice. J Cont Educ Nurs 13(6):13, 1982

23. Rerés ME: A message from the dean. UCLA Nursing 1(2):22, 1983

24. Harty MB: Accreditation, credentiating, and approval: What's it all about? In Cooper SS, Neal MC (ed): *Perspectives on Continuing Education in Nursing.* Pacific Palisades, CA, NURESCO, Inc., 1980

25. Millonig VL, Hazard ND: Considering pediatric nurse practitioner certification. Pediatr Nurs 12(4):268, 290, 1986

26. Clark KM: Recent developments in self-directed learning. J Cont Educ Nurs 17(3):76, 1986

27. Oliver SK: The effects of continuing education on the clinical behavior of nurses. J Cont Educ Nurs 15(4):130, 1984

28. Cooper SS: The past as prologue. In Cooper SS, Neal MC (eds): *Perspectives on Continuing Education.* Pacific Palisades, CA, NURESCO, Inc., 1980, p 15

VIRGINIA PETERSON TILDEN, RN, DNSc, FAAN

CHAPTER 13 *Graduate Education in Nursing*

Background and Overview

Graduate education in nursing has had a tremendous impact on the profile of the profession. Although a minority of nurses pursue graduate education, those who do greatly affect nursing education, nursing research, and nursing theory. As the twenty-first century approaches, there is now almost universal consensus on one point: graduate education is essential for nursing to be recognized as a credible scientific discipline capable of producing its own theory base.

Nursing is one of the few service occupations that calls itself a profession while educating the majority of its practitioners at less than the baccalaureate level. Most health professions, such as social work, clinical psychology, medicine, counseling, and dentistry, require a baccalaureate degree as basic college preparation before obtaining the first professional degree, which is at the graduate level. Nursing, on the other hand, allows its first generalist professional preparation to occur at associate degree, diploma, or baccalaureate degree levels, and reserves graduate education as specialty preparation. Nursing, compared to other disciplines, has been incredibly slow to bring its educational structure in line with the common standard of professions.

Historically, nursing's long climb through vocational hospital training has worked against educational advancement. Until the 1960s, the predominant mode of preparation for nursing was diploma training. Hospital-based diploma training, as opposed to academically-oriented education in university settings, created a trade school mentality that resisted innovations, risk taking, and questioning the status quo.[1] Trade school training curtailed a sense of autonomy in nursing and limited financial remuneration of nurses. Also, the predominant female membership of nursing made it more vulnerable to paternalism.[2] Low-level education in the context of "training" (versus "thinking") has been a major barrier to professionalism for nursing. Collegiality between nurses and other health-care professionals is unlikely to occur until nurses obtain commensurate amounts of education.[3,4] For this to be fully realized, the master's degree in nursing would be the first professional degree, an unlikely change in the near future in light of the current struggle within nursing to require the baccalaureate as the first professional degree.

THE NEED FOR GRADUATE EDUCATION

The need for graduate education in nursing is well documented in the extensive literature on the subject. Both the American Nurses' Association (ANA) and the National League for Nursing (NLN) have issued periodic statements urging nurses to pursue graduate preparation in high quality academic programs. The National League for Nursing's Council of Baccalaureate and Higher Degree Programs,[5] in particular, has taken a firm stand in its annual statement regarding master's preparation: ". . . contemporary nursing's most critical need [is] greater numbers of qualified teachers, administrators, and expert practitioners. To qualify for these leadership positions by today's standards requires graduate education in nursing." Master's and doctorally prepared nurses are needed as clinical specialists, educators, administrators, researchers, change agents, and spokespersons for the profession. A pressing need, indeed a need central to the survival of nursing as a profession, is the generation of practice-relevant theory, tested through scientific research, which constitutes the body of nursing knowledge. Graduate education is essential for the conduct of theory generation and testing.

HISTORICAL EVOLUTION OF GRADUATE EDUCATION

Few nurses obtained post-baccalaureate education until the second half of the twentieth century. A trend in society toward valuing education began in the United States after World War II. Many new master's programs (and a few doctoral programs) in nursing opened to meet the demand of nurses who sought higher degrees and often used service benefits to finance their education. In addition, federal funding for nurse training and education became plentiful in the postwar period. Beginning in 1941, Congress passed a series of laws, referred to as the Nurse Training Acts, which infused traineeships into both undergraduate and graduate programs.[6,7]

Master's programs in nursing in the 1950s and 1960s focused on preparing nurses to assume functional roles, such as educator, administrator, and supervisor roles. Nursing theory and practice were little mentioned in these programs, as nursing theory hardly existed and nursing practice was the focus of undergraduate education. By the mid-1960s a shift had occurred toward clinical specialization, and in 1969 an ANA statement on graduate education[8] proclaimed clinical specialization to be the major purpose of graduate education: "the major purpose of graduate study in nursing should be the preparation of nurse clinicians capable of improving nursing care through the advancement of nursing theory and science." In the ensuing years, as master's programs increased in number by 50 percent from some 50 in 1963 to 73 in 1972,[9] clinical specialization intensified within the four clinical areas of community nursing, maternal-child nursing, mental health nursing, and physiologic nursing. Currently, there is some indication[10,11] that the pendulum may be swinging away from extreme specialization and toward the master's prepared generalist who may be best suited to provide broad spectrum, comprehensive health care in multiple settings to diverse client populations. Andreoli[12] maintains that specialty nursing education belongs at the doctoral level, and master's degrees in nursing should prepare the nurse generalist with the first professional nursing degree.

Doctoral education in nursing has evolved along a similar functionalism-to-practice path. Grace[13] traced three phases of development of doctoral education: the era of functional specialists (1926–1959), the era of nurse scientists (1960–1969), and the era of nursing doctorates (1970 to the present). During the first phase, those few pioneers who obtained doctorates did so in teaching or administration, and therefore knowledge from those disciplines dominated nursing. During the 1960s, generous federal stipends under the Nurse Scientist Training Act subsidized nurses to study in the biological and behavioral sciences with the intent that nurses so prepared would bring knowledge from those related fields into nursing. By the late 1960s and early 1970s, more doctoral programs in the science of nursing had opened, and the profession was identifying nurse scholars with doctorates in nursing as best able to generate and test nursing theory related to nursing practice. The phenomenal increase in nursing doctoral programs, from a handful in the late 1960s to 46 in 1987,[14] attests to the demand for doctoral preparation and to the conviction that a body of nursing knowledge now exists at the doctoral level.

TYPES OF GRADUATE PROGRAMS

The nurse who chooses to pursue graduate education in nursing is faced with a broad array of master's and doctoral programs characterized by diverse foci, terminology, and degrees. Undoubtedly, so much diversity is a reflection of nursing as a young science, having engaged in building its own body of knowledge for only about 25 years.[2] No final consensus has been reached about the best degree designations for either the master's or the doctorate. On the other hand, there is general agreement,[10] that the master's of science in nursing with specialization in one of the four clinical areas (cited above) is the best level of education for the nurse practitioner and clinical specialist who practices in service settings as an expert clinician. The doctorate is generally considered necessary for nurse scholars who wish to be educators and researchers in academic or service settings and who intend to generate theory for nursing through the conduct of practice-relevant research. Not all agree with this distinction, however, with some arguing that the ND (nursing doctorate) should be the first professional degree required for entry into clinical practice.[15-18]

Master's in Nursing.   According to the NLN,[5] 144 accredited programs leading to the master's degree existed in the United States (including Puerto Rico) in 1986. The greatest number of programs lead to the master of science in nursing (MSN) or the master of science (MS), with fewer offering the master of nursing (MN) degree. This reflects the trend in nursing away from more technically oriented degrees and toward academic degrees that are better understood by the rest of the scientific community.

Other trends in program offerings apparent in the last decade are a decrease in the percent of programs that offer specialization in psychiatric-mental health nursing, and a sharp increase in both the number and percent of programs that offer gerontologic nursing as a clinical specialty.[19] Psychiatric-mental health nursing has experienced some identity diffusion as its content has been integrated into other clinical areas and as deinstitutionalization of the mentally ill has occurred. Concurrently, the aging of the population has triggered tremendous interest in the gerontological specialties.

Master's education includes core content in nursing science (usually conceived of as theory, research methodology, issues, and ethics), plus clinical specialization. Some programs require a secondary focus in a functional role (usually the educator or administrator role), while others make functional role preparation optional for the individual student. Responding to the periodic call for a common core of content in master's programs, McLane[9] surveyed deans of schools of nursing regarding their opinions of appropriate content. Subjects identified seven categories of essential role competencies: researcher, change agent, educator, humanist, interpersonal manager, spokesperson for the profession, and practitioner. These categories are congruent with the NLN[20] statement on the purpose of graduate education in nursing, which is to provide students with an opportunity to:

- acquire advanced knowledge from the sciences and the humanities to support advanced nursing practice and role development;
- expand their knowledge of nursing theory as a basis for advanced nursing practice;
- develop expertise in a specialized area of clinical nursing practice;
- acquire the knowledge and skills related to a specific functional role in nursing;
- acquire initial competence in conducting research;
- plan and initiate change in the health care system and in the practice and delivery of health care;
- further develop and implement leadership strategies for the betterment of health care;
- actively engage in collaborative relationships with others for the purpose of improving health care;
- acquire a foundation for doctoral study.

All master's programs include research content, but the requirement of independent research, traditionally called the thesis, varies considerably. One survey of 25 graduate programs containing both master's and doctoral components[23] found that only six required the traditional master's thesis, 16 had both thesis and nonthesis options (eg, clinical project, comprehensive exam), and three had no thesis requirement. Although, in general, expectations of master's students' research proficiency have increased, the trend within graduate programs where the doctorate is also offered seems to be a scaling down of the master's thesis. Schools that have a doctoral program are less likely to require a thesis of master's students than schools without a doctoral program.[19] This reflects a growing sentiment that the doctorate, not the master's, is the terminal research degree. Also, faculty in graduate programs that include master's and doctoral students have less interest in and energy for guiding master's theses.

Despite apparent consensus regarding the purpose of master's preparation, tremendous diversity in program offerings exists. Williamson conducted a content analysis of the descriptions of the 109 graduate programs listed in the 1982–1983 NLN publication, "Master's Education in Nursing." She found 23 different titles for these programs, which were described by 130 different phrases. Some programs offered 18 to 20 separate clinical areas within one graduate program. Williamson interpreted this extreme diversity as indicative of the profession's failure to reach consensus regarding the structure of the discipline. She concluded ". . . as long as nursing does not provide the structure, programs can and will continue to offer what they believe to be appropriate. And we will continue to have a lack of consistency and terminology and continue to ask, What is the domain of nursing?—a question raised from within and outside of nursing."[21] An additional problem is that the curricula of programs often lag behind the demands of the marketplace, leading to discrepancies between the real and the ideal content in master's curricula.[22]

Admission requirements of the great majority of master's programs include a baccalaureate degree in nursing from an NLN accredited program that includes an upper-division major in nursing; evidence of past scholarship ability as reflected in an adequate grade point average; test scores on such aptitude measures as the Graduate Record Exam or the Miller Analogies Test; data from a personal interview and/or personal references; course prerequisites, such as basic statistics; and licensure as an RN in the state of the institution. While most programs have cut-off points for quantitative admission data, such as 3.0 for GPA and 1000 for the combined quantitative and qualitative scores of the GRE, the present large number of master's programs and the relative drop in student enrollment per program has encouraged many admission committees to move to more lenient cut scores.

Improving access to graduate programs in nursing is a concept firmly supported by the National League for Nursing.[24] An effort to increase access and thereby improve career mobility has led to nontraditional master's programs that meet the needs of students in other than traditional situations. There is a range of types of nontraditional programs, such as external degree programs,[25,26] mobile outreach programs that serve nurses living in rural areas with great geographic distance from education centers, and programs within academic institutions that offer innovative pathways. For example, Yale University offers a master's degree program with three pathways, one for RNs whose baccalaureates are in fields other than nursing, one for non-RNs who have baccalaureate degrees, and one for traditional BSNs. Extensive evaluation over many years has found no significant differences among these groups on clinical or theoretical performance.[27,28]

Nurse practitioner preparation relative to master's education has been a topic of debate in the literature.[29-32] Nurse practitioner education began in the mid-1960s during a national push for improved availability of cost-effective primary care for all Americans. Nurses and physician assistants jockeyed for first place in the race to fill the role of physician-extender. Early nurse practitioner programs were primarily short-term certificate programs administered under continuing education auspices. Many nursing leaders argued that advanced professional nursing encompassed a domain of knowledge well beyond simply an extension of the physician's arm, and they spoke out forcefully for nurse practitioner programs to be offered within master's degree programs, a trend that has occurred in the past two decades.[29] A comparison of master's and nonmaster's prepared nurse practitioners[31] showed that master's prepared nurse practitioners performed more in-depth assessment, more management activities, and more leadership activities than their certificate nurse practitioner counterparts. These findings argue favorably for master's education for the nurse who wants nurse practitioner preparation.

Despite the broad array of master's programs in nursing, there seems to be agreement regarding indicators of the quality of programs, as outlined by the NLN Council of Baccalaureate and Higher Degree Programs in 1983.[33] The nurse considering pursuing a master's degree in nursing should review programs with the following criteria in mind: the curriculum should be logically organized and internally consistent; there should be opportunities for the attainment of advanced knowledge, the application of knowledge to a specialized area of nursing, the attainment of skills in research and scientific inquiry, opportunity for role development, and opportunity for development of leadership, management, and teaching skills; and instructional processes should support the philosophy and goals of the program. All of these criteria are important and, when taken together, provide indicators of high quality master's programs.

Doctorate in Nursing. Doctorally prepared nurses are a valuable resource in nursing's bid for professionalism and for the generation of its own theory base. Doctoral education in nursing began in the 1920s when Teachers College at Columbia University initiated an EdD in nursing. The first PhD program in nursing started in 1934 at New York University, and was followed during the next two decades by a small handful of nursing doctoral programs across the country. By the late 1970s, 22 programs leading to the doctorate existed, a number that increased to 29 by 1984, and to 46 by 1987.[14,34,35] Anderson and her colleagues[36] project that 73 doctoral programs in nursing will be in operation by 1988, a projected 115 percent increase in three years.

The recent increase in the absolute number of nurses who hold doctorates is encouraging, however proportionally, the number of nurses who hold doctorates is still infinitesimal (less than half of one percent of all nurses in the United States). Approximately 4000 of the 1.9 million American nurses hold doctorates, and about 200 nurses graduate from doctoral programs each year.[34,37,38] However, according to Kelly,[39] a survey by the American Nurses' Foundation projected a need for 14,000 doctorally prepared nurses by the year 1990, a figure that is unobtainable given the current rate at which doctoral preparation occurs. The supply of nurses with doctorates falls far short of the demand in both academic and service settings. Nurses with doctorates are urgently needed to serve as faculty, deans, directors, and chief administrators. However, a maldistribution of nurses with doctorates, whose numbers concentrate in desirable living areas, is beginning to close doors on tenure-track positions in major universities.

Consensus has not been reached on the most desirable doctoral degree designation. The nurse who wants a doctoral degree in nursing must decide between a PhD, a DNS, a DSN, a DN, or an EdD; the distinctions between these programs are often minimal or nonexisting. Theoretically, the **PhD in nursing** is a research-oriented academic degree intended to train students for scholarly research activities, including the generation of new knowledge via the conduct of original research. Theoretically, the **DNS (doctorate of nursing science)** is a practice-oriented, professional degree that prepares students for advanced clinical scholarship, including practice and practice-relevant research; its focus is the generation of clinical knowledge and the application of existing knowledge to the practice arena. In actuality, the differences between the PhD and the DNS are vague or absent; the designation of which degree to offer often is more of a political issue with a state legislature or university chancellor than it is an academic issue. Analyses of program content and dissertation requirements have shown no significant or even apparent differences between the PhD and the DNS.[40] However, because the PhD is considered the more desirable degree due to its public recognition and credibility, more programs offer the PhD and the trend in new programs is toward the PhD.

The purpose of doctoral education is to prepare nurse scholars to develop and apply new knowledge for the profession.[41] Therefore, essential content of doctoral education focuses on theory and research; undoubtedly there is less variance in doctoral program content than in master's program content. One survey of essential content of twelve doctoral programs[22] found that all programs required study of nursing theory, theory development, concept formulation, and quantitative analysis. In addition, half of the responding programs required content in experimental design, research methods, ethics, political issues, publications, and grants writing.

The rapid increase in programs leading to the doctorate in nursing has raised serious questions regarding the quality of programs and the adequacy of preparation for the demanding jobs that await new graduates. Holzemer and Chambers[34] conducted a program evaluation to analyze the growth and change in the quality of doctoral education between 1979 and 1984. Data were analyzed from 14 nursing doctoral programs, and overall findings suggested that quality had been maintained, that scholarly activities of nursing faculty had increased, and that a growth in scholarly maturity among nursing doctoral programs was evident.

Nonetheless, because the reputation of graduates is so important to the future public opinion about the profession, concerns about quality are still voiced and lead to position statements on indicators of quality in doctoral programs in nursing. A statement by a task force of the American Association of Colleges of Nursing[42] addressed indicators of the quality of PhD and DNS programs related to the preparation and accomplishments of faculty, the characteristics of students, the focus of the program, and the resources available to support the program (eg, library, computer facilities, laboratories, and student traineeships and assistantships). A program should be evaluated on the basis of the knowledge it contributes to nursing; faculty and student qualifications; student, faculty, and alumni research and other accomplishments; and the learning environment, including accessibility of faculty, the curriculum, learning resources, and other support systems.

Impacts on the Nurse, the Consumer, and Society

The structure of nursing education, which changed very little in the first 60 years of the twentieth century, has undergone rapid change in the past two decades. The impact of graduate education in nursing has reverberated throughout the profession, as well as beyond the profession. Nurses, consumers of nursing care, and society at large have all been affected.

THE NURSE

Career mobility in nursing is now tied in large part to graduate education. Positions once open to nurses with baccalaureate degrees are now almost exclusively open only to those with graduate degrees. Positions that require at least a master's degree include all education positions (staff development and in-service personnel positions, academic faculty, faculty, researcher, education coordinator, dean/director/chairperson); clinical specialist and nurse practitioner positions; and nursing service administration positions (supervisor, assistant/associate director, and director). The nurse who obtains the master's degree will be qualified for an array of responsible positions, and simultaneously will be overqualified for staff nurse positions.

While the focus of most master's programs is clinical specialization, the proportion of available clinical positions for new graduates is extremely small relative to positions in teaching and administration. Balint, Menninger, and Hurt[43] analyzed employment trends for master's prepared nurses and found that only 12 percent of positions available in 1980 were clinical specialist or nurse practitioner positions, compared with education positions (50 percent) and administration positions (25 percent; the remaining 13 percent of positions were miscellaneous roles, such as staff development and clinical coordinator). Therefore, paradoxically, while master's programs emphasize clinical specialization, the marketplace predominantly demands nurse educators and nurse administrators. The reason for this procrustean fit is that leaders in nursing[44] believe that knowledge for the profession is best generated by those prepared in the clinical specialties, even though the larger health care system has relatively few positions for such nurses.

A further complication in this absence of fit between graduate programs and jobs that await graduates is that many master's prepared nurses who take faculty positions feel completely unprepared for teaching. Although clinically expert, they are unfamiliar with the demands of transmitting their knowledge to students and are neophyte in the art of survival in academe.[45,46]

In the past, nursing schools have enjoyed a special dispensation compared to older, more established professions, which allowed nursing faculty without the doctorate to teach in universities. This era has essentially ended, so that the doctorate has become a prerequisite for tenure-track positions in all major universities. Master's prepared nurses who choose to teach can do so in associate degree programs, and can still find fixed-term teaching positions in universities. However, there is no doubt that one impact of graduate education in nursing has been an elevation in the degree requirement for the educator role.

The proliferation of doctoral programs has impacted the master's prepared nurse educator. When a doctoral program opens in a school of nursing, master's prepared faculty will likely experience pressure to pursue the doctorate. However, in an effort to prevent inbreeding,[47,48] most doctoral programs prohibit nurse faculty from simultaneously being students in the doctoral program and a faculty member. Therefore, master's prepared faculty must find other routes to the doctoral degree or find different jobs while being doctoral students.

Another consequence of the opening of a doctoral program in a school of nursing is intense competition between programs for scarce resources. Baccalaureate, master's, and doctoral programs often must compete for fiscal resources and access to clinical laboratories, computers, media services, and the like. A hierarchy of prestige, from the doctorate to the master's, and finally to the baccalaureate, usually means the allocation of resources in that same order. An important impact on baccalaureate programs when master's and doctoral programs exist within the same school is a "brain drain" toward the advanced degree programs. In other words, the most talented and best prepared faculty tend to be assigned to graduate level teaching. Nonetheless, despite this seemingly negative impact of graduate programs on undergraduate programs, benefits do occur when all three programs are offered within a school of nursing.[49] Faculty at all levels report using more research findings in their teaching, and they are more likely to encourage undergraduate nursing students to consider pursuing graduate education, and to encourage students to enter graduate school sooner as opposed to spending years in clinical practice first. Also, the position of nursing within the academic community is strengthened by the presence of nursing graduate programs. Faculty and students within the school of nursing enjoy new respect and increased collegiality with other disciplines on campus.[50]

In summary, the impact of graduate education on the nurse can have both positive and negative aspects. A graduate degree, whether the master's or the doctorate, prepares the nurse for positions of great responsibility and tremendous challenge. However, because it overqualifies the nurse for staff level positions, it may lead to a narrowed job market or a reduced fit between educational preparation and positions available.

THE CONSUMER AND SOCIETY

Graduate education in nursing has brought tremendous benefits to the consumer of health care, and, in most instances, without leading to new costs. Consumers enjoy new health benefits and improved quality of nursing care, as master's and doctorally prepared nurses conduct the research that leads to new clinical knowledge in the science of caring. Examples of improved nursing practice and reduced consumer costs, both monetary costs and human costs, abound in the nursing and medical literature. A recent example, published in the *New England Journal of Medicine*,[51] used a convincing research methodology to demonstrate that very low-birthweight infants could be discharged much earlier than previously believed, provided they are followed in the home by a hospital-based clinical nurse specialist who provides instruction, counseling, home visits, and daily on-call availability. The early discharge infants cared for in the home by the nurse specialist did not differ from those infants who remained in the hospital on the criteria of physical and mental growth, rate of rehospitalization, or acute-care visits. The only difference between the two groups of infants was in the net savings of $18,560 for each infant cared for in the home by the nurse. This study exemplifies the power and potential of nursing care as nurses move into expanded roles and as they use research to document the impact of their practice. Graduate education has made both of these accomplishments possible.

Graduate education in nursing has brought about an improvement in the image of nursing. The public's image of the nurse as either a mother figure or a sex kitten is gradually evolving into a more realistic picture of the nurse as clinician, administrator, and educator. It is difficult, however, for society to achieve a clear picture of the profession because of the great diversity of degrees, titles, credentials, and roles held by nurses. Society's confusion about who and what is nursing is unlikely to abate until the profession itself makes major changes in its entry and credentialing structure.

As more nurses obtain graduate degrees, the distinction between nursing at the graduate level and other professions, such as social work, counseling, rehabilitation therapy, and health education often becomes less clear. Thus, paradoxically, as graduate education prepares more nurses to develop and test nursing theory, thereby legitimating the scientific base of the profession, a simultaneous impact on society may be the lessening of differences between nursing and the allied health professions. This is a controversial point, however. Others maintain that the opposite effect occurs. Nurses with graduate preparation can articulate the domain of nursing, which serves to clarify the distinction between nursing and other professions.

Cost containment demands within health care have fueled interprofessional turf battles. As more nurses achieve graduate education, competition mounts between nurses and others for a legitimate piece of the health care pie. Although nurses with graduate degrees are able to be more assertive and thus more collegial with other professionals, they are also more competitive and thus more threatening. An oversupply of physicians in any geographic region tends to reduce the availability of positions for nurse clinical specialists and nurse practitioners.

Future Considerations

Nursing in the twenty-first century will be shaped by changes in society, in the consumer, in the environment, and in the health care system. All such changes have implications for graduate education in nursing. Societal changes have affected consumers of health care. Consumers are better educated and better informed; they are more knowledgeable about health matters and more interested in learning health behaviors that promote and protect their own health. While demanding to participate in their own health care, they are also less trustful of those who provide care, especially of government and other large organizations. The profile of the consumer has changed toward an aging population besieged with chronic and long-term health disorders.

The health care delivery system has changed dramatically in the recent past, and there is every indication that change will be constant into the twenty-first century. Cost-containment efforts have altered the nature of hospital care. The hospital acuity level is high and stays are short. The vast bulk of health care occurs in the home or elsewhere in the community. Cost-containment efforts are so apparent to the consumer that they have led to a crisis in confidence over quality. A recent *Wall Street Journal's* tips to readers on "Surviving a Stay in the Hospital" reflect this growing consumer concern. The new cost and quality consciousness has proven fertile ground for innovations in health care delivery methods. Investor-owned hospital chains, surgi-centers, emergi-centers, home health agencies, and other entrepreneurial efforts abound.

Ethical dilemmas increase at a geometric rate. New technologies bring new dilemmas for which previous moral decision rules fail to apply. The huge cost of these biomedical technologies in the face of increasingly scarce resources creates ethical dilemmas regarding who should benefit and who should pay. New diseases, such as AIDS, and old but little understood diseases, such as Alzheimer's, pose ethical challenges for both research and treatment.

In addition to ethical dilemmas, technological advances bring rapid changes in personnel job descriptions. Computers now perform such routine hospital nursing and medical tasks as admission assessments, analysis of test data, monitoring vital signs, and reaching a patient's diagnosis.

In light of these trends, then, the challenge before nursing education is to prepare new graduates to provide the highest quality nursing care in an environment in which change is the only constant. Graduate education in nursing must prepare leaders in nursing to be adaptive, futuristic, and proactive. Graduate education in nursing must consider the following specific points:

- Flexible graduate programs are essential in order to make graduate education accessible[52-54]; rising tuition costs and fewer federal traineeships will result in fewer students able to pursue full-time study during usual business hours.
- Graduate instruction in computer technologies and information storage, retrieval, and processing must increase.
- Courses in nursing research must emphasize research questions and methodologies that are relevant to practice, as well as the utilization of findings. In addition to research that builds nursing science, market research related to the delivery of nursing care is needed. Market research includes studies that demonstrate the cost-effective, positive health outcomes of nursing practice.
- Curricula must focus on students' acquisition of skills needed for coping and adaptation in highly complex situations fraught with ambiguities. A shift should occur from teaching methods of problem solving to teaching the methods of defining problems; nurses with graduate education must not only answer questions of the future, they must decide which questions to ask.[55]
- Nurse educators can ill afford their purist thinking of the recent past in which the master's and doctorate *in nursing* were the only desirable degrees. "Blended credentials," such as a dual MSN and MPH will increase nursing's marketability in the highly competitive marketplace.[53] The addition of other credentials outside of nursing should occur with or follow the acquisition of the master's degree in nursing.
- The trend toward upscaling in nursing education will continue, with

increasing numbers of AD nurses seeking the baccalaureate, of BSN nurses seeking the master's, and of MSN nurses seeking the doctorate.

In sum, graduate education in nursing in the future will continue in demand, provided that it is relevant to marketplace needs and accessible to a diverse student population. The product of graduate education in nursing must be individuals prepared and motivated to conduct credible research and incorporate findings into practice; able to develop and test practice-relevant theory; prepared to confront complex ethical dilemmas; familiar with new technologies and by-products of the information explosion; active in social policy formation; committed to humanism in health care; and capable of proaction in the face of certain change.

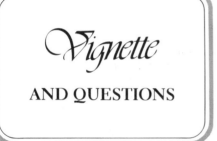

Vignette

AND QUESTIONS

Karen Anderson, a baccalaureate prepared head nurse, has been concerned about her future career options and is considering pursuing a master's degree in nursing. She is uncertain about what type of program to enter. Karen has arranged a meeting with Dr. Tolles, the associate dean of graduate studies in the school of nursing at the local university, in order to explore her questions.

Dr. Tolles greets Karen warmly, and commends her for being a wise consumer of graduate education by exploring her options carefully before making her decision. Dr. Tolles points out to Karen that a master's degree in nursing offers specialization with in-depth study usually in one clinical area, sometimes accompanied by one functional area (such as teaching or administration). Dr. Tolles explains that graduate education is different from undergraduate education in that the student is expected to be much more self-directed and internally motivated, ready to embark on innovative and independent thinking, to substantiate ideas with logical arguments, and to speak and write articulately. Dr. Tolles asks Karen to consider carefully her career goals; choosing a graduate program is a matter of matching one's own career goals with what a program offers. Does she plan to remain in the clinical setting as a master's prepared clinical specialist or nurse practitioner, likely to fill supervisory or primary provider roles? Does she want to explore an academic career, with teaching and research as her main roles?

Finally, Dr. Tolles outlines a series of steps Karen could take to determine her path to graduate education:

1. Start by exploring the broad range of master's program options throughout the United States. Knowing the range of options is valuable even if your mobility is restricted to the local university, because it allows you to place the local program in a broader context. The best source for this information is the National League for Nursing's annual publication, "Master's education in nursing: Route to opportunities in contemporary nursing." This pamphlet lists all NLN accredited programs with a brief description and information about cost and financial aid.

2. Write to those programs of interest and request the school's catalog, bulletin, program description, and application materials.

3. Carefully review these materials for their fit with your own goals and their evidence of program quality. Notice the qualifications of faculty, the availability of clinical, library, laboratory, and computer facilities, and the student-faculty ratio. After reading the written materials, don't hesitate to write or telephone the appropriate assistant dean or chairperson of a particular department with more specific questions about the program, such as whether financial aid is available or whether your career goals match well with their program. Ask specific questions about your qualifications for admission, such as whether you need to take additional prerequisite course work. You might ask what the characteristics are of students who do well in their program, and where their graduates find jobs after graduation.

4. If considering an academic career, consider choosing a program that combines the master's and doctoral degrees. The two degrees are often articulated together in a cost-effective and time-saving manner.

5. Consider the nurse practice act in the state in which future employment is planned. States differ in their credentialing requirements. For example, if you know ahead of time how many hours of supervised practice are required for nurse practitioner certification (and if that type of certification is a career goal), then match the program offering with the state's requirements.

Dr. Tolles encouraged Karen to continue her data gathering about graduate education, and asked her to consider several questions that she might discuss with a friend:

1. Consider the advantages of studying in a school of nursing that is located on a general university campus, versus the advantages of being on a campus that is strictly health sciences.

2. Consider the pros and cons of moving to a new location to obtain a graduate degree from a different school than the one from which the baccalaureate was earned.

3. Since doctoral programs are not accredited by the National League for Nursing, what indicators of quality could one assess in comparing the merits of programs?

4. What are the advantages of obtaining advanced degrees in nursing, versus the advantages of combining nursing with advanced degrees in other fields?

INFORMATION SOURCES

National League for Nursing publications:
   "Master's Education in Nursing: Route to Opportunities in Contemporary Nursing" (latest edition)
   "Doctoral Programs in Nursing" (latest edition)
   Write to the National League for Nursing, 10 Columbus Circle, New York, NY 10019

American Nurses' Association publications:
   "Preparing for the Future: Questions and Answers About Trends in Nursing Education"
   "Statement on Graduate Education in Nursing"
   Write to the American Nurses' Association, 2420 Pershing Road, Kansas City, MO 64108

US Government publication:
   "A Directory of Primary Care Nurse Practitioner/Specialist Programs for Registered Nurses"
   DHHS Publication OM 200683
   Write to the US Department of Health and Human Services, Public Health Service, Health Resources and Services Administration, Division of Nursing, Rockville, MD 20857

Acknowledgement

The author gratefully acknowledges Karen Anderson, RN, BS, master's student at the Oregon Health Sciences University, for her assistance in compiling material for this chapter.

REFERENCES

1. Ashley J: *Hospitals, Paternalism, and the Role of the Nurse.* New York, Teachers College Press, 1976

2. Meleis AI: *Theoretical Nursing.* Philadelphia, Lippincott, 1986

3. Christman L: Accountability and autonomy are more than rhetoric. Read before the Third Annual Innovations in Clinical Practice, Alpha Chi chapter, Sigma Theta Tau, Boston, April, 1977

4. Hawkins JW, Wang RY: Toward the future: Graduate education for professional nursing practice. J Nurs Educ 4:39, 1980

5. National League for Nursing Council of Baccalaureate and Higher Degree Programs: *Master's Education in Nursing: Route to Opportunities in Contemporary Nursing.* New York, National League for Nursing, 1985

6. Kalisch BJ, Kalisch PA: *Politics of Nursing.* Philadelphia, Lippincott, 1982

7. Hardy MA: The American Nurses' Association influence on federal funding for nursing education, 1941–1984. Nurs Res 36:31, 1978

8. American Nurses' Association: *Statement on Graduate Education in Nursing.* Kansas City, American Nurses' Association, 1969

9. McLane AM: Core competencies of master's-prepared nurses. Nurs Res 27:48, 1978

10. Reed SB, Hoffman SE: The enigma of graduate nursing education: Advanced generalist? Specialist? Nurs Health Care 7:43, 1986

11. Reichelt PA: The specialist/generalist dilemma in nursing practice, education, and research. Nurse Educ 3:29, 35, 1978

12. Andreoli KG: Specialization and graduate curricula: Finding the fit. Nurs Health Care 8:65, 1987

13. Grace HK: The development of doctoral education in nursing: A historical perspective. In Chaska NL (ed): *The Nursing Profession.* New York, McGraw-Hill, 1978, p 112

14. National League for Nursing Council of Baccalaureate and Higher Degree Programs: *Doctoral Programs in Nursing 1986–1987.* New York, National League for Nursing, 1987

15. Schlotfeldt RM: The professional doctorate: Rationale and characteristics. Nurs Outlook 26:302, 1978

16. Lutz EM, Schlotfeldt RM: Pioneering a new approach to professional education. *Nurs Outlook* 33:139, 1985

17. Newman MA: The professional doctorate in nursing: A position paper. Nurs Outlook 23:704, 1975

18. Cleland V: Developing a doctoral program. Am J Nurs 76:631, 1976

19. McKevitt RK: Trends in master's education in nursing. J Prof Nurs 2:225, 1986

20. National League for Nursing Division of Baccalaureate and Higher Degree Programs: *Characteristics of Graduate Education in Nursing Leading to the Master's Degree.* New York, National League for Nursing, 1979

21. Williamson JA: Master's education: A need for nomenclature. Image J Nurs Sch 15:99, 1983

22. Beare PG, Daniel ED, Gover VF et al: The real vs ideal content in master's curricula in nursing. Nurs Outlook 28:691, 1980

23. May KM, Holzemer WL: Master's thesis policies in nursing education. J Nurs Educ 24:10, 1985

24. National League for Nursing: Position statement on educational mobility. Nurs Health Care 3:213, 1982

25. Lenburg CB: Preparation for professionalism through regents external degrees. Nurs Health Care 5:318, 1984

26. Lenburg CB: An update on the regents external degree program. Nurs Outlook 32:250, 1984

27. Munro BH, Krauss JB: The success of non-BSNs in graduate nursing programs. J Nurs Educ 24:192, 1985

28. Slavinsky AT, Diers D: Nursing education for college graduates. Nurs Outlook 30:292, 1982

29. Dickenson-Hazard N: PNP/A education of the '80s. Pediatr Nurs 9:335, 1983

30. Lynaugh JE, Gerrity PL, Hagopian G: Patterns of practice: Master's prepared nurse practioners. J Nurs Educ 24:291, 1985

31. Glassock J, Webster-Stratton C, McCarthy AM: Infant and preschool well-child care: Master's and nonmaster's prepared pediatric nurse practitioners. Nurs Res 34:39, 1985

32. Hsiao V, Edmunds MW: Master's vs CE: The debate continues. Nurs Pract 7:42,46, 1982

33. National League for Nursing Council of Baccalaureate and Higher Degree Program: *Criteria for the Appraisal of Baccalaureate and Higher Degree Programs,* ed.5. New York, National League for Nursing, 1983

34. Holzemer WL, Chambers DB: Doctoral education in nursing: An assessment of quality, 1979–1984. Read before the International Nursing Research Conference, Edmonton, Alberta, May 7–9, 1986

35. Gorney-Fadiman MJ: A student's perspective on the doctoral dilemma. Nurs Outlook 29:650, 1981

36. Anderson E, Roth P, Palmer IS: A national survey of the need for doctorally prepared nurses in academic settings and health service agencies. J Prof Nurs 1:23, 1985

37. Murphy JF: Doctoral education of nurses: Historical development, programs, and graduates. Annu Rev Nurs Res 3:171, 1985

38. Kayser-Jones J: Doctoral preparation for gerontological nurses. J Gerontol Nurs 12:19, 1986

39. Kelly LY: *Dimensions of Professional Nursing*, ed 5. New York, Macmillan, 1985

40. Lancaster LE: Doctoral education in nursing, the Sisyphian concept, and Pandora's box. Crit Care Nurse 4:6, 1984

41. Jamann JS (ed): Proceedings of doctoral programs in nursing: Concensus for quality. J Prof Nurs 1:90, 1985

42. American Association of Colleges of Nursing Task Force on Doctoral Education in Nursing: *Indicators of Quality in Doctoral Programs in Nursing*. Washington DC, American Association of Colleges of Nursing, 1986

43. Balint J, Menninger K, Hurt M: Job opportunities for master's prepared nurses. Nurs Outlook 31:109, 1983

44. Murphy S, Hoeffer B: Role of the specialties in nursing science. Adv Nurs Sci 5:31, 1983

45. Karuhije HF: Educational preparation for clinical teaching: Perceptions of the nurse educator. J Nurs Educ 25:137, 1986

46. Fitzpatrick ML, Heller BR: Teaching the teachers to teach. Nurs Outlook 28:372, 1980

47. Miller M: Academic inbreeding in nursing. Nurs Outlook 25:172, 1977

48. Brown KC, Dashiff C, Henry BM et al: Faculty as doctoral students: Policies of doctoral programs in nursing. Image J Nurs Sch 17:27, 1985

49. Norris CM: The PhD in nursing program: A five-year projection. Nurs Educ 10:6, 1985

50. Brodie B: Impact of doctoral programs on nursing education, J Prof Nurs 2:350, 1986

51. Brooten D, Kumar S, Brown LP, et al: A randomized clinical trial of early hospital discharge and home follow-up of very-low-birth-weight infants. N Eng J Med 315:934, 1986

52. Aiken LH: Nursing's future: Public policies, private actions. Am J Nurs 83:1440, 1983

53. Forni PR: Nursing's diverse master's programs: The state of the art. Nurs Health Care 8:71, 1987

54. Conway-Rutkowski B: Future trends in post-basic nursing education. J Nurs Educ 21:5, 1982

55. Fahy ET: Keying in on the business of graduate education in nursing. Nurs Health Care 7:203, 1986

JACQUELINE F. CLINTON, RN, PhD, FAAN

CHAPTER 14

Influence of Nursing Research

Background and Overview

Like other health disciplines, nursing is responsible for generating a body of scientific knowledge on which its practice is based. Research is a uniquely human endeavor of searching for truths about the universe. It is a purposeful and systematic process used to create and test new knowledge. In the broadest sense, nursing research includes seeking answers to questions related to nursing practice, education, and administration, as well as the profession's historical development and impact on society.

Nursing has a long, yet uneven, history of scientific accountability. The roots of clinical nursing research go back to the beginning of modern nursing during the Crimean War, when Florence Nightingale skillfully documented her observations on matters affecting the health, efficiency, and hospital administration of the British army.[1] For well over a century since Nightingale, the majority of research conducted by nurses was targeted to nursing education, which was viewed as the principle means of improving practice.[2] Practice research in the first three decades of the twentieth century was predominantly geared to evaluation of nursing procedures, care plans, and case studies.[3] During and immediately after World War II, nurses focused their research on the supply of nursing personnel and resource management concerns that were linked to improving care.[3] Research relevant to practice again gained momentum in the late 1940s with the establishment of the Division of Nursing Resources within the United States Public Health Service.[4]

241

The focus of this chapter is on **nursing practice research** that is conducted to generate knowledge about human responses to actual and potential health problems. **Clinical nursing research** seeks answers to questions arising from nursing practice. Schlotfeldt[5] has identified six areas that are of particular concern to nurses and worthy of testing:

- What human phenomena, ie, innate human health-seeking mechanisms and innate and learned health-seeking behaviors, are of particular concern to nurses?
- How can those health-seeking mechanisms and behaviors best be named, classified, and characterized?
- What universals govern/regulate those mechanisms and behaviors?
- What factors promote and enhance and which ones disrupt and impede the regularity, function, and effectiveness of human health-seeking mechanisms and behaviors?
- What nursing strategies are effective in preserving, protecting, regulating, and promoting the normal functioning and effectiveness of human health-seeking and behavioral mechanisms?
- What nursing strategies are effective in bringing about constructive changes in the knowledge, beliefs, customs, commitments, motivations, and actions of human beings that lead them to avoid risks to their health status, assets, and potentials and to pursue life-styles and behaviors conducive to their attaining, retaining, and regaining optimal physical, physiological, social, and psychological function and comfort, and the personal productivity, self-fulfillment, and dignity that are appropriate to their humanity?

The broad scope of nursing science reflects the traditional holistic intent of nursing care, which includes consideration of the biological, cultural, social, developmental, behavioral, and emotional factors that influence how human beings maintain and restore health. The primary concerns in all practice-relevant research is quality of care and accountability for client welfare.[6]

Because scientific knowledge is cumulative, nursing research and practice are built, in part, on knowledge generated in the basic sciences, such as physics, chemistry, and biology. Nursing research, however, differs from more basic sciences in several important ways. First, nursing research is geared to problems particularly germain to nursing. Regardless of how fundamental or basic these discoveries, they may eventually lead to improvements in nursing practice. Second, because nursing phenomena and practice are complex, nursing research often requires more sophisticated and complex methodologies that allow for simultaneous investigation of multiple factors. Third, experimental research in nursing involves the manipulation of treatment conditions that are within the professionally and legally defined scope of nursing practice. That is, experimental studies in nursing include research of health responses that are amenable to independent nursing influence and expertise. Fawcett[7] warns that nurses must not rely on other scientists for knowledge that shapes nursing practice, but must be accountable for validating their own practices.

Research is vital to the advancement of nursing theory and practice. In any science, theory is invented for the purpose of explaining phenomena. **Nursing theory** seeks to explain human responses to actual and potential health problems by labeling (naming) such events, by describing their characteristics and relationships, and by predicting as well as mitigating their occurrence. Theory is used to guide practice in that it provides meaning and direction for nursing assessment, intervention, and evaluation of care. Theory also guides nursing research in that it helps scientists pose practice-relevant research problems, select appropriate variables to be measured, and determine relationships to be investigated. In turn, research is used to evaluate the validity of nursing theory when submitted to objective, systematic, empirical observations. As such, research is used to continually test and revise nursing theory. Both theory and research provide accurate information for decision-making in nursing practice.

Today there is consensus among nurses that, in order for nursing to advance and to improve the health of the public, some kind of involvement in research is expected from nurses at all levels of educational preparation.[8] The American Nurses' Association Commission on Nursing Research[9] (now the Cabinet on Nursing Research) provides guidelines for the investigative functions of nurses at various levels of preparation. Nurses with associate degrees are prepared to identify problem areas for research in nursing practice and assist in data collection. In addition, baccalaureate nurses are educated to interpret, evaluate, and communicate research in nursing and other health sciences for use in practice and to use practice as a means of gathering information and refining nursing care. Master's prepared nurses assist others in applying scientific knowledge in practice, enhance the relevance of research by providing expertise in clinical problems, analyze and reformulate nursing practice problems so that scientific methods can be used to find solutions, and conduct research geared to improving the quality of practice. Leadership in research is provided by doctorally prepared nurses who possess skills in: integrating scientific knowledge with other sources to advance practice; develop theoretical explanations of clinical nursing phenomena by empirical research; and develop and apply scientific methods to test, refine, and extend the existing body of nursing knowledge. Benoliel[10] pointed out that a scientifically based body of knowledge in nursing depends on the availability of a community of scholar-scientists who collaborate. This means that nurses at all levels of preparation must work together for the goals of nursing science and practice to be fully actualized.

Scientific work requires financial support to cover costs of personnel, equipment, supplies, library resources, data collection activities, and dissemination of findings. Funding sources for any science can be classified into two main categories: the public sector and the private sector. The public sector includes financial resources generated from tax dollars by federal, state, and local governments. Like other scientists, nurses have the right to compete for public research monies at all levels of government. In this process, a scientist submits a proposal to conduct research, which is then peer reviewed by a panel of scientists who make recommendations about funding based on the scientific merit of the proposal and its relevance to funding agency priorities. Federal support of nursing research has had a significant impact on the development of nursing science in the United States. It began in 1949 with the creation of the Division of Nursing Resources within the US Public Health Service, Bureau of Health Manpower, Health Resources Administration. In 1955 nursing research and research training gained momentum within the newly established Nursing Research Grants and Fellowships Program within the Division of Nursing.[4] The US Armed Forces have contributed significantly to the evolution of nursing research, first through supporting advanced educational preparation for nurses in the military, and later through the establishment of the first nursing research center located in an institute of research.[11] This center was initiated by Harriet Werley in 1951 at the Walter Reed Army Institute of Research, and the emphasis was on research in nursing practice.[12] In the early 1960s the Veterans Administration was the first institution to establish nursing service positions nationwide that centered on the development and conduct of nursing research.[13]

The most substantial gain for nursing science in the public sector occurred recently, in 1986, with the establishment of the National Center for Nursing Research (NCNR) within the National Institutes of Health. For the first time, nursing research is placed in the mainstream of health research in the United States.[14] The purpose of the NCNR is to "provide a program of grants and awards supporting nursing research and research training related to patient care, the promotion of health, the prevention of disease, and the mitigation of the effects of acute and chronic illnesses and disabilities."[15] The establishment of the center was due to organized lobbying efforts by individual nurses and nursing organizations to increase and stabilize federal support for nursing research.

The private sector refers to nongovernmental sources of research funding, such as voluntary organizations and foundations, as well as industry. Voluntary organizations that have made substantial contributions to health research include local and national offices of the American Heart Association, American Lung Association, American Association of Obstetricians and Gynecologists, and the Arthritis Foundation. Local citizen groups also provide funding for special projects, such as a mental health association.

A listing of such organizations can be found in most universities and, to a much smaller extent, in urban-centered public libraries. Nurses are becoming more influential in securing private sector funding for nursing research by serving on boards and scientific review panels of voluntary organizations.

Nurses themselves have made significant contributions to private sector support of nursing research through local and national nursing organizations. Sigma Theta Tau International Honor Society for Nursing has provided research grants to nurses continuously since 1936. The American Nurses' Foundation has awarded research grants since 1955.[16] Small grants awards are becoming more prevalent in other nursing organizations, such as the American Association of Critical Care Nurses and the Oncology Nursing Society.[17] In addition, many state level nursing organizations have established foundations that support nursing research and research training.

Impacts on the Nurse, the Consumer, and Society

THE NURSE

The essential element of all nursing practice is the nursing process, which requires astute observation, critical judgment, and decision-making. To perfect these skills, nurses need access to accurate information. Nursing research is essentially nursing's information system. It constitutes nursing's intelligence. Research is the most reliable and valid way of providing relevant and accurate information that helps the nurse make practice decisions.[18] As nursing is an applied science, one important goal in nursing research and theory is prediction—that is, advancing knowledge of those factors contributing to human responses to actual and potential health problems, as well as identifying and testing interventions designed to alter such responses. These goals go hand-in-hand with those of the nurse in practice, who is accountable for implementing care that has the highest probability of producing positive health outcomes for clients and their families.

Findings of nursing research are also useful to nurses in planning change and improvements in practice. Research findings provide the nurse with rationale and direction for proposing change in procedures and agency policy. There are four kinds of activities involved in research utilization in practice: 1) identification and synthesis of research in a problem area, 2) translating the knowledge into clinical protocol, 3) transforming protocol into specific actions or innovations that are implemented in practice, and 4) evaluation of new practice to determine if change produced expected results.[19]

Development of a scientific body of knowledge through research is the most critical factor in the advancement of professionalism in nursing. In all societies the privilege of being a profession is determined by the public, who ultimately authorizes what constitutes the scope of practice through social contact with the professions. The public expects, indeed demands, that those given the privilege of professional status in any human service discipline base their practice on research—extensive research that has been tested and retested. Hence the privilege of being a profession—of defining and controlling nursing practice, carries with it a prerequisite burden of responsibility to generate, test, apply, and communicate nursing's scientific base. In the past two decades, nurses and nursing organizations have become increasingly sophisticated in using political strategies to expand nurses' control over nursing practice. It is wise to remember, however, that no amount of politics can substitute for scientifically grounded knowledge. In essence, nursing research provides evidence that nurses do make a difference in the health of the American public. Thus it behooves nurses to become actively involved in undertaking research projects.

Another mark of an emerging professionalism is the extent to which a discipline influences public policy. In the case of a health discipline such as nursing, it is the ability to shape laws pertaining to how health resources are allocated in society. The strength of nursing's collective voice in influencing elected public officials who make these decisions is dependent on how well nursing argues its case. Legislators are accustomed to being presented with scientific evidence supporting how a proposed change in policy would benefit the public. Elected officials are not persuaded to make changes in laws or allocation of resources based on the needs or dreams of special interest groups seeking solely to improve their own economic or political situations.

THE CONSUMER

Nursing research has had a notable and measurable impact on the health care consumer. Research of numerous nursing innovations has led to many positive outcomes for a wide diversity of populations, such as lower costs for health care; greater selection of effective health care alternatives; better ways to maintain health and promote normal growth and development; lower incidences of complications, disabilities, and recidivism associated with chronic conditions; more effective means of coping with life transitions; decreased mortality in high risk groups; improved health conditions in the workplace; increased knowledge and skills in self-care; and increased quality of life.

SOCIETY

The full impact of nursing research on society, however, is yet to be fully actualized. This is due to two major reasons. First, not all practicing nurses use research findings as a basis for improving practice. Secondly, the majority of the public is not well informed about nursing research and how nurses apply it to everyday practice. Nor is the public generally aware of how it can use nursing research to promote better health. Citizens are not fully cognizant that nursing is a scientifically based discipline. This public image of nursing is in stark contrast to that of other health sciences, particularly medicine, whose name is virtually synonymous with science in western culture.

Concerted efforts to change these deterrents are being made by nurses. To increase nurses' skills in using research to improve practice, the vast majority of nursing curricula in the United States, as well as continuing education programs, include content on research and its utilization in practice. Nursing research positions, committees, and departments are becoming more commonplace in health care agencies. Nurses are making substantial progress in using public forums for communicating the importance of nursing research to the public.[20] More than ever before, nursing groups are encouraging public involvement and participation in nursing organizations and research committees. This provides consumers with a voice in determining priorities for nursing research and reflects nursing's respect for the consumer's self-determination in health.

The rapid growth of centers for nursing research in the past two decades is another way nursing impacts on the health of citizens. Such centers are commonly structural units within academic or service settings whose general purpose is to facilitate and support scientific inquiry in nursing. In a recent survey, the International Council of Nurses[21] identified at least 81 nursing research centers worldwide. The vast majority of these are located in the United States. Such centers encourage and support collaborative work among nurses in practice and those in research.

The public is interested in information, such as health research, that affects their everyday lives. As more citizens are made aware of nursing's contributions through research-based practice, they will be able to make better informed decisions about the kinds of health services they seek, as well as the kinds of health policy they promote. In a free society it is ultimately the voting public who decides what public funding is available for research in various areas. A public adequately informed about nursing research is highly likely to elect public officials who allocate resources for nursing research. This is also true in the private sector. As nurses involve more of the public in their research activities, citizens will be more likely to advocate increasing financial support for nursing research.

Nurses have given careful thought to future expectations of nursing relative to research-based practice. Priorities for nursing practice research are based on the projected needs of the public and include: 1) the study of health practices that prevent or alleviate actual or potential health problems; 2) evaluation of innovative interventions geared to vulnerable populations, including children, adolescents, senior citizens, culturally diverse groups, the technologically dependent, the homeless, the developmentally disabled, the mentally ill, and the economically deprived; and 3) evaluation of the effectiveness and cost benefits of alternative health care delivery models. To meet these priorities, the American Nurses' Association Cabinet on Nursing Research[22] has identified the following major goals for nursing research for the twenty-first century:

- to ensure an increased supply of nurse scientists by the year 2000;
- to generate knowledge about the well-being and optimum functioning of human beings, the effective delivery of nursing services, and the impact of the profession on health policy;
- to develop environments that support nursing inquiry, including opportunities to initiate and implement nursing investigations and access to subjects, personnel, research facilities, and equipment;
- to disseminate the results of nursing research to clinicians, the scientific community, the general public, and health policymakers, and to increase use of the results.

Future advances in nursing research will also be greatly accelerated by Sigma Theta Tau International's recent creation of its Center for Nursing Scholarship. This center will provide nurses worldwide with access to resources for research and opportunities to develop nursing as a scholarly discipline.

Future Considerations

The quality of studies conducted by nurses in the future is dependent on several critical factors. One is the extent to which educational opportunities for nurses are expanded, especially in regard to doctoral and postdoctoral research training. This includes nurses pursuing advanced degrees in nursing as well as other fields, particularly information technology, health policy, health services administration, and the basic sciences. The American Nurses' Association Cabinet on Nursing Research[22] predicted a minimum of one percent of the total nurse population should be doctorally prepared by 1995 in order to meet society's needs for nursing research in the next century.

Human health is complex and health research requires the talents of many disciplines in addition to nursing. As more nurses pursue doctoral level preparation, nursing will be better able to contribute to and assume leadership in interdisciplinary health research that contributes to the welfare of the public. Nursing's newly established presence within the National Institutes of Health will greatly enhance nursing's role in interdisciplinary research.

Baccalaureate students and nurses in practice are primarily the consumers of nursing research. Hence, the quality of future nursing research also depends on how well undergraduate programs foster critical thinking and a spirit of inquiry in nursing students. This includes nurturing young scholars by providing opportunities to challenge current practices, to identify problems needing research, and to be directly involved in research and its utilization in clinical practice. The same is true for continuing professional education programs for practicing nurses.

An equally salient factor affecting the quality of future nursing research is the availability of funding. Between 1965 and 1983, there was essentially no increase in the amount of federal support for nursing research, which remained at five million dollars. In 1984 it was increased to nine million dollars, which is still negligible compared to the total federal budget for biomedical research. The recent creation of the National Center for Nursing Research within the National Institutes of Health is no guarantee that support for nursing research will stabilize or increase, particularly in times of extreme austerity within the federal government. The nursing profession remains vigilant on Capitol Hill and has well organized lobbying strategies geared toward increasing the allocation of federal funds for nursing research.

Also affecting the evolution of nursing as a profession is the extent to which research discoveries are disseminated. No study is complete until its findings are communicated to members of the profession, as well as the public. Since the 1950s there has been noteworthy growth in the number of scientific journals in nursing, including: *Nursing Research, Advances in Nursing Science, Research in Nursing and Health, Western Journal of Nursing Research, Annual Review of Nursing Research*, and the *International Journal of Nursing Studies*. Nurse scientists are also making their research findings more accessible to practicing nurses by reports in practice-oriented publications. More than ever before, scientific sessions are being integrated into professional nursing meetings at the local, state, national, and international levels. Nurse scientists are increasingly more active in presenting their research results at interdisciplinary health conventions.

Nurse scientists are fully aware that the mass media is the most predominant way citizens gain access to information in modern societies. In the 1980s nurses have greatly accelerated the public's knowledge of nursing research findings through newspapers, television, radio, and health-oriented lay publications. Nurse scientists are becoming increasingly more sophisticated at writing news releases describing their research for widespread distribution. In turn, these efforts have enhanced the public image of nursing as a legitimate scientific discipline.

While this chapter has focused primarily on the relevance, development, and future directions of clinically oriented research, it should be noted that advancing other kinds of research in nursing is crucial to nursing's evolution to full professional status. This includes research in nursing education particularly related to recruitment and retention of nursing students, levels of practice, and practitioner roles. Research into professional issues, such as reimbursement mechanisms, work conditions, quality of care in different settings, and resource acquisition are also high priorities.

For nursing research to achieve its full impact and purpose, there must be widespread application of findings by nurses in their everyday practice. Now and in the future, all nurses, including those in administration, education, practice, and research, are required to collaborate more closely to create a clinical environment where nurses can raise questions about current policies, seek out research solutions to such problems, and develop protocol for testing research innovations geared to improving nursing care.

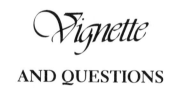

Vignette

AND QUESTIONS

Nurses belonging to the local Critical Care Nurses' Association observed that various intensive care units in their area have different standards and procedures for endotrachial suctioning. None are sure how any of these protocol originated, nor are they sure if one is more beneficial to clients than another.

1. Where would this group of nurses turn for more information about the effectiveness of different endotrachial suctioning protocol?

2. Whom should they consult to help them improve standards of care in this area?

3. How would nurses go about collaboratively testing research findings in endotrachial suctioning?

4. Where would nurses go for securing funding for clinical trials in endotrachial suctioning?

5. How would nurses communicate research-based standards to the profession and the public?

INFORMATION SOURCES

Advances in Nursing Science
Aspen Systems Corporation
20010 Century Boulevard
Germantown, MD 20767

ANA Directory of Nurses with Earned Doctorates
Center for Research
2420 Pershing Road
Kansas City, MO 64108

Annual Review of Nursing Research
Springer Publishing Company
536 Broadway
New York, NY 10012

Directions for Nursing Research:
Toward the Twenty-First Century
American Nurses' Association
2420 Pershing Road
Kansas City, MO 64108

Directory of Nurse Researchers
Sigma Theta Tau
International Honor Society of Nursing
1100 Waterway Blvd.
Indianapolis, IN 46202

Image: Journal of Nursing Scholarship
Sigma Theta Tau
International Honor Society of Nursing
1200 Waterway Blvd.
Indianapolis, IN 46202

Midwest Nursing Research Society (MNRS)
P.O. Box 9117
Cincinnati, OH 45209

National Center for Nursing Research
National Institutes of Health
Lister Hill 3B
Bethesda, MD 20892

New England Organization for Nursing (NEON)
55 Chapel Street
Newton, MA 02160

Nursing Research
555 W. 57th Street
New York, NY 10019-2961

Research in Nursing and Health
John Wiley & Sons
605 Third Avenue
New York, NY 10016

Research in Nursing: Toward a Science of Health Care
American Nurses' Association
2420 Pershing Road
Kansas City, MO 64108

Southern Regional Educational Board (SREB)
130 Sixth Street, NW
Atlanta, GA 30313

Western Journal of Nursing Research
Sage Publications, Inc.
275 South Beverly Drive
Beverly Hills, CA 90212

Western Society for Research in Nursing
P. O. Drawer P
Boulder, CO 80301-9752

REFERENCES

1. Beckingham AC: History, trends and planning for research in nursing. Nigerian Nurse 2:36, 1974

2. Gortner SR: The history and philosophy of nursing science and research. Advances in Nursing Science 1:1, 1983

3. Gortner SR, Nahm H: An overview of nursing research in the United States. Nurs Res 26:10, 1977

4. Abdellah FA: US Public Health Service's contribution to nursing research. Nurs Res 26:244, 1977

5. Schlotfeldt RM: Defining nursing: A historic controversy. Nurs Res 36:64, 1987, pp 66–67

6. Houser D: Research committee membership: Roles and responsibilities. In Lieske AM (ed): Clinical Nurs Res Rockville, MD, Aspen, 1986, p 91

7. Fawcett J: A declaration of nursing independence: The relations of theory and research to nursing practice. J Nurs Adm 6:36, 1980

8. Wilson HS: Research in nursing has a history. J Nurs Adm 12:4, 1984

9. Commission on Nursing Research. *Guidelines for the Investigative Function of Nurses.* Kansas City, MO, American Nurses' Association, 1981

10. Benoliel JQ: Collaboration and competition in nursing research. In Batey M (ed): *Communicating Nursing Research: Collaboration and Competition*, ed 6. Boulder, CO, Western Interstate Commission for Higher Education, 1973, p 1

11. Kalish PA: Weavers of scientific patient care: Development of nursing research in the United States Armed Forces. Nurs Res 26:253, 1977

12. Werley H: Promoting the research dimension in the practice of nursing through the establishment and development of nursing in an institute for research. Milit Med 127:219, 1962

13. Cross ED: Nursing research in the Veterans Administration. Nurs Res 26:250, 1977

14. Jacox A: The coming of age of nursing research. Nurs Outlook 34:276, 1986

15. Merritt DH: The national center for nursing research. Image: J Nurs Scholarship 18:84, 1986

16. Hyde A: The American Nurses' Foundation's contributions to research in nursing. Nurs Res 26:225, 1977

17. Stevenson JS: Forging a research discipline. Nurs Res 36:60, 1987

18. Hinshaw AS, Chance HC, Atwood J: Research in practice: A process of collaboration and negotiation. J Nurs Adm 2:36, 1981

19. Haller KB, Reynolds MA, Horsley JA: Developing research-based innovation protocol: Process, criteria, and issues. Res Nurs Health 2:45, 1979

20. Clinton J: Informing the public about nursing research. Image: J Nurs Scholarship 18:121, 1986

21. International Council of Nurses. Survey of nursing research units. Int Nurs Rev 31:116, 1984

22. Cabinet on Nursing Research. Directions for Nursing Research: Toward the Twenty-first Century. Kansas City, MO, American Nurses' Association, 1985, p 3

R I T A M. C A R T Y, RN, DNSc, FAAN

B R E N D A J. C H E R R Y, RN, PhD

National Center for   CHAPTER 15
Nursing Research

Background and Overview

On April 18, 1986, Secretary Bowen of the Department of Health and Human Services (DHHS) announced the establishment of the National Center for Nursing Research (NCNR) at the National Institutes of Health (NIH). Authorized under the Health Research Extension Act of 1985, P.L. 99–158, the NCNR is charged with conducting a program of grants and awards supporting basic and applied nursing research and research training.

HISTORICAL EVOLUTION

As early as 1978, the American Nurses' Association (ANA) supported the concept of a separate institute of nursing to be located at the NIH. It was believed that the establishment of an institute would increase nursing's capacity and capabilities in nursing research, elevate nursing research into the mainstream of health care science and research, and increase the visibility and prestige of nursing research.[1] Legislative support for this to occur was not readily available and therefore the idea of an institute was not widely discussed within the nursing profession until late 1982. From this time to early 1983, the ANA Cabinets on Nursing Research and Nursing Education considered the institute concept and determined to continue exploration of the political realities and nursing policies required to initiate the institute concept.[2]

254

About the same time, the Institute of Medicine (IOM) report *Nursing and Nursing Education: Public Policies and Private Actions* recommended that the federal government establish an organizational entity to place nursing research in the mainstream of scientific investigation. Recommendation 18 of this report stated: "an adequately funded focal point is needed at the national level to foster research that informs nursing and other health care practice and increases the potential for discovery and application of various means to improve patient outcomes."[3]

While the preceding activities were taking place, a political battle was occurring in the House of Representatives over legislation for the NIH. Representative Henry A. Waxman (D-California), chairman of the subcommittee that oversees the NIH, pressed for legislation that would give Congress considerable influence over the operation of NIH. Representative Edward R. Madigan (R-Illinois) and James T. Broyhill (R-North Carolina) offered a competing bill supporting scientific decision-making by NIH officials.[4]

Through the efforts of the ANA Cabinets on Nursing Research and Nursing Education, recommendation 18 of the IOM report, and battles over the NIH legislation, a political opportunity developed that promoted the concept of a national institute of nursing at NIH. Representative Madigan amended HR 2350 to include an institute, and the nursing profession attained an initiative to establish an institute of nursing at NIH. This was a significant landmark for the nursing profession, but it was not without controversy.[5]

The controversy that surrounded the establishment of an institute of nursing stemmed more from the process of professional organizational decision-making and communication than from opposition to the concept. Dumas and Felton (1984) indicated that there was little disagreement among nurses that an adequately funded national focal point for nursing research was needed, but questioned the profession about how the decision to determine the most appropriate organizational placement of the focal point was to be made.[6] Concerns ranged from the primary goals of NIH, basic biomedical research and the cure of disease, to a grave concern over the effects of an institute of nursing on the existing Division of Nursing. The Division of Nursing located within the Bureau of Health Professions, a component of the Health Resources and Service Administration, Public Health Service, Department of Health and Human Services, served as the principle focus for nursing education, practice, and research. Some nurse leaders expressed the concern that nursing research was not receiving the resources, visibility, and prestige it could if it were removed from the Division of Nursing and placed within NIH. Other leaders thought that such a move would greatly diminish the viability of the Division.[6]

The preceding concerns, and an eagerness to have HR 2350 enacted without delay, fired the controversy within nursing. The **Tri-Council**, a committee consisting at that time of elected presidents and appointed executives of the American Nurses' Association (ANA), the National League for Nursing (NLN), and the American Association of Colleges of Nursing (AACN) supported the Madigan Amendment to HR 2350. Because of the perceived need for the immediate enactment of HR 2350, the general memberships of these organizations were consulted only after the enactment, and then mainly with requests for support.

Professional activities and discussions related to an institute of nursing continued during the remainder of 1983 and into mid-1984. Much concern was focused on limitations of the NIH goal of basic research toward the cure of disease as related to nursing research needs. Views were expressed that past nursing research proposals reviewed at NIH were often disapproved, or approved with low priority scores, because they focused more on disease prevention and improving the quality of care than on disease cure.

Nurses comprised only 67 percent of the membership of NIH review groups or advising councils.[6] On the other hand, the Division of Nursing administered programs had a great impact on all aspects of nursing, including research. The broad purpose of the nursing research program in the Division of Nursing provided an extramural program of support for nursing research to enlarge the body of scientific knowledge underlying nursing practice, education, and administration and to strengthen these areas through the utilization of such knowledge.[7] In 1984 the Division of Nursing received 5 million dollars for nursing research. Under HR 2350, nursing research funds would increase to 9 million dollars in the institute for nursing. Although much of the 9 million dollars would go to the administration of the new institute, there was a designated increase in funding for nursing research. In fact, many in the profession doubted that the number of nurses prepared to do research was sufficient to support an institute and utilize the funds. In 1983 approximately 3000 of the nation's 1.3 million nurses were doctorally prepared. On the other hand, if funds were not available to support nursing research, who would prepare at the advanced levels demanded for researchers?

There was much concern that the Division of Nursing would be weakened if the Research Branch was removed and transferred to NIH. In September 1983 the Virginia/Carolinas' Doctoral Consortium strongly recommended that nursing research, education, and practice programs remain under a single organization and that the current Division of Nursing be immediately strengthened to serve as their nucleus.[8]

Nurses of the Washington Roundtable, at its November 1983 meeting, presented the proposed institute of nursing to a capacity gathering of nurses from all aspects of the profession. This forum, and discussions held by various professional organizations, helped answer questions about the proposed institute, dispelled fears about future outcomes, and generally consolidated the profession in its support of nursing research.

In July 1984 the NIH Bill HR 2350 passed the Senate and was sent to the House of Representatives. The House version of the bill was then sent to the President for his signature. In August 1984, for a variety of political reasons, the President vetoed the NIH reauthorization bill ten days after Congress had adjourned. This veto was accompanied by a memorandum of disapproval for the institute of nursing.

During the remainder of 1984 and in spring and summer of 1985, efforts continued for an institute of nursing. The 1985 NIH reauthorization legislation HR 2409 included the institute of nursing and passed the House in May 1985. In October 1985 it became clear that a second presidential veto would result if the NIH Bill contained provision for an institute of nursing. Negotiations with the support of Congressman Madigan led to a compromise position that would create a center, instead of an institute, for nursing research at NIH. The center would be modeled on the Fogarty Center, and nursing research would be removed from the Division of Nursing. The center director would be approved by the Secretary of Health and Human Services and report to the Director of NIH. The center for nursing research would provide a focal point for promoting the growth and quality of research related to nursing and patient care, provide leadership to expand the pool of experienced nurse researchers, and promote closer interaction with other bases of health care research.

That same month the Senate and House passed HR 2409, including the Center for Nursing Research. On November 11, 1985, the President vetoed HR 2409. However, with strong constituent and professional support, the Senate overrode the presidential veto on November 20, 1985, making the Center for Nursing Research a reality.

THE NATIONAL CENTER FOR NURSING RESEARCH AT THE NATIONAL INSTITUTES OF HEALTH

The concept of the National Center for Nursing Research became a reality through the political process, but staffing became a reality through a transfer of personnel from the Health Resources and Service Administration, Division of Nursing, HRSA/DNS, to the NIH Department of Health and Human Services. Six professional nurse scientists were transferred to NIH and became the core staff of the National Center for Nursing Research. Under Dr. Doris Merritt, Acting Director, this reestablished group was to create a research program as mandated by the HR 2409 legislation. The purpose of the Center under Sec 483 of HR 2409 is the conduct, support, and distribution of information respecting basic and clinical nursing research, training, and other programs in patient care research.[9]

The Director of the National Center for Nursing Research reports to the Director of the NIH. Figures 15-1 and 15-2 depict the organizational structures of DHH and NIH.[10]

Under Dr. Merritt the NCNR staff defined the **scope of nursing research** as "covering scientific inquiry into fundamental biomedical and behavioral processes relevant to nursing and investigations relating to nursing interventions in patient care. The perspectives employed in the design and conduct of nursing research are multidisciplinary; the outcomes are for either short term or eventual improvements in nursing practice to enhance disease prevention and promote the speed of recovery and maintenance of health."[11]

NCNR PROGRAMS AND ACTIVITIES

The Division of Extramural Programs (DEP) serves as the administrative branch of the NCNR and is responsible for program management of research and research training activities. Program activities fall under four branches:

- Health Promotion and Disease Prevention Branch
- Acute and Chronic Illness Branch
- Nursing Systems and Special Programs
- Research Development and Review Branch

Each branch is directed by a branch chief, who reports to the NCNR Director. See Figure 15-3 for the organizational management of the Center.

Health Promotion and Disease Prevention Branch. This branch is primarily concerned with research that reduces the risk of illness and disability for individuals and families. Studies that promote health throughout the lifespan, such as those investigating growth and development needs and variables, are applicable to the health promotion focus. On the other hand, the disease prevention focus includes research that identifies methods and measures to prevent the onset of an illness or disability.[11]

Acute and Chronic Illness Branch. The research focus of this branch is on human responses to illness and disability. Factors that contribute to the causes, prevalence, alleviation, and remediation of illness and disability are specifically considered. Studies addressing technological developments in rehabilitation therapies, adherence to therapeutic regimens, and nursing interventions are selected examples of research advocated and supported by this branch.[11]

Nursing Systems and Special Programs. The nursing care delivery environment is the focus of research within the Nursing System and Special

Programs Branch. Nursing care approaches that enhance patient outcomes in different settings are emphasized. Research in methods to assess cost, increase collaboration, and facilitate nursing care delivery in underserved areas are selected examples.

This branch is also responsible for issues. Ethical and bioethical issues related to death and dying, transplantation, and prolongation of life are selected examples.[11]

Research Development and Review Branch. The responsibility of this branch is to advocate and support preparation of nurse scientists. Emphasis is placed on assuring availability of an adequate quantity and quality of nurse scientists to meet future research needs. Predoctoral and postdoctoral research training are supported.[11]

Support for research that addresses the foci of the four branches is provided by the National Center for Nursing Research through the following mechanisms:

- Research Project Grant
- Academic Research Enhancement Award
- Research Demonstration Project
- First Independent Research Support and Transition Award
- Small Business Innovation Research Award
- Method to Extend Research in Time
- Program Project Grant
- NRSA Institutional Training Grant
- NRSA Individual Predoctoral Fellowship
- NRSA Individual Postdoctoral Fellowship
- NRSA Senior Fellowship
- Academic Investigator Award
- Clinical Investigator Award
- Cooperative Agreements[10]

Individuals seeking funding from the National Center for Nursing Research identify the appropriate program category that relates to their particular interest and topic area. Consultation is available from the nurse scientists assigned to the various programs. Applications are available from the Center and should be precisely followed. Submission dates should be strictly adhered to.

Once a grant application is submitted, the initial scientific and merit review is conducted by the Division of Research Grants, NIH. Within this division a nursing Research Study Section has the responsibility for review of nursing grant applications. Responsibility for scientific and technical appraisals of the nurse scientist development and special program activities lies specifically with the Nursing Science Review Committee of the National Center for Nursing Research.

FIGURE 15-1

Department of Health and Human Services

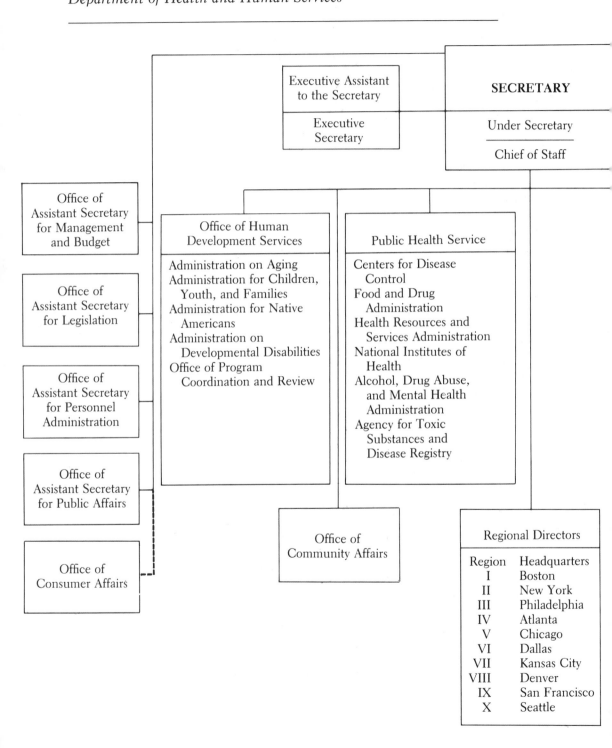

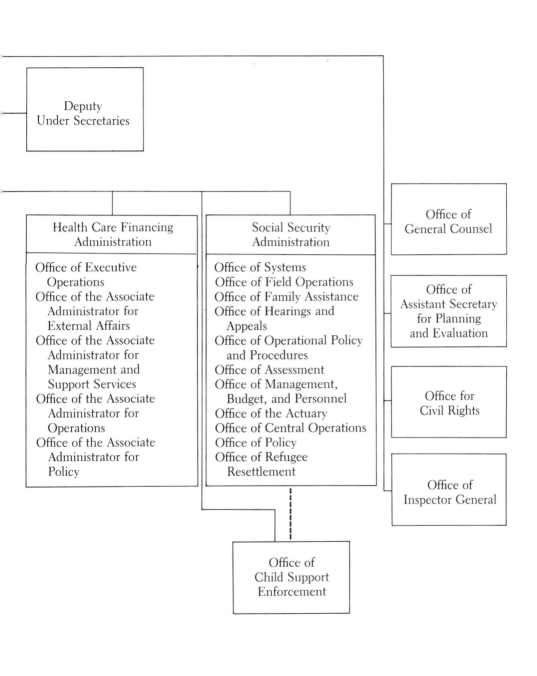

Deputy
Under Secretaries

Health Care Financing
Administration

Office of Executive
    Operations
Office of the Associate
    Administrator for
    External Affairs
Office of the Associate
    Administrator for
    Management and
    Support Services
Office of the Associate
    Administrator for
    Operations
Office of the Associate
    Administrator for
    Policy

Social Security
Administration

Office of Systems
Office of Field Operations
Office of Family Assistance
Office of Hearings and
    Appeals
Office of Operational Policy
    and Procedures
Office of Assessment
Office of Management,
    Budget, and Personnel
Office of the Actuary
Office of Central Operations
Office of Policy
Office of Refugee
    Resettlement

Office of
General Counsel

Office of
Assistant Secretary
for Planning
and Evaluation

Office for
Civil Rights

Office of
Inspector General

Office of
Child Support
Enforcement

FIGURE 15-2

National Institutes of Health

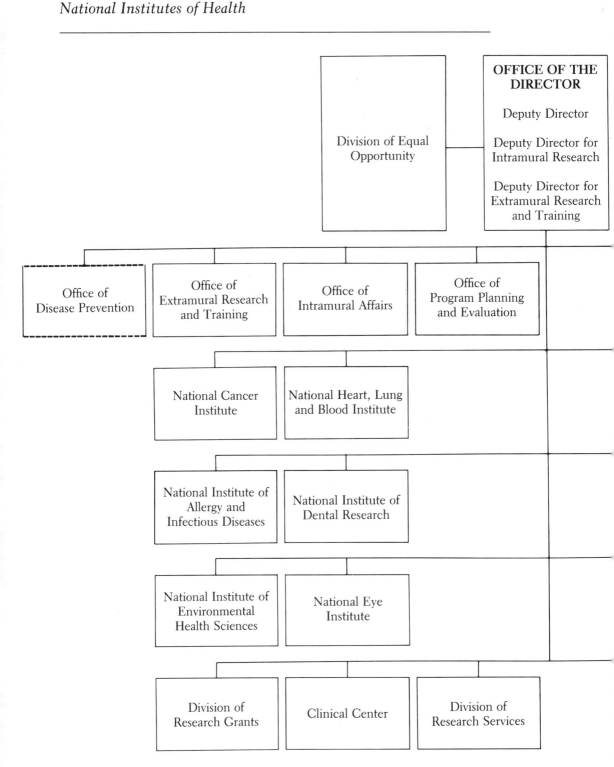

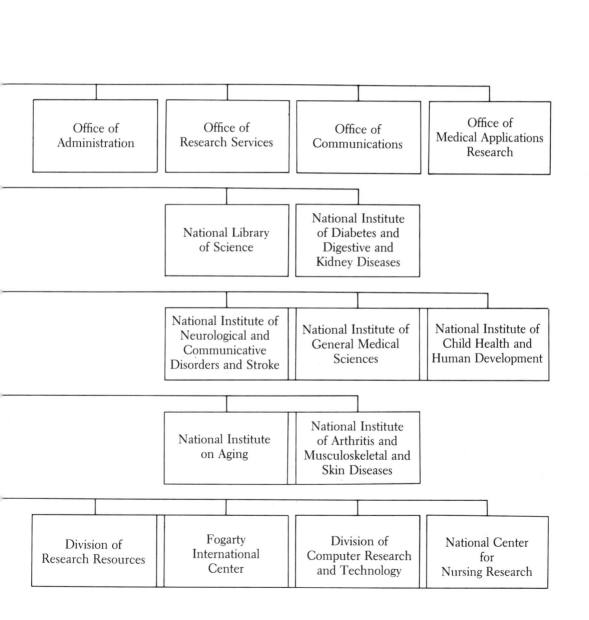

FIGURE 15-3

National Center for Nursing Research

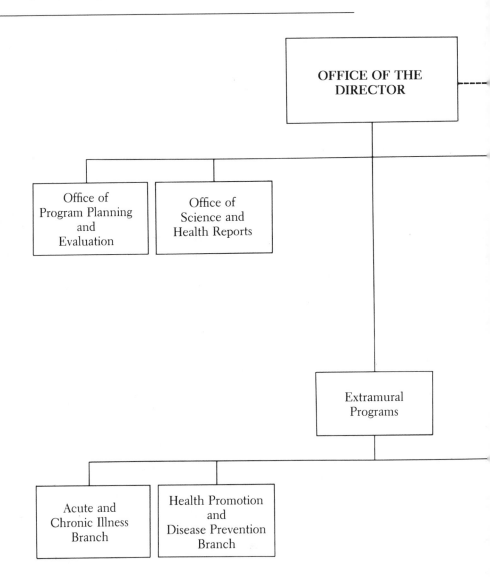

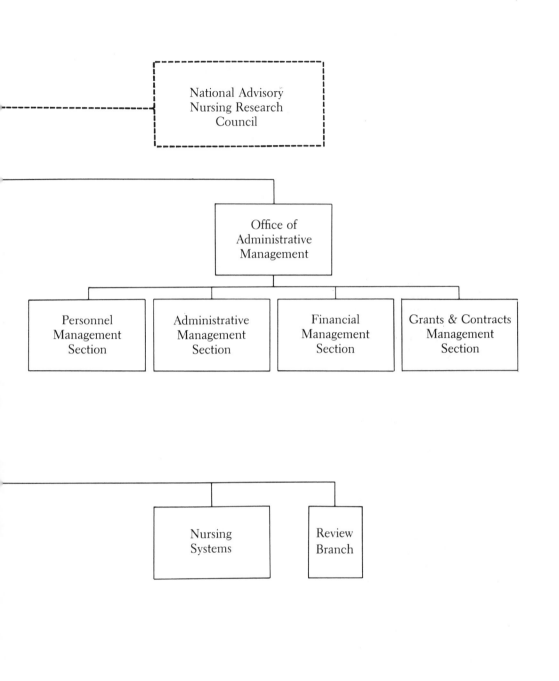

A National Advisory Council, under Public Law 99–158, provides secondary review and advises the Secretary of Health, the Director of NIH, and the Director of the National Center for Nursing Research on programs and directions of the Center.

ADVISORY COUNCIL

Hinshaw, Ada Sue, PhD, RN, FAAN (Chairperson)
Director
National Center for Nursing Research
National Institutes of Health
Bethesda, MD 20892

Affonso, Dyanne S., PhD, FAAN 1988*
Associate Professor of Nursing
Department of Family Health Care Nursing
School of Nursing
University of California
San Francisco, CA 94143

Burgess, Ann W., DNSC, RN 1988
van Amerigan Professor of Psychiatry/Mental Health Nursing
University of Pennsylvania
Philadelphia, PA 19104

Conway, Elaine W. 1988
9 Rittenhouse Road
Bronxville, NY 10708

Cordes, Donald W. 1990
President
Cordes and Associate, Inc.
Des Moines, IO 50309

Damus, Karla H., PhD, RN 1989
Director, Division of Community Health and Epidemiology
Department of Obstetrics and Gynecology
Albert Einstein College of Medicine
Bronx, NY 10461

Howell, Doris A., MD 1987
Professor
Department of Pediatrics
University of California
San Diego Medical Center
San Diego, CA 92093

Kirchhoff, Karin T., PhD, RN 1987
Associate Director of Nursing
University of Utah Hospital
Salt Lake City, UT 84112

Kjervik, Diane K., JD, RN 1987
Associate Professor
School of Nursing
University of Minnesota
Minneapolis, MN 55455

Matthaei, Frederick C., Jr 1990
Chairman
Arco Industries Corporation
Bloomfield Hills, MI 48013

Pender, Nola J., PhD, RN 1989
Professor of Nursing
School of Nursing
Northern Illinois University
Dekalb, IL 60115

Trofino, Joan, MSN, RN 1990
Vice President
Patient Care Services
Riverview Medical Center
Red Bank, NJ 07701

Heller, Leonard E., EdD Vice President - Health Illinois Diversatech Manteno, IL 60950	1989 * Year term of service ends

EX OFFICIO

Abdellah, R/Admiral Faye G., RN, EdD,
  ScD, FAAN
Deputy Surgeon General and Chief
  Nurse Officer
US Public Health Service
Parklawn Building
Rockville, MD 20857

Cournoyer, Paulette, DNSC, RN, CS
Chief, Nursing Research, Psychiatry/
  Mental Health, and Career Development
Veterans Administration Central Office
Washington, DC 20420

Elliott, Jo Eleanor, MA, RN, FAAN
Director, Division of Nursing
Bureau of Health Profession
Health Resources and Services Administration
Rockville, MD 20857

Hernandez, Gloria A., MSN
Colonel, USAF, NC
Senior Policy Analyst
  for Quality Assurance
Office of Assistant Secretary
  of Defense for Health Affairs
Washington, DC 20301-1200

Hinshaw, Ada Sue, PhD, RN,
  FAAN
Director
National Center for Nursing
  Research
National Institutes of Health
Bethesda, MD 20892

Merritt, Doris H., MD
Special Assistant to the
  Director, NIH
National Institutes of Health
Bethesda, MD 20892

Executive Secretary

Aladj, Ruth K., MA, RN
Office of the Director
National Center for Nursing Research
National Institutes of Health
Bethesda, MD 20894

Under Public Law 99–158 the Advisory Council has the following membership:

- Six ex-officio members, including the Secretary of the Department of Health and Human Services, the Director of NIH, Director of the National Center for Nursing Research, the Assistant Secretary of

Defense for Health Affairs, the Director of the Division of Nursing HRSA, and the Chief Nursing Officer of the Veterans Administration (or their designees).

- Twelve members from the leading health and scientific disciplines:
    a. Seven of the 12 will be professional nurses recognized as experts in clinical practice, education, and research.
    b. Four of the 12 will represent the general public and include leaders in the fields of public policy law, health policy, economics, and management.

Under the direction of Dr. Doris H. Merritt, the first Acting Director, the National Center for Nursing Research was established at the National Institutes of Health. NCHR staff was expanded with a new allocation, bringing the total to 28 full-time staff positions from the original six. Peer review panels and the first National Advisory Council were named under Dr. Merritt's guidance. At least three review cycles will have occurred by the time this chapter is published. Dr. Merritt's goals for the NCNR included working toward the establishment of research programs independent of, but complementary to, the research activities currently supported by NIH. Focus was placed on encouraging nurse investigators to establish their own research programs and collaborate with active researchers at institutions throughout the country funded by various NIH Institutes.

Impacts on the Nurse, the Consumer, and Society

Dr. Ada Sue Hinshaw has been named the first Director of the National Center for Nursing Research. Extremely qualified for this position, she no doubt will lead the NCNR to emerge and firmly take its place within the NIH.

The 1987 budget of NCNR was approximately $16,200,000 in support of research and research training. It is difficult at this writing to analyze the full impact of the Center on patient care, nursing, and society in general, due to the newness of its existence. However, it can be assumed that in accomplishing its mission, the Center will have a positive impact on nursing, the consumer, and society.

The mission of the NCNR is to augment the nursing science base that underlies effective patient care and efficient delivery of nursing services to all people of our country.[11] Accomplishment of this mission will impact the nurse, the consumer, and society in a number of significant ways. In general there will be an increase in the quality of care, based upon empirical findings, which will benefit all who need nursing care in our country. This quality care will increase the visibility of nursing to other health care researchers and ultimately increase the status of nursing research and nurse researchers. Nursing will gain recognition as a learned science and a major societal force.

The impact of the National Center for Nursing Research on the nurse, the consumer, and society can be viewed as a cyclical phenomenon. Due to the nature of nursing, changes in one area will ultimately affect the others. The NCNR is projected to produce positive changes in nursing and, consequently, to have positive effects on society.

The viability and perceived value of nursing to society is based on how well it meets the nursing care needs of society. The type, quality, and quantity of nursing research can be key factors in how well these needs are met.

THE NURSE

As a entity within the National Institutes of Health, the NCNR should stimulate the quantity and quality of nursing research, increase competency and commitment to research within the profession, and enhance the visibility and credibility of nursing research within the health care community.

By supporting basic and applied nursing research and research training through grants, consultation, leadership, and environmental opportunities, the NCNR should become a potent catalyst in establishing an effective balance in the quality and quantity of nursing research. Although increased financial support will enhance research opportunities for neophytes and experienced researchers, perhaps the greatest motivator in the proliferation of quality nursing research will be the Center's concerted effort to initiate change. By providing guidance, leadership, and encouragement to persons in all areas of nursing, the base of nursing research can be broadened and appreciation of individual contributions enhanced. Thus, nursing's value system will be expanded to incorporate research as an important vehicle in providing quality nursing care.

A commitment to increased competency in nursing research must be made by the critical mass of nurses. It is not enough that the profession has a select cadre of well trained and productive researchers. Research questions must be posed by those having the need to know and utilize answers in direct patient care. Innovations in nursing care generated by research must be valued by those responsible for directing nursing care and distributing nursing care resources. Realistic application of research findings in practice settings must also receive greater emphasis by those planning and conducting research. Developing a commitment to increase research competency will depend on the perceived relevance of this ability in influencing the quality of patient care. By effectively implementing its charges, the NCNR will promote these accomplishments and thereby enhance nursing's commitment to and competence in research.

The increased visibility and credibility of nursing research within the health care community can produce positive outcomes of increased commitment to and competence in research. The NCNR can also have a more direct influence on the achievement of these outcomes. As the center develops and gains the respect of researchers from other health care disciplines within NIH and the larger community, its products (sponsored research and research programs) will receive greater attention and consideration. Nursing research in general would consequently receive recognition and esteem and move into the mainstream of research.

THE CONSUMER AND SOCIETY

The benefits society, the consumer of nursing care, will receive from the NCNR are indirect, but significant. As the quality of nursing care is improved through nursing research, the health status and quality of life of society should improve. As nurses become more knowledgeable, sensitive, and innovative in assessing risk factors, identifying needs, and delivering care, consumers shall begin to experience improvements in primary, secondary, and tertiary health care. Health education should become more relevant and effective, the reliability and validity of health assessment tools should improve, nursing technologies should become more efficient and effective, strategies for delivering care should become more organized, flexible, and efficient, and the consumer should experience greater satisfaction with care received.

Advancements in nursing research generated by the support and guidance of the NCNR will effect changes in the type, quality, and quantity of nursing care provided society. As the status of nursing research is elevated, so will the status of nursing in the eyes of potential members of the profession, other health care disciplines, and society in general. Through the efforts of the NCNR, society will also gain greater insight as to what nursing research is and how it enhances the quality of life.

Future Considerations

The next 25 years should see the NCNR well established within the National Institutes of Health, given a traditional progressive socioeconomic environment. There should be a modest to moderate increase in funding, which would enable the NCNR to expand its support of research within the scope of its charges. There is also a good possibility that charges of the NCNR will be broadened to incorporate more interdisciplinary research, increased emphasis on team efforts in research studies, and a focus on enhancing staff nurses' and nursing administrators' ability to utilize research within health care delivery settings. Greater emphasis in these areas will assist nurses and administrators to increase their ability to read, critique, synthesize, and apply research finding in the workplace.

Another desirable possibility is that the NCNR will become a mainstream institute within NIH. Although this would provide additional research resources, opportunities, and recognition, another benefit would be the establishment of ideal environmental settings in which nursing care research and collaboration can occur under expert guidance and leadership. As a center, the NCNR can pave the way for the accomplishment of this initial goal.

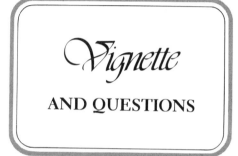

Dr. Kathleen Jones, a nontenured assistant professor in a large school of nursing of a private university, has been teaching for four years and conducting nonfunded research in her clinical speciality area of gerontological nursing. She has identified what she believes is an important research question in the delivery of nursing care to elderly patients. Some of her preliminary research has had an educational focus and is the outgrowth of teaching graduate nursing students gerontological nursing. Some is a follow-up of her doctoral dissertation, with a gerontological nursing care focus. She thinks she is ready to undertake a major research project to answer the identified question and is seeking support from the school of nursing dean.

Although clearly supportive of Dr. Jones's research and her search for funding to obtain release time for research, the dean feels that Dr. Jones has not clearly delineated her research as educational or clinical in terms of external funding. Consequently, the dean has referred Dr. Jones to information on the National Center for Nursing Research and the categories of research to be funded by the NCNR. Dr. Jones has reviewed the NCNR categories and contacted a nurse scientist at the Center for consultation. Following consultation, she has concluded that her research question really involves an educational question that impacts the delivery of quality care to the elderly and would most adequately fall under the Academic Investigator Award of the NCNR. This is a three- to five-year award providing salary and fringe benefits of up to $40,000 per year and a modest sum for the partial defrayal of research costs to be made to junior faculty beyond the postdoctoral stage who have demonstrated evidence of research potential. These awards are designed to allow promising investigative nursing faculty release time from administrative and teaching duties to establish their research programs and mature into independent investigators.

Dr. Jones has obtained an application kit from NCNR, which contains written instructions on how to prepare her proposal, submission dates, and review-cycle dates. Dr. Jones has prepared her proposal, strictly adhering to the instructions. When she experienced a major difficulty, she consulted the nurse scientist who had originally assisted her, who was able to solve her problem. Dr. Jones has submitted the proposal on time and is awaiting notification from the NCNR of results from peer and National Advisory Council reviews.

Individuals considering the NCNR as a source of research support should obtain answers to the following questions.

1. Does the research question meet criteria for funding at the NCNR?

2. Which category does the question best fit under?

3. Who can help with questions or problems?

4. How do you contact a resource person?

5. Are there guidelines for proposal applications?

6. Will submission dates be strictly adhered to?

7. Who reviews the proposal?

8. How will the applicant be notified of the outcome of peer review?

INFORMATION SOURCES

General information about the NCNR may be obtained from the following address:

National Center for Nursing Research
National Institutes of Health
Building 38A, Room B2E17
Bethesda, MD 20894
(301) 496-0526

Specific information and applications for grants may be obtained from the following:

Office of Grant Inquiries
Westwood Building, Room 449
National Institutes of Health
Bethesda, MD 20892
(301) 496-7441

Opportunities for Postdoctoral Research Training

Certain laboratories at the National Institutes of Health (NIH) in Bethesda, MD, will provide a research environment and supervision for nurses holding the doctorate and wishing to spend one to three years in postdoctoral research training. The training will be funded by individual National Research Service Awards (NRSA) supported by the NCNR.

Individuals interested in applying for individual National Research Service Awards (NRSA) postdoctoral fellowships should contact one of the persons listed below to discuss the research training opportunities available. If an appropriate sponsor for proposed research can be identified, applications for an individual NRSA postdoctoral fellowship and related materials may be requested from the Office of Grants Inquiries.

CLINICAL CENTER INTRAMURAL LABORATORIES

National Cancer Institute
Dr. Richard H. Adamson
Division of Etiology
Building 31, Room 11A11
(301) 496-6618

Dr. Bruce Chabner
Division of Cancer Treatment
Building 31, Room 3A52
(301) 496-4291

National Eye Institute
Dr. Robert Nussenblatt
Laboratory of Immunology
Building 10, Room 10N202
(301) 496-3123

National Heart, Lung, and Blood Institute
Dr. Jack Orloff, Director
Division of Intramural Research
Building 10, Room 7N214
(301) 496-2116

National Institute on Aging
Dr. Robert P. Freidland
Laboratory of Neurosciences
Building 10, Room 12AS235B
(301) 496-4754

Dr. Kathleen McCormick
Baltimore, Laboratory of Behavioral Sciences
Gerontology Research Center
Francis Scott Key Medical Center
4940 Eastern Avenue
Baltimore, MD 21224
(301) 955-1791

National Institute on Alcohol Abuse and Alcoholism
Dr. Markku Linnoila
Clinical Director
Building 10, Room 3B19
(301) 496-9705

National Institute of Allergy and Infectious Diseases
Dr. Michael Frank
Laboratory of Clinical Investigation
Building 10, Room 11N228
(301) 496-5807

Dr. Robert Chanock
Laboratory of Infectious Diseases
Building 7, Room 100
(301) 496-2024

Dr. Clifford Lane
Laboratory of Immunoregulation
Building 10, Room 11B09
(301) 496-7196

National Institute of Arthritis and Musculoskeletal
  and Skin Diseases
Dr. John Klippel
Arthritis and Rheumatism Branch
Building 10, Room 9N218
(301) 496-3374

National Institute of Child Health and Human Development
Dr. Arthur Levine
Building 31, Room 2A50
(301) 496-2133

National Institute of Dental Research
Dr. Michael Roberts
Clinical Investigation and Patient Care Branch
Building 10, Room 6S255
(301) 496-6241

National Institute of Neurological and Communicative
  Disorders and Stroke
Dr. Mark Hallett
Clinical Director
Intramural Research
Building 10, Room 5N226
(301) 496-1561

National Institute of Mental Health
Dr. Frederick K. Goodwin, Director
Intramural Research Program
Building 10, Room 4N224
(301) 496-3501

CLINICAL CENTER DEPARTMENTS

Dr. Ron Elin
Clinical Pathology (Chemistry)
Building 10, Room 2C306
(301) 496-5668

Dr. Harvey Gralnick
Clinical Pathology (Hematology)
Building 10, Room 2C410
(301) 496-6891

Dr. Thomas Fleisher
Clinical Pathology (Immunology)
Building 10, Room 2C410
(301) 496-9565

Dr. Joseph Parillo
Critical Care Medicine
Building 10, Room 10D48
(301) 496-9565

Dr. John Doppman
Diagnostic Radiology
Building 10, Room 1C660
(301) 496-5080

Dr. David Henderson
Hospital Epidemiology
Building 10, Room 11N223
(301) 496-2209

Dr. Joseph Gallelli
Hospital Pharmacy
Building 10, Room 1N257
(301) 496-4363

Dr. Steve Larson
Nuclear Medicine and Positron Emission Tomography
Building 10, Room 1C401
(301) 496-6455

Dr. Lynn Gerber
Rehabilitation Medicine
Building 10, Room 5D37
(301) 496-4733

Dr. Harvey Klein
Transfusion Medicine
Building 10, Room 1E33
(301) 496-9702

All addresses are National Institutes of Health, Bethesda, MD 20892,
unless otherwise indicated.

REFERENCES

1. Jacox A: Science and politics: The background and issues surrounding the controversial proposal for a national institute of nurses. Nurs Outlook 33:76, 1985

2. Riker E: National Institute of Nursing Amendment to HR 2350. Office of Minority Council, Health and Environment Subcommittee. July 1983

3. Institute of Medicine Science Nursing and Nursing Education: *Public Policies and Private Actions*. Washington, DC, National Academy Press, 1983, p217

4. Culleton BA: Nursing Institute for NIH. Science 222:1310, 1983

5. Program information. The National Center for Nursing Research. National Institutes of Health, October 27, 1986

6. Dumas R, Felton G: Should there be a national institute for nursing. Nurs Outlook 32:16, 1984

7. Block D: A conceptualization of nursing research and nursing science. In McCloskey JC, Grace H (eds): *Current Issues in Nursing*. Boston, Blackwell, 1981, p81

8. Virginia/Carolinas' Doctoral Consortium in Nursing. Report of meeting, Fairfax, VA, September 12, 1983 (mimeographed)

9. Conference report on HR 2409. *Congressional Record-House*, October 11, 1985, p8760

10. National Center for Nursing Research. Briefing materials for candidates for director, NCNR, August 1986

11. Merritt D: The national center for nursing research. Image 18:84, 1986

JANE LYNNE ECHOLS, RN, PhD

Nursing Education and Nursing Service: A Common Goal

CHAPTER 16

Background and Overview

Nursing service and nursing education in the United States, although inextricably bound together during most of their evolution, have only intermittently shared a common goal. Their interwoven history has its origin in the nature of the relationship between the nursing profession and the society from which it has evolved. Nursing, as noted in the American Nurses' Association *Social Policy Statement*,[1] is like all other professions in that society, consistent with its socio-political and cultural values and conditions and varying levels of economic and technological development, determines the professional knowledges and skills it needs and desires. When society has acknowledged a need and desire for a professional service, institutions have emerged in which individuals could be trained or educated to meet those needs. It is in this context that the intertwined history, present, and future of nursing service and nursing education must be viewed.

Arthur Schlesinger, in *The Cycles of History*,[2] suggests that American history has occurred in 30-year cycles in which there have been alternating patterns of an average of 15 years of conservatism, during which society strongly supports private interests, and 15 years of liberalism, during which there is a turn toward a strong public purpose. These eras of "private interest" and "public purpose," according to Schlesinger, usually gain impetus first at the local level and then reach the national scene three to four years later around a presidential election time. People, according to Schlesinger's theory, crystalize their political value systems by the time they reach 18 to 20 years of age. The pervading local and/or national focus present when they reach their age of social awareness is usually adopted and generally continues to be reflected in their political views throughout their adult life. Thus leaders who come of age in a local and early public purpose period tend to be more liberal, and those coming of age during a local and early private interest period tend to be more conservative.

During "private interest" periods, society has consistently sanctioned a major focus on private enterprise, profits, and consolidation of gains. To achieve greater profits, means have been found to increase productivity without a concurrent increase in critical resource expenditures. To consolidate gains made, means have been found to legitimize the right of the most economically successful to retain more of their gains than the less successful. Thus as private enterprise flourishes, professions become more specialized, gaining or increasing their monopoly on the economic values and scope of their practice.

"Public interest" periods, on the other hand, have been characterized by society's focus on growth, innovation, and attempts to more equitably distribute available resources. Thus more jobs have been created, more people have moved into the work force, higher education has become more available to more people, more semiprofessions have emerged, and the middle class has expanded. In addition, privileges and luxuries such as work, education, environmental safety, health care, and housing have been increasingly viewed as rights and necessities.

By examining these 30-year cycles of history, it is possible to gain a clearer perspective about the evolution of the relationship between society and the nursing profession and of the resulting sometimes calm, sometimes turbulent relationship between nursing education and nursing service. The cycles most relevant to nursing's history and future extend from 1860 to 1890, 1890 to 1920, 1920 to 1950, 1950 to 1980, and, if the pattern continues, 1980 to 2010.

HISTORICAL EVOLUTION OF THE RELATIONSHIP BETWEEN NURSING EDUCATION AND SERVICE

Cycle I: 1860–1890. The Civil War necessitated a major expansion in the number and size of hospitals in the United States.[3] Because the number of trained nurses available to care for the hospitalized sick and injured was negligible, most of the skilled observations were provided by physicians. All other care and housekeeping needs were provided by untrained women who were often societal rejects.

TABLE 16-1

Cycles of American History

CYCLE	FOCUS	PRESIDENT
	1857–1861 Public Purpose—local	
CYCLE I	*1861–1869 Public Purpose - national*	*A. Lincoln*
1860–1890		*A. Johnson*
	1867–1870 Private Interests - local	
-----------	*1870–1900 Private Interests - national--*	*U.S. Grant -----*
CYCLE II		
1890–1920	*1897–1901 Public Purpose - local*	
	1901–1920 Public Purpose - national	*T. Roosevelt*
-----------		----------
	1918–1921 Private Interests - local	
	1921–1931 Private Interests - national	*W.G. Harding*
CYCLE III		*C. Coolidge*
1920–1950	*1928–1932 Public Purpose - local*	
	1932–1947 Public Purpose - national	*F.D. Roosevelt*
	1945–1948 Private Interests - local	
--------	*1948–1960 Private Interests - national--*	*D.D. Eisenhower--*
CYCLE IV	*1958–1961 Public Purpose - local*	
1950–1980	*1961–1972 Public Purpose - national*	*J.F. Kennedy*
		L.B. Johnson
	1969–1973 Private Interests - local	
--------	*1973–1988 Private Interests - national--*	*R. Nixon--------*
CYCLE V	*1986–1989 Public Purpose - local*	
1980–2010	*1989–2000 Public Purpose - national*	
	1998–2001 Private Interests - local	
--------	*2001–2012 Private Interests - national----------------*	

Responding to the needs of the wounded and to the media image of nursing created by Florence Nightingale, many well-bred society women volunteered to serve as nurses during the Civil War. Although appalled by the patient care conditions they found in the military and civilian hospitals, these society women were impressed with the contributions of the few trained nurses among them. After the war, many returned to their private lives as social matrons with a strong belief that patient care in the hospitals could no longer be left in the hands of untrained women and physicians. They quickly formed or joined philanthropic and educational societies and began efforts to establish training schools for nurses.

Within two years after the Civil War, a strong private interest mood began to appear at the local level and reached the national level with the election of President Ulysses S. Grant. The conservatism of the period made finding financial backing for such enterprises as training schools for nurses difficult. The social leaders, therefore, turned to major public hospitals, which agreed to finance the schools in exchange for the services provided by the students during their clinical practice experiences.

By the end of 1873, four training schools for nurses in the US had been established. As in the Nightingale schools, women accepted for training had to be 25 to 35 years of age and meet standards, set by the founders, of intelligence, diligence, and high moral character.[4] The focus of those early schools was to be education. Separate superintendents of the school were to direct their studies and clinical experiences, and physicians were to provide the needed "theory" lectures.

The semi-autonomy of these early schools was short-lived. Hospital administrators immediately recognized the increased quality of care provided by the nursing students and perceived the economic advantages of their free labor. They moved quickly to absorb the schools into the hospital structure.[5] The superintendents of the schools and their students thus became the nursing services for their respective hospitals. Physicians saw the students and graduate nurses as sorely needed assistants, but also as potential threats.[6] Because there were few physician practice acts at the time, physicians were fearful that graduate nurses would leave the hospital and practice medicine. They, therefore, with the cooperation of hospital administrators, very carefully defined the exact limits of the nursing students and graduate nurses' duties. This early delineation of what nurses could do, and the hospital's and ultimately society's acceptance of it, did much to prevent nursing from developing professionally at the same rate as did medicine. The alliance of the early schools of nursing with hospitals and medicine also tied the history of nursing more directly to the growth and development of these two groups and somewhat less directly to the public's health needs and sociopolitical and cultural values and conditions.

As the nation moved into a period of capitalistic expansion in the 1880s, an accelerated growth in the number of hospitals occurred.[3] Planners of these hospitals, cognizant of the patient care and economic advantages of nursing students, began to open their own training schools. By 1890, 35 hospital schools of nursing had been established. During this period, nursing education in the US became firmly placed within the hospital, where it would essentially remain for the next 79 years.

Graduates of these early programs had limited career options. Of the approximately 77 percent who stayed in nursing, 73 percent did 24-hour private duty in individuals' homes, 23 percent were employed as superintendents and supervisors in hospitals and schools; and 3.5 percent worked as visiting nurses.

Cycle II: 1890–1920.   After a decade of unprecedented capitalistic growth, a period of consolidation and a sense of economic conservatism swept across the nation. During the 1890s the growth of large public and private hospitals began to ebb. Small private hospital growth, such as "doctors'" hospitals, however, gained momentum. To insure higher productivity and profits, many of these hospitals also opted to have their own schools of nursing and the free labor of their students. By 1900 there were 432 hospital schools of nursing.

This continued growth of training schools quickly depleted the available applicant pool. To meet the growing hospital need for nursing students, admission standards were often lowered or sacrificed. Some hospitals began to extend their training programs to three years, thereby retaining for an additional year their most experienced student workers. Other hospitals began to offer postgraduate courses, in which minimal additional course work was actually provided, as another way to gain the services of experienced nurses.

The student's life in the average hospital training school during this period was one of systematic socialization to a rigid, autocratic hospital hierarchy, strict discipline, hard work, respectful submission to the absolute authority of the physicians and the nursing superintendent, and unquestioning loyalty to the hospital. Any attempt to find new or innovative ways to do the prescribed procedures was quickly squelched.

Many physicians objected if the nursing students received "too much theory," contending that an overtrained nurse had too many ideas of her own about how to do things and was thus less respectful and more prone to get into trouble. To many physicians, a "good nurse" was one who restricted herself to keeping the environment clean, cared for the bodily needs of the patients, carried out the physicians' orders promptly and without question, and simply but completely recorded her observations of "vital patient phenomena." It was believed that repetition could best insure the development of "good nurses." Thus the average student workday was 12 to 15 hours, six and a half to seven days a week for a period of two years. Evening lectures presented by physicians or the head nurses (who were themselves senior students) were offered once a week. Attendance at class was not mandatory. Any time missed from work duties, however, had to be made up before graduation. Some hospitals further exploited their students by contracting them out as 24-hour private duty nurses and calling the practice "field experience." The income generated from the nursing services of students was more often than not used to develop other parts of the hospital rather than for the improvement of student courses and learning experiences.

In all hospitals in which there was a training school for nurses, the superintendents and supervisors of nursing carried dual accountability for the training of students and the provision of nursing services for patients.

When they sought ways to improve education standards for the students, they found themselves in conflict with the economic practices of hospital administrators and physicians. When they gave priority to the goals of the hospital and their own need for job security, they did so at the expense of the students. The resultant role dilemma was the basis for the first schism that began to appear in the late 1880s and 1890s between nursing service and education leaders.

Some of these nursing service and education leaders chose to resolve their role dilemma through total identification with the hospital goals rather than with nursing. They formed an absolute allegiance to their hospitals and the administrators and physicians who managed and controlled them. They justified their actions by contending that patient care needs would best be served by maintaining an economically sound hospital enterprise. The quantity of patient care provided thus became their major focus.

Other nursing service and education leaders, many of whom had graduated from the early, more prestigious training schools, and had come of age prior to or during the Civil War and thus absorbed a public purpose political outlook, resolved their role dilemma by developing a strong concept of nursing as a vital public service, which they believed could only be insured by well educated, competent nurses. The quality of patient care and nursing education became their primary focus.

Believing that the power of nursing and its potential for meeting the public's nursing needs was dependent upon its ability to organize its members to influence public opinion, leaders from this latter group succeeded by 1900 in establishing the American Society of Superintendents of Training Schools for Nursing (ASSTSN), which later became the National League of Nursing Education (NLNE), as well as the Nurses' Association Alumnae of the United States and Canada, which later became the American Nurses' Association (ANA).[4] Forming a separate association for superintendents of training schools did indeed provide a means for organizing this group to influence public opinion. It also succeeded, however, in dividing them from superintendents in hospitals in which there were no training schools. This division set the stage for many future nursing education and nursing service conflicts.

Postgraduate courses for nurses also came under the scrutiny of these pronursing, proeducation leaders.[5] For some time nurse superintendents had found it difficult to find competent assistants and supervisors to assist with student training and the supervision of nursing services. Believing that advanced courses in the management of the various hospital departments would enhance nurses' administrative competencies and aware that the hospital based graduate courses were not providing this critical content, the ASSTSN turned to higher education. A one-year course in hospital economy was subsequently established in 1899 at Teachers College in New York.[7]

Another major goal set by these early leaders was licensure for nurses. Without such laws, anyone could advertise themselves as nurses and be hired for private duty in homes.[3] The abysmal care provided by these incompetent and sometimes unscrupulous, untrained nurses created a very negative public view of nursing. In addition, there was great variability in the quality of training provided in the established hospital schools of nursing. The licensure law drive was an attempt to protect the public and nursing, as a profession, by limiting membership to only those who had achieved, through approved educational programs, a designated minimum level of competence.

Strong opposition to licensure laws for nursing came from trained nurses fearful of jeopardizing their job security, from managers of hospitals who were exploiting the students in their own training schools, and from physicians, many of whom were the owners of hospitals with schools of nursing, who feared such laws would shift the control of nursing practice and education from the hospitals and physicians to state governments.[4] By 1901, however, the pendulum had swung once again toward a strong public purpose. With it came passage, in 1903, of the first licensure laws for nursing in North Carolina, followed quickly by similar laws in New Jersey, New York, and Virginia. By 1923 all states had passed licensure laws for nurses. These laws, however, were what is known as permissive licensure laws. That is, they provided for voluntary registration of nurses and allowed anyone else to practice as a nurse, whether licensed or not, as long as he or she did not claim to hold the title of registered nurse.

The next two decades of national growth and expansion stimulated an increase in the growth of hospitals and hospital diploma schools of nursing. The number of diploma schools increased from 432 schools in 1900 to 1755 by 1920. The needs of the hospital, however, continued to take precedence over those of the school. Efforts by nursing leaders to improve the standards of these schools were largely ignored.

The Flexner Report in 1910, sponsored and funded by the Carnegie Foundation, stimulated major reforms in medical education.[3] Poorer schools closed, instructional standards were raised, and, as medical education moved into institutions of higher education, medicine became more scientifically oriented. The emergence of scientific medicine brought major changes to hospitals. Advances in immunology, surgical asepsis, and laboratory and x-ray diagnostic procedures prompted hospitals to provide the necessary labs, equipment, and supplies. Physicians began to admit more patients to these well-equipped hospitals and to shift the focus of their practice to the more scientific aspects of clinical and laboratory diagnosis and surgery.

While the Flexner Report was stimulating major reforms in medical schools and, ultimately, medical practice, nursing leaders were proposing major reforms in nursing education.[3] When the ASSTSN approached the

Carnegie Foundation for assistance, however, they were told that the foundation's resources were already directed elsewhere. Indeed, a considerable amount of the foundation's funds were subsequently directed toward similar studies of dental, legal, and teacher education. The education committee of the ASSTSN, therefore, conducted their own survey, "The Educational Status of Nursing (1912)," which highlighted the need for educational reform in nursing and the need for schools of nursing to be independent of hospital control. The report stimulated much controversy, but minimal changes. Perhaps the poor condition of the many thousands of abused workers in factory sweatshops captured the public's attention and spirit of reform more dramatically than did the plight of the few thousand exploited nursing students. Gradually, however, the workday in hospital diploma schools was reduced to nine hours, with an average of 56 hours per week. The discipline and strict rules of the past, however, continued to be the norm and all physician orders had to be followed immediately and fully. The superintendent of nursing continued to be all powerful, second only to the physicians and hospital administrators.

The women's movement, which gained momentum during this period, began to open higher education to women. By 1916 there were 16 colleges and universities that had nursing courses, departments, or schools.

The acute need for better-educated nurses capable of assuming civilian and military leadership positions during World War I, however, provided the strongest incentive to move nursing education into colleges and universities.[3] In a somewhat bold move to attract mature, female college graduates into nursing, an experimental program was initiated at Vassar College. Over 439 college graduates, many of whom were experienced teachers, social workers, librarians, newspaperwomen, and secretaries who had come of age during the early years of the public purpose period, attended an intensive summer school for nurses at Vassar. The curriculum included courses in chemistry, anatomy and physiology, bacteriology, hygiene and sanitation, nutrition, elementary nursing, hospital economics, and, for those who had not had prior course work in the subjects, psychology and social economy. Following completion of the summer program, students chose from among 33 cooperating hospital schools of nursing in which they completed the balance of their training over the next 27 months. The success of these students, many of whom filled key leadership roles in nursing over the next four decades, prompted many other hospital schools to give college graduates credit for eight to ten months of their usual three-year diploma program. It also stimulated a few other universities to offer prenursing and preparatory courses such as those given at Vassar.

This modest move toward higher education assisted in raising nursing education and practice standards and in the preparation of more competent teachers and administrators. At the same time, however, it further widened the schism between education and service as graduates from these programs emerged with very different ideas from their contemporaries in the hospitals about how to educate students and supervise the practice of nursing, as well as how to constructively respond to societies' changing health care needs.

Cycle III: 1920–1950.   The end of World War I ushered in a decade-long private interest period. Consistent with this conservative mood, physicians waged major campaigns for physician licensure laws and restriction of hospital admission privileges to only those physicians who held membership in state medical societies.[3] The move of health care into the hospitals, where physicians could more easily employ the more advanced medical care modalities discovered and/or perfected during WWI, also continued. Hospitals accordingly moved to consolidate their gains. To defray the cost of providing increasingly sophisticated, costly medical diagnostic and treatment facilities, they created new or expanded hospital schools of nursing and reorganized their management of hospital services for greater efficiency. Hospital surveys during this period indicated that 73 percent employed no graduate nurses for unit level charge or staff duty.

The women's movement, and achievement of voting rights for women with the passage of the 19th Amendment to the Constitution in 1920, greatly increased women's options and changed their public image.[8] Women in the 1920s shed their Victorian inhibitions and became more fashionable, adventuresome, and active in their personal and social pursuits. The image of nurses, however, was at odds with that of the "new woman." Nurses retained their altruistic image as faithful, dependent, cooperative, long suffering, and subservient women. This image of the nurse, combined with increasing enrollment in expanding hospital diploma schools, attracted more applicants from lower socioeconomic backgrounds and fewer from the middle and upper-middle class backgrounds than the previous two decades. Exploitation by others was not a new experience for most of these new recruits to nursing who had come of age during a private interest period.

The stock market crash of 1929 brought the private interest era to a resounding halt. In its wake a critical oversupply, unemployment, and maldistribution of graduate nurses was found.[3] Although salaries for graduate nurses were exceptionally low and working conditions for both students and nurses were poor and exploitive, a survey of nurses, patients, and physicians indicated that patients, physicians, and many superintendents of nursing were quite satisfied with the nurse services that were being provided. Nursing's altruism was benefitting everyone but nurses.

By 1930 countless nurses had joined the seemingly unlimited lines of the nation's unemployed as America entered the Great Depression and a two-decade long public purpose era. This serious unemployment situation, however, greatly reinforced the moral persuasion of two reports on nursing during the early 1930s. These reports, "An Activity Analysis of Nursing" and

"Nursing Schools Today and Tomorrow," cosponsored by nursing associations, other health professional associations, and private foundations and individuals, recommended the closing of all hospital schools that were unaccredited, had less than 50 hospital beds, employed fewer than four registered nurses (including one instructor with at least a high school education), worked students more than 56 hours a week, used students to carry head nurse and supervisory duties, or contracted students out as private duty nurses for the profit of the hospital. A third study, "A Curriculum Guide for Schools of Nursing," published by the NLNE in 1937, provided the "state of the art" in curriculum development and instructional strategies for the preparation of professional nursing students.[4] This publication was so timely and practical that it served as a guide for schools of nursing for the next two and a half decades.

Most states, consistent with the public purpose mood in the country, responded to these reports and the unemployment situation by raising their accreditation requirements. In response to these requirements, many hospitals, finding their schools to now be an economic liability, began to close their schools. The number of schools that had reached an all-time high of 1885 in 1929 fell to 1311 by 1940.

At the same time many unemployed graduates were sent to work in hospitals and public health settings under the Federal Emergency Relief Administration (FERA), the Civil Works Administration (CWA), and the follow-up Works Progress Administration (WPA) programs initiated by President Franklin D. Roosevelt to stem the tide of unemployment. In 1929 there had been only 4000 graduate nurses in hospitals. By 1937 that number had increased to 28000. Employment of graduate nurses for ward duty and the higher accreditation standards began to draw to a close the era of student nurses as head nurses, charge nurses, and staff nurses.

The discovery of sulfa drugs during the 1930s and penicillin in the 1940s made many infectious diseases curable and gave physicians their first true power to cure.[1] The admission of infectious patients to hospitals, rather than treating them at home under the care of private duty nurses, became an increasing norm. These developments accelerated the shift of the principal employment setting for graduate nurses from the home to the hospital and further tied the evolution of nursing to that of hospitals.

As more nurses entered the employ of hospitals, a critical need for better qualified nursing service and nursing education administrators was recognized. At the same time, it was recognized that the more autonomous practice of public health nurses necessitated advanced educational preparation. This need for better qualified teachers and administrators in hospitals and nurses in public health settings motivated several collegiate nursing programs, particularly baccalaureate programs for diploma graduates, to offer specialized degrees in administration, education, and public health. By 1940 there were 76 baccalaureate programs in nursing. Graduate education also began to be made available to nurses. Although most of the graduate programs open to nurses were in education, a few schools, such as Yale, Western Reserve, Vanderbilt, and Catholic University began to offer graduate courses in nursing during the 1930s, with others following suit in the 1940s.

The modest gains in the quality of nursing education and nursing practice were added to significantly by the Labor Federal Security Appropriations Act, 1941, the Community Facilities Act, 1941, and the Bolton Act of 1943.[4] These acts, designed to insure an adequate supply of qualified nurses to meet both military and civilian nursing service needs during WWII, provided federal funding for hospital and baccalaureate schools of nursing. In addition, the Bolton Act, under which the Cadet Nurse Corps was established, resulted in the development of the Division of Nursing Education, which, after several reorganizations over the next two decades, became the Division of Nursing in the Department of Health, Education, and Welfare (HEW), thereby legitimizing nursing at the federal government level.

The need to insure an adequate supply of qualified nurses during WWII also fostered the growth of a standardized licensing examination for nurses in all states.[4] The State Board Test Pool with tests prepared by the NLNE for use by state boards of nurse examiners provided this standardization. By 1950 all state boards of nursing in every state in the US had joined the State Board Test Pool. Nursing thus became the first profession to employ the same licensing examination nationally.

During this same period, several states began to change their nurse licensure laws from permissive to mandatory. These mandatory licensure laws were compulsory for all nurses and prohibited anyone without a license to practice nursing in the state on pain of fine or imprisonment. The move toward mandatory licensure, however, was slow, taking almost four more decades to become a national norm for professional nurses.

As had happened after the Civil War and WWI, the ending of WWII introduced a period of conservatism during which the nation attempted to consolidate its resources and stabilize the economy through the stimulation of private enterprise. Government and business, following the war, faced two serious domestic problems.[9] The first problem was how to politically contain the labor and domestic reform movements begun in the 1930s and escalated during the war. The second problem was how to prevent another economic collapse similar to that of 1929. The weight of these concerns preempted any new efforts to continue major federal funding for nursing education and practice.

The postwar period witnessed a tense struggle between business and labor and between conservative and liberal interest groups. Business, requiring labor's support to stabilize the economy, and with encouragement from the federal government, agreed to enter into collective bargaining agreements with the labor unions and to increase wages and fringe benefits, particularly health care benefits. In return labor gave business a free hand in introducing newer, highly productive labor-saving machinery. The resulting economic expansion of business assisted in stabilizing the economy. Also, from this basic labor-business agreement, billions in tax-exempt employer and employee payments to Blue Cross and other commercial health insurance companies were ultimately won by labor.

As more workers gained health benefits, there was an increased demand for hospitals as well as other health services. The construction of hospital facilities, however, had been severely curtailed during the Depression and WWII. In addition, of the existing hospitals, only one-third met minimum standards of approval. Furthermore, there were approximately 1200 counties, mostly rural and in the South, in which there were no hospitals at all.

In designing a response to the need for more health care facilities, the federal government saw an opportunity to meet the needs of several strong constituent groups as well as to stimulate the economy. The compromise program that was forged was the Hill-Burton Hospital Survey and Construction Act of 1946. Passage of this bill achieved several significant political, social, and economic purposes: 1) it redirected organized labor and other liberals' attention away from the national health insurance they were advocating and thereby appeased the American Medical Association (AMA), AHA, and the conservative coalition in Congress; 2) it provided jobs for organized labor in hospital construction, as well as hospital facilities for their use; 3) it bolstered the economy by stimulating construction and subsidizing the private business sector; 4) it provided critically needed rural hospital facilities, which particularly pleased southern politicians; and 5) it maintained private dominance of health services, thereby gaining the support of the increasingly influential conservative groups and state governments.

In addition to the Hill-Burton Program, the government also began to put more funds into biomedical research under the auspices of the National Health Institutes (later combined under the National Institutes of Health—NIH). Research funds from NIH stimulated increasingly complex medical technologies and medical specialization that required more high technology hospitals and an increasing number of nursing and allied health professionals.

The entire US health care system, subsequent to the Hill-Burton Act and the major support given to biomedical research, assumed dimensions that continue to characterize it today: labor intensive, specialized medical care provided predominantly in hospital settings. It had not seemingly been the intent of the proposers of the postwar plan to have "health care" shift to "medical-illness" care or to legitimize a monopoly of the health care system by hospitals and physicians. Nonetheless, these were the inevitable results of a compromise achieved during a private interest period.

When nursing leaders realized that the federal government had no interest in continuing its wartime support for nursing, they turned to private foundations for help.[2] The outcome was the report, *Nursing for the Future* (also called the Brown Report), published in 1948, which stimulated considerable controversy by noting that society was not assisting nursing education as it was teacher education and that nursing was unable to attract the needed numbers of young women to a career in which the authoritarianism in hospitals and the dilemma of being forever caught between the demands of physicians and administrators precluded any self-determination of their own practice.[4] This report was also the first to propose that all, not just the elite part, of nursing education should be in higher education. Many nurses, including diploma school faculty and nursing service administrators, hospital administrators, and physicians felt threatened by the report and, fearing its implications for the economic security of hospitals and nurses, considered it to be a subversive document.

Immediately following the report, nursing organizations initiated an accreditation program for schools of nursing.[3] To prepare for accreditation, they appointed a committee that studied and attempted to classify all schools of nursing in the US. Each school was evaluated and rated on a 100-point scale based on standards of nursing recommended by the nursing organizations. Schools in the upper 25th percentile were classified as Group I, the middle as Group II, and the lowest 25 percent as Group III. All college controlled schools that were rated were classified in Groups I and II.

The classification project stimulated an immediate reaction among diploma schools, who believed they were in a struggle for their very existence. They quickly formed the National Organization of Hospital Schools of Nursing (NOHSN) to aid hospital-based schools in their fight for what they perceived would be the transfer of control and administration of nursing education from the hospital to educational institutions. The NOHSN contended that accreditation and the collegiate nursing education movement would have to be financed by federal funds, which would lead to more federal control and be tantamount to denying free enterprise and freedom of choice.

The controversy created by the Brown Report and subsequent accreditation efforts changed the nature of the schism that had been gradually developing between nursing service and education over the last 70 years. The polarization of diploma schools and collegiate schools drove nursing service and diploma school administrators and faculty back together as they mobilized to fight the "menace" of the "ivory tower" collegiate school faculty, students, and graduates.

Cycle IV: 1950–1980. The government-business alliance during the private interest period 1948–1960 enabled medicine to consolidate the medical advances made during WWII and to continue the development of increasingly more scientific practice in new and expanded public hospital facilities. By 1954 it was estimated that the role demands on nurses in these increasingly complex, scientific health care settings necessitated 20 percent prepared at the master's level and 30 percent at the baccalaureate level. In reality, only one percent of all nurses at that time held master's degrees and seven percent had bachelor's degrees.

Rapid growth of an increasingly complex, specialized hospital based health care system also led to a proliferation of allied health professions and the use of an increasing number of nonprofessional health care workers. By 1952 approximately 56 percent of all hospital nursing personnel were nonprofessionals, primarily practical nurses.[4]

The increasing demand for more knowledgeable and skilled nurses in the highly technological medical-hospital system of the 1950s encouraged the development of more collegiate programs and the preparation of clinical specialists at the master's level.[3] The rate of growth of these programs, although facilitated by the receipt of some federal funds under the Health Amendment Act of 1956, could not keep pace, however, with the steady demand for highly skilled nurses. Consequently, associate degree nursing (ADN) programs in community colleges emerged. The ADN programs, pioneered by Mildred Montag, were designed to prepare competent nurse technicians who could concentrate on the more technical, curative aspects of patient care (which were under the control of the physician), while the practice of the baccalaureate nurse would be focused on the more independent nursing care role. No adjustment in the licensure laws to distinguish between these two types of registered nurses occurred. Nursing service administrators, therefore, responding to the daily pressures of the growing shortage of nurses, failed to make any distinction in how they utilized the ADN and BSN graduates in the provision of nursing services. Polarization of diploma schools and nursing service on one side with collegiate schools on the other found expression in the subsequent technical versus professional nursing practice debate. The nature of the issue became apparent in 1960 when the ANA House of Delegates set their goal to have all nursing education placed within institutions of general education. The distinction between technical and professional nursing practice was formalized by the ANA in 1965 when it issued a position paper endorsing the baccalaureate degree as minimum preparation for professional nursing practice and the associate degree for technical nursing practice.[10]

When 1961 ushered in another public purpose period, newly elected President John F. Kennedy directed the surgeon general to analyze and make recommendations concerning nursing needs and the appropriate federal government role in assuring adequate nursing services in the US.[3] The report of this 1963 study, *Toward Quality in Nursing: Needs and Goals*, recommended federal action: 1) to increase the number of nursing schools, particularly in colleges and universities; 2) to increase the number of basic and master's prepared nursing graduates for effective teaching, supervision, and practice; and 3) to increase the amount of nursing research needed for the advancement of nursing practice. The report further stated that a baccalaureate degree in nursing should be the minimum preparation for all nurses who carried leadership responsibilities.

The assassination of President Kennedy in 1964 and the assumption of office by Lyndon B. Johnson created an anomalous period in American politics. Public policy had consistently been made (and continued to be after this unique period) through "incrementalism," a process uniquely suited to our American democratic system. **Incrementalism** consists of slow but regular marginal changes in policy that give all participants in the system time to adjust, reanalyze, and redefine their positions. The collective public guilt engendered by Kennedy's assassination and the assumption of office by a president who was a consummate politician and the epitome of liberalism, served to focus and activate society's "silent majority."[11] A ground swell of social awareness joined the government forces activated by President Johnson. A landslide reelection victory by Johnson and the concurrent defeat of the Republican candidate, also strengthened the coalition of liberal groups and Democratic legislators and broke the alliance that had existed since the post-WWI period between the AMA and Republicans. The result of these combined events was a six-year period of sweeping and unprecedented major public policy reforms and social programs. Millions of federal and state dollars were poured into the health care and education systems through new and continuing programs such as Medicare, Medicaid, Hill-Burton, and the Public Health Service Act (which included major funding for medical, nursing, and allied health education). Predictably, the late 1960s and the 1970s saw an explosion of growth in hospital construction and use, rapid increases in the size of and admissions to medical, nursing, and allied health schools, and major medical research breakthroughs that resulted in the advent of intensive care units and trauma centers as a norm in hospitals.

A major flaw in the Medicare and Medicaid programs, pass-through payments, guaranteed hospital and physician payment based on their "customary" fees. They were thus free to, and indeed did, set their fees at whatever rate they wished. This flaw quickly made the federal government the leading purchaser of health care services. By the late 1970s, when a strong private interest era was reaching its peak, US health care expenditures were increasing at a rate of 13 percent annually. A variety of federal efforts to contain the escalating costs of health care during the 1970s were unsuccessful. Not until the advent of Medicare DRG's (see Chapter 18) in the early 1980s did federal health spending begin to moderate.

Federal funding for nursing education between 1940 and 1960 primarily assisted in providing better prepared nursing educators, administrators, and public health nurses. Over one-third of the master's graduates, supported by federal traineeships between 1951 and 1961, went into education positions and another third into nursing service administration. Funding through the next two decades, however, was targeted toward the development of master's prepared clinical nurse specialists. Graduate schools of nursing, to qualify for these funds, increasingly dropped their master's programs in nursing administration and in education and started or expanded clinical specialization programs.[12] Federal funds were also made available for the doctoral preparation of nurse researchers.

The nature and evolution of basic nursing education programs and of nursing practice, since the 1960s, have been significantly affected by federal support of nursing. For example, diploma schools of nursing decreased from 908 in 1960 to 303 by 1980, baccalaureate schools increased from 172 in 1960 to 393 by 1980, and associate degree programs dramatically increased from 57 in 1960 to 726 by 1980.[14] For nursing practice, federal support enabled nurses to respond to increasingly complex patient care situations demanding exceptional decision-making and practice skills, to focus on comprehensive, holistic, and primary care, and, for nurses with advanced degrees, to advance in status and autonomy of practice without having to move into teaching or administrative positions.

Two unforeseen outcomes of federal funding for nursing, however, occurred. First, since the early 1970s, faculty members and nursing service administrators have had to be increasingly drawn from among the cadre of clinical nurse specialists who have had minimal preparation in their academic programs for education and administration roles. At the same time, the early doctorally prepared nurses were diverted from research to academic administration in an attempt to increase nursing's credibility with the rest of the academic community as it moved its educational programs more steadily into the higher education system. The latter slowed the profession's progress toward the development of its own theory and science. The former created a shortage of highly qualified, academically prepared nurse administrators for health care agencies that were becoming increasingly complex and experiencing a critical need for more competent, innovative administrative leaders.[13] It also created a shortage of competent faculty knowledgeable in the development of relevant curriculums and the use of effective teaching-learning strategies.

The master's prepared clinical nurse specialists thus assumed administrative roles in nursing service for which they found themselves ill prepared.[14] Having marginal self-concepts as nurse administrators and finding themselves faced with the need to increase technical nursing productivity without a concurrent increase in critical nursing resource expenditures, placed these nurse administrators in conflict with their contemporaries remaining in clinical nurse specialist practice roles and in academe. Many of these nurse administrators, as had their predecessors in the 1890s, 1920s, and 1950s, turned from their own professional members to hospital administrators and the medical staff to satisfy their need for endorsement of their role enactment.[15] Gradually reinstating majors and minors in nursing administration in master's programs in the late 1970s and 1980s did little to facilitate the realignment of these nurse administrators with the community of nursing. Rather, the nurse administrator tended to see graduates of nursing administration programs as threats to the status quo.

Clinical nurse specialists entering academe also experienced profound role dilemmas.[13] Unprepared as educators and frequently unable to make a distinction between what they had mastered as clinical nurse specialists and the basic nursing concepts and clinical skills needed by beginning practitioners, these faculty members often overloaded their students with so many unneeded scientific facts that the students had difficulty learning to process and use them in clinical practice settings. These faculty members also became increasingly territorial about the amount of time during the nursing program that should be spent in each area of clinical specialization. The unending changes and curriculum revisions seen in schools of nursing across the country were as often territorial wars among these faculty members as they were attempts to make the curricula more relevant to society's changing nursing care needs. The increasing recruitment of doctorally prepared faculty, especially those with nursing doctorates, did little to mitigate these problems. On the contrary, these doctorally prepared faculty's desire to concentrate on their research and publications often led them to overlook these instructional problems, the resolution of which would take them away from their more scholarly research activities.

At the same time, hospital administrators and physicians, responding to health insurance and Medicare/Medicaid reimbursement systems that consistently paid more for "intrusive" than for "nonintrusive" procedures and "cognitive services," increasingly stressed the reimbursable tasks associated with patient care.[16] Nursing service leaders who followed suit increasingly alienated their most highly prepared nurses.

As the 1970s drew to a close, greater numbers of the better educated nurses began to leave the restrictive hospital and frustrating academic settings and to practice as autonomous entrepreneurs, providing more affordable direct nursing care to consumers in their homes and community. This movement was aided in 1977 when the Rural Health Clinics Act authorized reimbursement for nurse practitioners serving in rural districts.[17] Other nurses left nursing and entered the growing number of professional and business fields that had increasingly opened to women. Still others began to experience "burnout."

Throughout the 1970s, nursing service leaders had chastised nursing educators for not preparing their graduates for the "real world."[18] To nursing service leaders, the flight from hospital nursing to other practice settings and other fields and the increasing incidence of burnout supported their charge that educators were not adequately preparing new graduates for the realities of hospital nursing. Nurse educators, on the other hand, saw movement by nurses to more autonomous practice settings as an appropriate response to changing consumer health needs and saw the disillusionment with high task hospital nursing as an indication that nursing service needed to employ more nurses with advanced preparation and utilize them more appropriately. The initiation of faculty practice, joint appointments, and the use of clinical preceptors may, in part, have been attempts to deal with the faculty dilemmas and rapid staff turnover of this era.

Cycle V: 1980–2010.   The 1980s saw a continuation of what became the longest private interest era in this century. Perhaps the duration of this era was what finally brought the full attention of the federal government, the public, and health care professionals to the perils of an unchecked inflationary health care industry. Consequently, federal initiation of Medicare DRGs in 1983 to control the high cost of health care joined with three other social trends: an oversupply of physicians and hospital beds; a new philosophy of health care based on preventing illness and keeping patients out of the hospital, and an emphasis on "free market thinking" and "market driven" health care, in which consumers bargain for less costly health care services.[16] DRGs and these trends, as evidenced by the growth of corporate, for profit hospitals, hospices, outpatient surgery centers, health maintenance organizations (HMO), preferred-provider organizations (PPO), and independent-practice associations (IPA), brought competition to traditional hospitals. The net result was an increase in the acuity of illness level of hospitalized patients and a shorter time period in which they could receive care. The complexity and intensity of the patient care situations thereby created, increased the need for staff level nurses who could consider patient events from multiple views and make rapid, accurate clinical judgments. This then necessitated greater levels of cognitive development and more advanced nursing preparation than ever before.[19]

Hospital administrators and physicians initially attempted to find an economic solution to the loss of revenue anticipated in the wake of DRGs by telling nurses and the public that nursing budgets were too high due to escalating nursing salaries and would have to be cut. Nurse resarchers, however, conducted studies to cost out nursing from other hospital charges and invalidated that assumption.[20,21] Nevertheless, many hospitals began to retrench, cut back on their nurse staffing patterns, and employ proportionately more unskilled workers. Some of these hospitals, still unable to maintain their economic viability, closed. Others, however, by improving their management practices, employing strategic planning, and recognizing the profitability of a well-educated, expert nursing staff, experienced an increase rather than a decrease in their profits.[16]

In those hospitals that erroneously assumed that general care units could be converted to special and critical care areas without changing the professional/technical nurse staffing patterns, without legitimizing more autonomous practice for professional nurses, and without forming an alliance with nursing education to collaboratively assist nurses to expand and refine their special/critical care practice competencies, the current acute, escalating shortage of critical and special care nurses has reached crisis proportions. Both inadequate recruitment of nurses and inadequate attention to the retention of currently employed nurses contributed significantly to this shortage.[22,23]

At the same time DRGs were being introduced, federal support for nursing education was being drastically reduced.[24] This reduction in educational grants to nursing programs and students combined with a reduction in nursing positions in many hospitals, increasingly stressful hospital work environments, and the opening of all professions and disciplines to women (in response to the Women's Movement of the 1960s and 1970s), ultimately led to declining enrollments, a shrinking applicant pool, and increasing difficulty in attracting qualified applicants to every type of nursing education program: diploma, associate degree, and baccalaureate. By 1986 baccalaureate programs, while experiencing a significant increase in the enrollment of RN students, still experienced a 10.7 percent reduction in enrollment (their biggest annual loss since 1983).[24] Full-time enrollments in master's programs were offset by part-time enrollments. Full and part-time enrollments in doctoral programs, however, although numbering less than 2000, were slightly increased.

The economics of private interest periods was the most critical factor contributing to this shortage of nurses and declining enrollments in schools of nursing. Shortages and declining enrollments have consistently been the rule in nursing during periods of depressed wage rates.[25] Depressed wage rates for nurses have consistently been the norm when hospitals and physicians attempt to consolidate their economic gains and increase productivity without a concurrent increase in critical resource expenditures. During the late 1970s and increasingly during the 1980s, general care units in hospitals were converted to special and critical care units without significantly changing the professional/technical nurse staffing patterns. At the same time, wage growth for nurses fell to almost a vanishing point. When nurses and nursing service leaders acquiesced to this exploitation of nurses, the percentage of young people interested in nursing careers decreased. When nurses and nursing leaders aggressively resisted, exploitation decreased and enrollments increased. The norm, for most of the 1970s and 1980s, however, was the former.

The changing social values that accompanied the private interest era of the 1970s and 1980s—a shift from humanitarianism toward materialism—also contributed to the current nursing shortage and decline in student enrollments.[26] Individuals coming of age during this period looked for careers in which they could derive the greatest economic benefit and achieve the greatest autonomy, power, and status. They were well aware that human service careers such as nursing were increasingly requiring advanced training while remaining relatively low-paying with dwindling status. They were also aware that the income-generating capacity in business and formerly traditional male professional careers such as medicine and dentistry had steadily and markedly increased, as had the power and status associated with these careers. The dramatic increase in enrollments in these courses of study and the concurrent decrease in human service careers such as nursing were consistent with society's values during this private interest period.

As was seen in the private interest periods of the 1890s, 1920s, and 1950s, hospital administrators and nursing leaders more frequently chose a "quick-fix" route to combat the dwindling applicant pool and the shortage of nurses. Two approaches that reappeared during the mid-1980s were the reduction of admission standards to schools of nursing and the employment of increasingly larger numbers of nonprofessionals, such as practical nurses and unlicensed "nurse extenders." The latter was frequently done even though evidence was available that in settings where proportionally more of the patient care was directly provided by practical nurses and aides, the quality of nursing care was substantially diminished. In 1976 Christman warned nursing service administrators that nonprofessionals and unlicensed personnel could not apply knowledge they did not possess and that although a professional nurse might design an excellent nursing care plan to guide the nonprofessional's practice, "telling others what to do does not transmit the competence needed to do it with professional skill."[27] Nonetheless, this approach to reducing the nursing shortage continued and indeed is beginning to show signs of escalating in 1989 with the AMA's Registered Care Technologist proposal.[28]

Although some health care leaders are still seeking a "quick-fix" for the nursing shortage, recognition of the indispensability of well-educated, expert nurses for the economic viability of American health care enterprises has recently led the AHA and AMA to join the major nursing organizations in publicly supporting the baccalaureate as the entry level for professional nursing practice. This support, and the subsequently unimpeded final movement of nursing education into institutions of higher education it will facilitate, has done much to reduce the schism between service and education.

Impacts on the Nurse, the Consumer, and Society

THE NURSE

The schism between service and education, although potentially reduced, has not been eliminated. The economic constraints of the 1980s have impacted all health science schools in institutions of higher education, as well as hospitals and other health agencies in the US health care system. All health science educators, particularly nursing, medical, and dental faculty, as well as hospital and nursing administrators and physicians, have been challenged to find more cost effective ways to produce their products and alternative ways to increase their revenues. How they have responded and continue to respond to these economic demands can either create additional stress and strain for the practicing nurse or create the potential for a stimulating and professionally and economically rewarding career for nurses.

If nursing service administrators choose a "quick-fix" approach and continue to rely on high control tactics and traditional management styles such as close supervision to insure more productivity with fewer resources, then staff conflicts, absenteeism, loss of career commitment, and staff turnover will become the norm. In addition, nurses who were educated in community college and university nursing programs and who incorporated the beliefs and values of the educated technical and professional experts who taught them might be less tolerant of this close, high task, regimented supervision.[29] They may be more inclined to "buck the system" or to change jobs until they find a working environment in which their expertise is more valued and rewarded. An escalation in turnover with its concomitant recruitment and orientation costs can dramatically increase the economic pressures on hospitals.

If nursing programs lower admission standards, yet maintain their instructional standards, the student failure rate will increase and the nursing shortage will continue. If admission and instructional standards of schools of nursing are lowered, individuals graduating from these programs will be less likely to resist being exploited and less likely to provide the level of professional nursing care needed to respond in today's complex patient care situations. If admission standards are maintained, but academic nurse administrators attempt to offset the economic deficit created by the last decade of drastically reduced federal support for nursing education by shifting their primary focus from teaching to research, future graduates may also be impacted. The risks are great of focusing too exclusively on the acquisition of grant funds and the accompanying status as a research university such grants generate. Replacement of the most expert translators and disseminators of new nursing knowledge (the teaching, practicing faculty who are essential for the preparation of new clinicians and the ongoing development of current nurse clinicians) with research and publication generators who have lost contact with the realities of clinical practice is a very real risk with long-term consequences. The outcome can be less time spent by faculty in instructional and expert clinical role modeling activities, increased professional conflict and competitiveness among faculty, and the relegation of students and their learning to a low priority position. Students in such an environment will have no exposure to the essential collaborative professional nursing role, will learn to compete for grades rather than strive for clinical competence, and learn to be successful students rather than lifelong learners. As graduates they will be at high risk for "reality shock."

Where nursing service administrators recognize that bedside/chairside nursing decisions are clearly linked with the cost effectiveness of their agencies' operations, major efforts will be directed toward developing new administrative practices that encourage and reward quick and accurate nursing care decisions, legitimize professional nurses as autonomous colleagues equal to other professional members of the health team, and provide opportunities and financial support for their ongoing professional development. Nursing service leaders such as these will increasingly collaborate with college and university nursing education leaders who have acknowledged the short- and long-term advantages of maintaining a balance between faculty who are scholarly teacher/clinicians and those who are scholarly theoretician/researchers. From such collaborative relationships have, and will continue to, come expanded preceptor programs, joint appointments, faculty practice, and clinical nursing research. All have been proven to assist in the professional socialization and clinical development of nursing students[30] and new and experienced staff nurses. The common recruitment and retention needs of service and education since 1983 have and will continue to stimulate even greater collaboration. Research on collaborative staff development programs for administrative and clinical staff and patient-care delivery systems to cost out nursing services and to assess the impact of advanced preparation of nurses on hospital and community based care will also begin to accelerate.

The new graduate entering the hospital nursing service of today will face the most rapidly changing, highly technological patient care environment in the history of the US health care system. Moreover, there is a greater diversity of health care professionals with whom the new nurse must interface in the provision of patient care than ever before. The "reality shock" experienced by new graduates who must make an immediate transition from a relatively predictable student role to a practitioner role in an environment in which the only constant is change will, for many, be a profound shock. Frisch[19] suggests that the "reality shock" experienced by new graduates is increasingly associated with the level of cognitive development demanded by today's complex patient care conditions, which exceeds that which can usually be attained by the average 20 to 22-year-old associate or baccalaureate graduate. Perhaps this explains, in part, why many other professions that require a baccalaureate degree for entrance into professional level schools are less often heard to complain about "reality shock" among their new graduates. Joint nursing education and nursing service efforts to expand preceptor programs, to develop faculty practice programs, to maintain a balance among teaching, practice, and research among faculty and clinical staff, to reinstate internship programs for new graduates, to initiate alternative nursing delivery systems such as primary nursing, and to utilize more master's prepared clinical nurse specialists and nursing administration specialists will all provide tangible means for enhancing the cognitive development levels of newer nurses and for minimizing the stressful effects of their transition to the "real world" of clinical practice.

Experienced nurses will also continue to be subjected to a form of "reality shock" in that the rapidity with which their roles are changing will exceed, in many instances, the available time and resources they have to learn and gain the clinical competencies their changing roles demand. The role strain and concomitant professional self-doubt engendered by such role overload has prompted many staff nurses to increasingly employ personal and reactive coping strategies, such as overlooking some of their role demands, changing their attitudes toward their roles, working harder and longer with less and less efficiency, and, in some instances, changing jobs or leaving nursing practice.

Nursing services that have developed or are beginning to develop active retention programs that include ongoing collaborative administrative and staff development programs with nursing education, joint clinical nursing research to test the impact of alternative nursing practices, delivery systems, and computer based information processing systems, and joint efforts to respond to the consumers' needs rather than the physicians' and the organizations' needs will reduce the incidence of "burnout" and facilitate the growth of professional competence and career, rather than merely occupational, commitment among these nurses. The increased incidence of creative partnerships between education and service for "work-study" programs (which facilitate the attainment of advanced nursing degrees while maintaining full-time employment) will also move practicing nurses closer to a full-time, lifelong career commitment.

THE CONSUMER AND SOCIETY

Education's continued efforts to prepare more nurse practitioners and clinicians with baccalaureate and higher degrees and the increasing willingness of many nursing services to employ these graduates in inpatient and outpatient settings have provided more cost-effective and higher quality care for patients. Nursing's various levels of education and levels of professional expertise, however, have continued to be confusing to the consumer. A united stand on the baccalaureate degree for entry into professional practice will do much to lessen this confusion.

The relationship between nursing education and service has been, to date, tied more directly to the growth and development of hospitals and medicine than to the public's recognized need for nursing. Collaborative nursing research, however, has begun to validate that nursing is a revenue producing, critical quality enhancement center, rather than a cost center. Nursing's basic commitment to prevention of disease and restoration of health places nursing in a strong position to respond to society's need for cost-effective, quality health care. Numerous studies have documented the impact nurses have on the quality and quantity of care in a variety of health care settings.[31,32,33] As these nursing research results become known by health professionals, consumers, and society, nursing will be able to extricate itself from its symbiotic relationship with the hospital and medicine and become truly responsive to and supported by society at large.

Nursing began the 1980s with its *Social Policy Statement*, in which it affirmed its responsibility to society and noted that nursing ". . . can be said to be owned by society, in the sense that nursing's professional interests must be perceived as serving the interests of the larger whole of which it is a part."[1] As the nation begins its movement into a public purpose era in 1989, nursing service and education have a unique opportunity to use this period of increased social awareness to form a lasting, mutually beneficial joint partnership with society to address some of the disparities in the quantity and quality of health care that will inevitably occur from changing disease patterns and the introduction of market forces into the health care delivery system. Nursing service and education must forge a common goal directed toward meeting society's needs. In so doing, they can better achieve nursing's needs. When nursing's professional service to society is legitimized and publicly acknowledged, by reimbursement comparable to its worth, recruitment of nursing students to nursing education programs and recruitment and retention of clinically competent career professional nurses will be assured.

Future Considerations

Where should service and education direct their efforts to achieve their common goals? First, nursing practitioners, leaders, and professional associations need to stop "playing it safe" by echoing the AMA's and the AHA's positions and take the lead in speaking out candidly and forthrightly about the magnitude of social and sexual diseases, such as elder parent abuse, drug abuse, and AIDS. Nursing education and service need to pool their resources and develop straightforward, factual programs to help citizens prevent and effectively and humanly deal with these and other widespread and public health threatening diseases. Nurses in all education and practice settings need to actively publicize and work to achieve health insurance coverage for the 37 million working poor whose employers do not provide adequate coverage, to do away with the "preexisting condition" clauses in health insurance plans, to decrease higher reimbursement for "invasive" procedures and bring them in line with "noninvasive" procedures, and to increase reimbursement for "cognitive services" that enable people to learn more healthful lifestyle behaviors.

Nursing education and service also need to publicize, in the public media, research results that indicate nursing's impact on health care maintenance and quicker recovery and seek and accept direct economic rewards for the success this nursing practice engenders. Nursing needs to unite in an effort to obtain legal legitimization, through nurse practice acts, of the baccalaureate degree as the entry level for professional nursing practice. Only by going public and assuming an active, participative partnership with society can nursing service and education unite as a profession and fulfill its social responsibility.

Nursing education and service can, through a variety of service-education partnerships and unification models, conduct joint clinical research, clinical staff development, and quality assurance programs, as well as support joint administration and practice roles.[18] Collaborative curriculum development for basic and graduate level programs that would be more germane to the practice roles of new clinicians and faculty would be a natural outcome. For example, in basic education programs, a curriculum based on nursing rather than medical diagnosis, and one in which critical thinking skills are coupled with more clinical decision situations would assist in moving new graduates to a higher cognitive development level by the time they graduate. The inclusion of graduate core courses in both education and administration would do much to reduce the role dilemmas faced by clinical specialists in service and education settings. In addition, the inclusion of computer, health policy, economics, and organizational competence in graduate programs in nursing administration would prevent our future leaders from having to seek this information by obtaining business administration degrees that socialize them away from nursing and into a private enterprise value system.

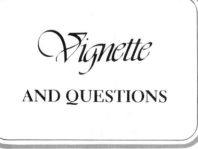

Vignette

AND QUESTIONS

Ms. Ashley, a master's prepared (in nursing administration) head nurse, has been working on 3 South, a 32-bed oncology unit in a major academic health center hospital for two years. Over the last year, the acuity of illness of the patients admitted to the unit and the admission of AIDS patients has steadily increased. The staffing pattern, however, has not been changed in total number or in the ratio (1:2:2) of professional, technical, and nonprofessional nursing staff. Nursing administration has just mandated that within one year all units will be converted to a primary care patient care delivery system.

Students from the university's baccalaureate program and one graduate student in nursing administration, in addition to students from two neighboring associate degree programs, have their clinical practicums on her unit. Recently faculty in the university school of nursing developed a faculty practice plan.

The mandate from nursing administration and the role overload her staff are having to carry convinced Ms. Ashley that she must do something soon. Ms. Ashley assesses her unit level needs and resources, as well as the resources available from nursing service. She decides that she has two major unit level needs: to provide counseling and staff development for the nursing staff, who are showing signs of increasingly nonproductive levels of role stress, and to determine if 3 South is indeed a candidate for primary care. When she reviews the staff development resources available, she is reminded that the clinical specialist position she shares with two other units has not yet been filled and that the staff development department is currently tied up with new staff orientation and new graduate internship programs. Ms. Ashley decides to call her school of nursing faculty contacts and explore options for exchanging resources. She contacts her university school of nursing faculty contact in the graduate program in nursing administration and also one in mental health-psychiatric nursing. Both, she knows, are doctorally prepared and are seeking clinical practice and clinical research settings for themselves and their graduate students.

1. How realistic is this vignette? Give the rationale for your answer.

2. In what ways might Ms. Ashley and her two faculty contacts develop a mutually advantageous exchange of resources?

3. How do you think Ms. Ashley's assistant director and director of nursing will respond to her collaboration with the school of nursing faculty?

INFORMATION SOURCES

For those wishing to go beyond the references cited in this chapter, the four reports from the American Academy of Nursing Faculty Practice Symposium are recommended.

Barnard KE (ed): *Structure to Outcome: Making it Work.* Kansas City, MO, American Academy of Nursing, 1983

Barnard KE, Smith GR (eds): *Faculty Practice in Action.* Kansas City, MO, American Academy of Nursing, 1985

Feetham S, Malasanos, LJ (eds): *Translating Commitment to Reality.* Kansas City, MO, American Academy of Nursing, 1986

Leadership in Practice: Taking Advantage of the Times. Kansas City, MO, American Academy of Nursing, 1987

REFERENCES

1. American Nurses' Association: *Nursing: A Social Policy Statement.* Kansas City, MO, 1980

2. Schlesinger A Jr: *The Cycles of History.* Boston, Houghton Mifflin, 1986, p23

3. Kalish P, Kalish B: *The Advance of American Nursing*, 2nd ed. Boston, Little, Brown, 1986

4. Kelly LY: *Dimensions of Professional Nursing*, 5th ed. New York, Macmillan, 1985, p38

5. Ashley JA: *Hospitals, Paternalism, and the Role of the Nurse.* New York, Teachers College Press, 1976

6. Ingles T: The physician's view of the evolving nursing profession—1873–1913. Nurs Forum, 152:139, 1976

7. Bullough VL, Bullough B: *History, Trends, and Politics of Nursing.* Norwalk, CT, Appleton-Century-Crofts, 1984

8. Kalish P, Kalish B: Anatomy of the image of the nurse: Dissonant and ideal models. In Williams CA (ed): *Image-Making in Nursing.* American Academy of Nursing, 1983, p3

9. Feshback D: What's inside the black box: A case study of allocative politics in the Hill-Burton program. Int J Health Services, 9:314, 1979

10. Quinn CA, Smith MD: *The Professional Commitment: Issues and Ethics in Nursing.* Philadelphia, Saunders, 1987

11. Litman TJ, Robins LS: *Health Politics and Policy.* New York, Wiley, 1984

12. Creason NS: *Effects of External Funding on Instructional Components of Baccalaureate and Higher Degree Nursing Programs.* New York, National League for Nursing, 1978

13. Ezell AS: Future social planning for nursing education and nursing practice organizations. In Chaska LN (ed): *The Nursing Profession: A Time to Speak.* New York, McGraw-Hill, 1983

14. Feathers DK: Relevance of Graduate Education Programs to the Role Enactment of Nurse Administrators. Unpublished Master's Thesis, Medical College of Georgia, Augusta, 1986

15. Halsey S: The queen-bee syndrome: One solution to role conflict for nurse managers. In Hardy ME, Conway ME (eds): *Role Theory: Perspectives for Health Professionals*. New York, Appleton-Century-Crofts, 1978

16. Easterbrook G: The revolution in medicine. Newsweek, January 26, 1987

17. Baer ED: Making the most of today's economic climate. Nurs Health Care, 8:143, 1987

18. Ford LC: Organizational perspectives on faculty practice: Issues and challenges. In Bernard KE (ed): *Structure to Outcome: Making it Work*. Kansas City, MO, American Academy of Nursing, 1983, p13

19. Frisch NA: Cognitive maturity of nursing students. Image, 19:25, 1987

20. Walker DD: The cost of nursing in hospitals. In Aiken LH (ed): *Nursing in the 1980s: Crises, Opportunities, Challenges*. Philadelphia, Lippincott, 1982

21. McKibbin RC, Brimmer PF, Clinton JF, Galliher JM, Hartley SS: *DRGs and Nursing Care*. Kansas City, MO, American Nurses' Association Center for Nursing Research, 1985

22. Nursing shortage symptomatic of changes in health care. *American Nurses' Association, Inc. News*, January 27, 1987, p1

23. BSN enrollments are falling at a faster rate. Amer J Nurs 87:529, 1987

24. Downturn in aid puts new pressure on students. Am J Nurs 87:532, 1987

25. UCLA study sparks debate over nursing's enrollment ups and downs. Amer J Nurs 87:531, 1987

26. National study shows sharp drop in the number of college freshmen planning nursing careers. Amer J Nurs 87:530, 1987

27. Christman L: Where are we going? J Nurs Admin 6:15, 1976

28. Maraldo, PJ: AMA hegemony in decline produces the RCT. NLN Executive Director Wire, 1–4, 1988

29. Poteet GW, Hodges LC: The future of nursing. In Vestal, KW (ed): *Management Concepts for the New Nurse*. Philadelphia, Lippincott, 1987

30. Kramer M, Polifroni EC, Organels N: Effects of faculty practice on student learning outcomes. J Prof Nurs 1:289, 1986

31. Freund CM: Nurse practitioners in primary care in Meazy, MD. In McGiven DD (ed): *Nurses, Nurse Practitioners: The Evolution of Primary Care*. Boston, Little, Brown, 1986

32. Knaus WA, Draper EA, Wagner DP, Zimmerman JE: An evaluation of outcome from intensive care in major medical centers. Ann Intern Med, 104:410, 1986

33. Master RJ: A continuum of care for the inner-city: Assessment of the benefits for Boston's elderly and high-risk populations. N Engl J Med 301:1434, 1980

UNIT III *Sociopolitical Perspectives in Nursing*

This unit presents various societal and political components of our environment that influence nursing's ability to meet the demands of today's health care needs. The chapters in this section address the existing inequalities of health care delivery; how diagnostic related groups have attempted to control rising health care expenditures; the diversification and decentralization of various health care delivery systems; how nursing is obtaining financial equity for services rendered; the development and delivery of home health care; who is responsible for paying for society's health and illness care; what deinstitutionalization of the mentally ill has done to health care delivery; nursing's participation in public policy formulation; and nursing's involvement in the political arena. It must be kept in mind that each chapter is written by a different author(s) and, as a result, the styles of writing will vary. The reader might find it helpful to read the chapters on inequalities in health care delivery and deinstitutionalization of the mentally ill as a set, to read the chapters on diagnostic related groups and the payment of health and illness care as a set, and the chapters on public policy formulation and political involvement as a set, since the contents of these sets of chapters tend to complement one another. After reading each chapter in this unit, the student should have a better understanding of the various types of societal and political issues that influence the delivery of nursing care within the health care system.

TRUDY KNICELY HENSON, PhD

CHAPTER 17   *Right or Privilege?: Inequalities in Health Care Delivery*

Background and Overview

In sociological terms, **stratification** refers to a system in which ranked categories of people have unequal access to desirable goods or services. In a social class system such as the one in the United States, inequality is based on different amounts of wealth, power, and prestige. This stratification of society as a whole then carries over into such specific areas as health care. The result is that people do not start life with the same level of health and they do not receive the same levels of treatment and maintenance during their lifetimes. In all societies some categories of people experience shorter lives, more illnesses, higher rates of specific diseases or injuries, and higher mortality rates than others. Some differences are genetically determined, but many are the result of the society's social structure and culture.

Prior to socialization into their professions, nurses and physicians are taught to be members of a society. That means learning the society's culture—beliefs, values, and norms. When a person enters the health care field, occupational beliefs, norms, and values are superimposed on the earlier cultural socialization. Professional education changes some values, beliefs, and perceptions, but not all. Consequently, it is not surprising that society's views are reflected in the performance and attitudes of health care professionals. They are reflected in the specialties pursued and in interaction with patients. Social attitudes and values are also reflected in administrators' decisions about locating care facilities and spending funds on particular kinds of medical research, training, and care. The following discussion examines some of the factors that influence differential delivery of health care and the consequences that it has for nurses, patients, and society.

FACTORS INFLUENCING STRATIFICATION OF HEALTH CARE

None of the factors influencing health care stratification acts totally independently of the others. Factors may reinforce each other or one may negate the usual impact of the other.

Race and Ethnicity. It is well documented that a patient's race or **ethnicity** (cultural identity) has an impact on the responses of nurses and physicians. Both race and ethnicity are frequently associated with social class, also. If the patient and caregiver are of different cultural/racial backgrounds, the possibilities for misunderstanding and stereotyping are abundant. Ethnic and racial categories may differ from each other on such factors as language, openness to being touched, willingness to seek care, amount of eye contact in interaction, home lifestyles, and even explanations for illness. Two of the best known studies of ethnicity and illness are by Zola[1] and Zborowski[2].

Zola studied Catholic, male Italian, and Irish ethnics. Patients in the two ethnic categories responded very differently to being ill. The Italians were more emotional and reported more symptoms than did the Irish, who were likely to ignore and understate physical symptoms. He concluded that both reactions were tactics employed by the patients to deny or dissipate possible consequences of their conditions.

Zola also found that physicians responded differently to the Irish and Italian patients. The Italians were more often assessed as having psychological problems in addition to, or instead of, physical problems. Since the patients were matched for actual illness and no other characteristic explained differences in patient behavior or physician response, it appears that the patients' behaviors and manner of conveying information to their physicians explain the differences in analysis by physicians. Patients diagnosed with psychological problems are often treated as if their physical complaints were imaginary.[3] So this response to ethnic Italian patients could have serious implications for their medical treatment and health.

Zborowski compared illness behaviors of male Italian-Americans, Jewish-Americans, and "old" Americans. Both the Italian and Jewish patients responded in a highly emotional way to physical pain, but with different motives. The Italians used emotional outbursts to get medical attention and analgesics, pain relief being their primary goal. Jewish patients, however, used emotional displays to get information from the caregivers about the future consequences of their conditions and medications. Immediate pain relief was not desirable if the analgesics contributed to future risks.

Finally, "**old**" **Americans** (whites with no ethnic self-identity other than American) were unemotional in front of others. Their concern about the implications of their illnesses and treatments was tempered by a desire to cooperate with the staff. They "reported on their pain," neither understating nor overstating it.

Just as culture shapes patients' responses to illness, pain, and hospitalization, it has also shaped the expectations of caregivers. If patient and caregiver hold different views, their interaction is likely to be unsatisfactory. A caregiver who believes that pain should be born stoically will not respond sympathetically to a woman in labor, even though her cultural background led her to expect sympathy and painkillers.

Zborowski also suggests that cultures create differing reactions to pain, depending on whether it is self-inflicted, other-inflicted, or spontaneous. Self-inflicted pain results from voluntary actions, such as tattooing or coming-of-age ceremonies, and is often a mark of status. In the United States, the reaction to self-inflicted pain is often one of "you did it, now suffer the consequences," or "it won't hurt long." Other-inflicted pain is caused by a second party, and may occur in a socially approved or socially disapproved manner. The quarterback who breaks a leg in the game is treated with social approval and sympathy, but a delinquent's knife wound, the result of gang warfare, is not honorable and earns little sympathy from society. (Within the gang subculture, however, it may have high status.) Spontaneous pain results from disease or injury that is not seen as intentional or self-inflicted, and thus warrants sympathy and treatment.

Cultural background and socioeconomic factors, such as loss of wages, affect decisions about whether and where to seek assistance.[4] Mexican-Americans often preferred folk medicine to hospitalization. The importance they place on being with their families leads them to avoid hospitals because patient and family are separated.[5]

In addition, culture affects communication between patient and caregiver. Federal statistics indicate that native American Indians have the poorest health of all groups in the United States.[6] Lifestyle and availability of health care are relevant factors in this, but communication problems between Indians and the usually white "American" caregivers exacerbate the problem. Native Americans feel "talked down to" when health personnel chide them about their personal hygiene and behavior patterns. Thus they defer seeking care unless the condition is severe. Such subtle cues as maintenance of eye contact, degree of physical closeness, and perceived level of respect all affect patient-caregiver relationships and subsequent health care.[7] For example, US culture views eye contact as a mark of respect for the speaker, but Japanese and Mexican ethnics show respect by looking down or away. The resulting potential for misunderstanding is obvious.

While **race** refers to perceived biological characteristics, rather than cultural ones, it is also often a minority status.[8] Race and ethnicity are frequently confounded by connection with social class. Studies suggest that blacks are less likely than whites to seek medical care, and that they are more likely to seek it from a clinic or emergency room than from a private physician.[6] Emergency room personnel see those who seek routine care at the emergency room (ER) as nuisances, and often respond with brusqueness, less than average care, and delays. These punitive responses in turn make the patient even more reluctant to return the next time.[9]

Nurses and physicians also carry the racial and ethnic stereotypes from the society into interactions with patients.[10] Higher status patients are asked more questions about their complaints and are taken more seriously than minority patients and this may result in inaccurate diagnoses. Such biases have the most impact on segments of minority populations most at risk, such as infants and children.[11]

In general, ethnic and racial minorities are likely to be received differently by the health care system than are members of the majority category. Study after study reports that minority patients seek health care less frequently and are likely to receive less than average quality of care when they do seek it.

Sex/Gender.   Although they have longer life expectancies, lower mortality rates at most ages, and lower rates of chronic illnesses than males, when it comes to health care, women are treated much the same as the minorities mentioned above. Women use preventive medical services more than men do, and are more perceptive of their physical symptoms.[12] Since women appear more attuned to their bodies and health than men, and seeking care early is valued by caregivers, it would seem they would be appreciated by medical personnel. After all, such health habits increase the probable success of treatment. Instead, Weaver and Garrett contend that women, like other minorities, "are exploited, abused, and discriminated against"[13] by the health care industry, both as consumers and providers. A glimpse of the differences in treatment of males and females can be found by comparing the self-descriptions of treatments given Sally Macintyre and David Oldman, both migraine sufferers who sought help from a number of doctors in different settings over several years.[14] Some treated Ms. Macintyre's headaches as a legitimate medical problem, but others viewed her as a mentally disturbed female who brought the headaches on herself. Her physicians recommended that she quit graduate school and undergo psychoanalysis, or get married and start a family. Mr. Oldman was also seeking an advanced degree, but no physician suggested that he marry and become a parent to relieve his migraines. Instead, they prescribed medication, acknowledged the link between stress and his headaches, and commiserated with him over this negative side-effect of a prestigious occupation.

Research on larger numbers of patients substantiates the differences in treatment of male and female patients. Armitage and her colleagues studied the medical workups of 90 male and 91 female patients by a group of male physicians.[15] (The patients had been matched on a variety of factors, including levels of health, and all patients were married.) The complaints studied were limited to dizziness, lower back pain, fatigue, headache, and chest pain. Although the only significant difference between the two categories was their sex/gender, physicians gave the males more extensive workups, especially for symptoms of lower back pain and headache. The authors suggest that since these females had visited their physicians more frequently than had the males, the physicians might have felt more knowledgeable about the females' conditions. However, the researchers suggest it is more likely that the male physicians perceive males and females differently, and that they share the cultural stereotype of female hypochondriacs and male stoics. Therefore, they take females' complaints less seriously than those of males. There is a substantial body of research to support the position that physicians view female patients as submissive and neurotic.[6,16] Research also indicates that physicians are likely to recommend unnecessarily extreme treatments for females (eg, an hysterectomy when antibiotics would do).

When health care stratification is based on sex/gender differences, caregiver-patient communication is often a major part of the problem. Women, especially minority women, may avoid seeking care from a system dominated by males. And when they do seek care, information exchange between the parties may be inadequate or misleading. Many of the complaints for which females seek medical care involve gynecological or obstetrical matters.[17] Even though these areas are limited to female patients and the problems of male-female communication are well known, these fields continue to be dominated by male physicians. So, not only is health care delivery unequal, so is the system.[18]

Women make up just over half of the total US population, but only about 25 percent of physicians are female. Female medical students disproportionately specialize in areas associated with women patients—gynecology, pediatrics, and psychiatry—and are under-represented in high pay, high prestige specialties such as surgery. In nursing, which has been stereotyped as "women's work," men have increasingly taken over the higher levels of supervision.[13] Studies continue to find that gender role stereotypes of health care positions persist among male medical students.[18] This stereotyping and associated communication problems pose numerous problems for women's health care.

Education.   Level of education is a factor closely bound up with socioeconomic status and its effects on care. Higher levels of education are related to longer life expectancies, lower mortality at most ages, and fewer illnesses and injuries. These are tied to differentials in lifestyles, knowledge of prevention, and exposure to environmental hazards. Educated patients ask more questions of caregivers and expect more specific information than do less educated patients. Less educated patients are more likely to settle for general assurances that they will recover.[19] Cockerham[6] reports that physicians treat less educated people more like objects than like humans who might ask questions and benefit from answers.

Social Class.   Social class in the United States involves access to wealth, power, and prestige, so it is not surprising that those in the higher social classes have better access to health care. A major factor in health care access and quality is ability to pay. Nationwide, over three-fourths of middle- and upper-class people have health insurance, but less than half of lower-income people have health insurance, or they have it only some of the time.[8] The elderly have some support from Medicare, but it is not sufficient for long-term treatment of the chronic illnesses they often suffer.[20] Medicaid, the federal health support for the poor, covers only 6.1 percent of the total population. Connections between social class and race are evidenced when 86.1 percent of whites have private health insurance, but only 61.3 percent of blacks and 58.6 percent of Hispanics are covered by private programs.[6]

Given today's cost of health care, particularly hospitalization, only higher income patients can afford to pay for care from their own resources, without help. At the same time, for-profit facilities are taking over an increasingly larger share of the health care market, and they are likely to be more interested in patients who can pay their bills than in those who cannot.[21] Consequently, public and charity hospitals, which have had paying patients to subsidize those who could not pay, risk losing their financial base. And even those who can pay initially, with insurance or Medicare, may not have enough coverage. Patients who cannot pay may be transferred ("dumped") from the for-profit facilities to public, nonprofit ones when the money runs out. (**Indigents,** needy or poor, are sent there initially.) Those who are uninsured and whose ability to pay is suspect are often required to pay in advance of treatment, even in emergency situations.[8,22]

Some physicians offer free or reduced-fee treatment for poor patients, but they provide a limited amount of such care and it must fit in around their paying patients.[23] Hospitals, even for-profit operations, have varying degrees of obligation to treat low-income patients, but the patients who need it may not have ready access to the facility. Hospitals in low-income neighborhoods are often teaching facilities that focus on specialties other than those needed by the community. For-profit hospitals prefer to locate in affluent neighborhoods, not poor ones.[21] Even general care physicians tend to locate offices in more affluent areas. A study of Boston[24] found only half as many general practice physicians located in lower-income neighborhoods as in higher-income areas.

These care conditions result in "second rate" care for the poor. They make fewer physician visits per year, have higher infant mortality, see specialists less often, and have little or no insurance. At the same time, they are more likely than other classes to suffer from more than one disorder at a time, to have more chronic illness, to lose more days from work due to illness, to be disabled, and to exhaust their insurance coverage before discharge, if hospitalized. In addition to costs and location, health care barriers to lower-income groups result from the structure of the system and complexity of facilities. Hospitals and clinics are large, complex physical structures where the personnel often at least "seem" impersonal and unfriendly. Lower-income patients are doubly handicapped by low levels of education and information, which increase the problems of coping with the care system.[8] Also, low-income patients have more child care problems, less access to transportation, and more difficulty and expense related to taking time off from work. These conditions are aggravated by long waits and the need for return visits. While the complexity of the system can also be a problem for higher-income patients, they usually have the advantage of a private physician to smooth the way for them by making admissions arrangements, and they have more skill at maneuvering in formal organizations.[25]

Problems of access are intensified by interpersonal barriers between lower-income patients and middle- and upper-class medical personnel. Physicians stereotype the poor as dirty and smelly, living unhealthy lifestyles, and not following up on medical instructions.[26] Lifestyle differences between higher-status physicians and lower-status patients result in miscommunications as physicians assume a three-meal-a-day lifestyle when patients have a different reality.[9] This barrier might be reduced if more lower-income persons pursued medical careers, especially as physicians and hospital administrators, but few lower-income people go to medical school. Those who do tend to specialize in primary care areas rather than surgery and other high status specialties that are positions from which to change the structures and procedures.[21]

Given this situation, many lower-income patients exhibit behaviors that further decrease their probability of getting adequate care. They respond passively and submissively and are shy about asking questions or challenging directions. They express hostility or are evasive or withdrawn. Such behaviors undermine effective communication and have a negative effect on caregivers.[9] The less affluent in the US tend to see their health as a matter beyond their control and, consequently, take little action to maintain or correct their own conditions.[27] More affluent persons, however, take considerable responsibility for their own health, in both maintenance and cure. A result of these class differences is that physicians often identify more personally with their higher-status patients and attend to their complaints and reports of symptoms more than to those of the poor, who are less like the physician.[28] This is in line with well-known basic principles of social interaction for society in general. We tend to like people who are like us more than we like those who are different. Here again, the dynamics of the larger society are acted out in the institutions of health care.

Social and Medical Worth.   Yet another factor that influences the level of care given patients is the staffs' perceptions of the social and medical worth of individual patients. Age, occupation, family ties, race, speech, dress, degree of cleanliness, sobriety, smell, and insurance coverage are used by caregivers as indicators of social worth.[26,29] Those personnel who encounter the patient first pass their perceptions on to other staff members. Ambulance drivers may signal a first impression by the length, loudness, and tone of the emergency siren and by comments made on arrival at the ER. A police officer who delivers a patient with the comment that the patient was drunk in a gutter sets the tone for others' perceptions.[26,30] Drunks are rather consistently devalued, and as a result their verbal reports are treated as untrue, they are shunted into side rooms and ignored, and "They [are] frequently handled as if they were baggage."[26] Shabby dress and absence of friends or family further devalue drunken patients. Valued patients—the young; those with families, especially young children; and those in valued occupations such as medicine and law—have been observed to receive better care from both nurses and physicians.[29]

Patients are also evaluated for medical worth; rare or interesting cases may get more attention because the staff can learn or gain experience from them.[30] Millman[3] observed that residents and interns in emergency and operating rooms often tried time-consuming or unusual procedures on patients for the practice. Extra attention can be beneficial, but in some cases it leads to injury or even death. Millman notes that conflict sometimes arises between residents/interns and private attending physicians, because the residents/interns want experience working with certain patients. They complain that the private physicians keep all the interesting cases for themselves and send only the commonplace cases to them. This may be especially true of patients suffering from common chronic illnesses. The residents/interns feel that treating these patients is a waste of their time, because it is not a learning experience and the patient is unlikely to ever recover. In fact, chronically ill patients, who are more likely to suffer from multiple disorders, may affect the mood of the entire medical staff. As the patient's stay drags on with no improvement or with furher complications, nurses and physicians spend less and less time with the patient, effectively cutting off even the emotional support of interaction.[31]

Even less medical worth is assigned to patients who are perceived to have no actual physical illness.[32] Such patients waste staff time and take beds away from other patients. Often they are further disvalued by being labeled mentally ill, a diagnosis that may result in failure to treat very real physical ailments.[3]

Overall, patient categories thought to have little social or medical worth may include elderly patients with chronic illnesses, alcoholics whose problem is chronic and thought to be self-inflicted, the poor and less educated who are not expected to follow orders once they go home, and those who have no detected physical illness.

Young emergency patients and those of high status receive more immediate and extensive care than do the elderly, welfare recipients, drunks, or those labeled "immoral" (eg, a young, unwed, welfare mother). Sudnow[30] observed a young child and an elderly woman, in roughly the same clinical conditions, who were brought to the same emergency room within a few hours of each other. A large team of caregivers gave the child immediate mouth-to-mouth resuscitation and used extraordinary lifesaving measures to revive him. The same staff left the elderly female unattended for a period and later she was pronounced DOA. The intern who resuscitated the child commented that he could not bring himself to do that to the "old lady."

Among renal failure patients, those who survive are more likely to be insured, "respectable" people with families and stable employment records.[33] Young, unmarried black females with lower-class appearance and speech patterns are likely to be diagnosed with pelvic inflammatory disease (PID) if they complain of abdominal pains and fever. The PID diagnosis in such cases includes physicians' assumptions of promiscuity, premarital pregnancy, venereal disease, or illicit abortion.[26] Such stereotyping often results in failure to give prompt and considerate treatment.

Neighborhoods of devalued people, such as the Haight-Ashbury section of San Francisco, are avoided by physicians opening offices, nurses looking for jobs, and administrators making decisions about hospital and clinic locations. Lack of medical services in such neighborhoods further intensifies the health consequences of drug use, poverty and malnutrition, and injuries from assault. When treatment is available it is often accompanied by lectures about morals and lifestyle, long waits, or police reports. Thus, patients postpone seeking help until their conditions are serious, or they treat themselves or seek out unqualified "healers."[34]

Even after death, disvalued patients are treated with less care than valued patients. Staff members practice inserting endotracheal tubes and other procedures on bodies of devalued patients, but not on children and others with valued traits. Note, however, that when a combination of valued and disvalued traits occurs, the valued trait may win (eg, when an elderly person is admitted to a *private* hospital, the financial cue may dominate).

Also, extraordinary steps may be taken to revive some highly valued patients, even after it is obviously too late. The extraordinary efforts made to revive President John F. Kennedy after he was shot are an example.[30,34]

In summary, disvalued traits indicate low social or medical worth and earn the patient minimal care. But valued traits result in average or extraordinary care.

"Good" Patients Versus "Bad" Patients.   "Good" patient-"bad" patient is one of the most frequently referred to sets of nonclinical labels for patients. Both in ER and inpatient services, hospital personnel expect patients to act in a certain way. Those who fail to conform do not receive the same care as those who do. But there is a catch. The rules "are seldom clear and unambiguous. You should help other patients but not try to do nursing work; you should have insight into your own condition, but you are not entitled to all the information; you are expected to be a competent patient, but in all matters medical you are assumed to be incompetent."[35]

This leaves patients to figure out on their own what is expected of them. And patients who ask too many questions may be labeled troublesome or uncooperative. They may earn the same label by innocently violating staff expectations.

Standards for good patients do vary slightly from the ER to inpatient treatment. By definition, emergency conditions should be seen in the ER. Patients using the ER as a clinic for routine problems are bad patients, and the ER staff is limited to more obvious and immediate characteristics for judgment. Inpatients have longer contact and personnel have a wider range of patients' behaviors on which to judge them good or bad. But in both settings, behavioral traits and such factors as appearance are used as guidelines for labeling. One intern described a bad patient who died in the ER as "an obese, alcoholic woman of Irish extraction who was very uncooperative and used very abusive language."[3] Her loud physical complaints were perceived by the staff to be the ravings of a drunken woman. She died before her negative blood alcohol test came back.

In his study of British Casualty Departments (ERs), Jeffrey[36] suggests that good patients are those who 1) make appropriate demands; 2) allow less experienced physicians to practice their skills or 3) to practice their specialties with quick results; and 4) present a challenge to test the general preparedness and efficiency of the staff. Severe head injuries or bilateral abdominal bruising are good for learning. Surgical cases allow specialty practice, including practice for highly experienced nurses who may be allowed to perform procedures usually reserved for physicians. A case requiring rapid treatment, possibly a team effort, is a challenge. British caregivers use the same criteria as their US counterparts to label patients as "bad" or "rubbish," the British term for "crocks."

A study of nurse and physician attitudes toward admitted patients concluded that patient behavior is even more important in the long-term care situations than in short ones. Staff members were asked to classify their discharged patients as good, average, or problem.

> Patients who were considered cooperative, uncomplaining, and stoical by the physicians and nurse were generally labeled good patients, no matter what their procedure or postoperative complications.
>
> In contrast, patients whom the physicians and nurses felt were uncooperative, constantly complaining, over emotional, and dependent were frequently considered problem patients, whether they had routine or very serious surgery.[37]

For example, a highly emotional and uncooperative 30-year-old female admitted for gallbladder removal was labeled "bad." A 63-year-old woman with terminal cancer was a good, even model, patient. She knew her prognosis and was matter-of-fact about it. The staff cited her cooperation and cheerful attitude as reasons for the positive label.

British social scientist Ann Holohan[38] learned the consequences of a bad patient label firsthand during her own maternity experience. Holohan was negatively labeled when she insisted on natural childbirth, although her physician preferred to do an epidural and episiotomy. After complications arose and a caesarean section was required, the label came into play. Holohans' great discomfort and high fever were put down to "feverish neurotic allergy," a psychological problem. When another physician later accurately diagnosed puerperal fever, bad patient Holohan was near death. Had Holohan died, Millman's research suggests that her physician probably would have rationalized that uncooperative, know-it-all, neurotic females are known to be unreliable reporters of symptoms. (The physician was a woman.)

Lorber concluded that nurses' and physicians' expectations of patients are products of the caregivers' own backgrounds. Their traditional middle-class expectations are rooted in white, Anglo-Saxon, Protestant (WASP) values. Thus, a good patient cooperates, does not self-inflict illness, respects staff authority, is stoic about pain, and does not make trivial or unnecessary demands. In short, a good patient is easy to manage. The patient who fails to meet the criteria for a good patient risks consequences that run from minor discourtesy to life-threatening.

Impacts on the Nurse, the Consumer, and Society

THE NURSE

The impact of health care stratification on nurses is a result of **role conflict,** the simultaneous occurrence of two (or more) sets of pressures such that compliance with one will make it difficult to comply with the other, involving three social statuses relevant to the care setting. As members of society, nurses are socialized to accept cultural norms and values. At the same time, they are patient advocates *and* members of a care team working within a formal organization—the hospital or clinic. The problem is that the expectations associated with any one of these statuses may be at odds with the expectations of one or both of the others. Then the nurse experiences stress until the conflict is resolved.

As a member of society, the nurse has learned a set of values, norms, and stereotypes. Nurses bring these values, behaviors, and prejudices with them to nursing. Yet, if patients are to be given equal care, all members of the care team must put their personal stereotypes and prejudices away and treat all patients on the basis of clinical indications, not extraneous social factors. In order to do this, nurses must first develop self-awareness. Once they know what their prejudices are, they can monitor their reactions to patients. This may prevent such judgments from affecting medical treatment. In this sense, nurses will operate like anthropologists who must try to keep their personal biases from distorting their research.

Over and beyond self-awareness and reaction monitoring, nurses must be informed about specific differences that result from ethnicity, gender, social class, and the like.[39] If Hispanic patients are common in the area, nurses should be aware of Hispanic culture. Where Jewish patients are common, nurses would benefit from understanding the future anxiety characteristic of hospitalized Jewish patients. A prepared nurse with knowledge of relevant subcultures and with good interpersonal skills is more likely to provide effective and equal care to all patients. Nurses who lack self-awareness and who apply the same set of expectations to all patients contribute to health care inequality with all its ethical implications.

Nurses are also socialized to be members of a health care profession. As such they take on the profession's dedication to patient advocacy, and pledge to protect the rights and dignity of patients.[40] This often puts nurses in direct conflict with physicians and administrators. Conflict with physicians is further increased by stratification of the health care team in which physicians have higher status, and stereotype nurses as submissive, associating them with the female stereotype.[41] (Ironically this puts male nurses in a double bind. Because male nurses work in a field stereotyped as female, male physicians in particular see them as deviant.)[42] Just as patients face the need to learn the health care game rules, nurses have to learn how to negotiate with others on the health care team.[43]

As nursing becomes increasingly professionalized, nurses face another impediment to patient advocacy. Professionalization is raising the status of nurses, but it also may be removing them from close contact with patients, contact that effective advocacy requires. In its place, nurses move into more powerful administrative roles and patient care is left to less qualified staff members and volunteers. Nurses may face the dilemma of deciding between higher status, power, and pay or continued close patient contact.

Finally, nurses are health care team members within a formal organization. And increasingly that organization is a private, for-profit operation. In this role nurses have specific tasks to perform as part of the division of labor. The goal is efficient management and care of patients. But what happens to "sentimental work," the emotional support provided to patients?[44] Taking time to talk to a patient and calm anxiety interferes with the work flow, disrupts routine, and puts an extra burden on colleagues. There is also the possibility that nurses will be given a disproportionate share of responsibility for certain undesirable patients, such as "crocks" and the chronically ill.

As a team member, nurses are both employees and representatives of the facility. If that organization implicitly or explicitly practices treatment inequality, nurses face an ethical dilemma—cooperate with the organization and compromise individual and professional values, or try to change the rules. How will nurses respond when a woman in labor is turned away because she has no medical insurance, or an injured child is refused treatment because the parents have no insurance or money?

THE CONSUMER

The impacts of stratified health care on consumers—the patients—has been described throughout the chapter. These impacts fall into one of two categories: access and treatment. Accessibility includes both location of care facilities and ease of use. As noted earlier, physicians and hospitals often avoid locating in poor neighborhoods. In addition, residents of rural areas may not have health care available without traveling long distances.[24] Relatively small populations in rural areas make these communities less attractive for large medical facilities and offer physicians less of a chance to specialize.

If a medical facility is available, patients must then negotiate the organization itself. Lower-income, less educated consumers have considerable difficulty finding their way around the medical organization and negotiating a maze of corridors.[9,24] In fact, anyone who is not already familiar with care facilities is likely to experience confusion and frustration at first, but better educated, more self-confident consumers are more likely to have the necessary coping skills.

If the patient's sociocultural background differs from that of the largely white, middle-class staff, miscommunication is likely to result in a "bad" patient label with all its consequences.[1,3,38] Once past these barriers, the consumer must possess legitimacy—valid medical need—and a means of paying. Without these the consumer risks being turned away. Even then, some patients initially admitted will later be "dumped" once their insurance, Medicare, or Medicaid is exhausted.

The consequences of treatment affect independence of action and self-esteem, as well as health and later return to normal functioning. The consumer must decipher the appropriate patient role, with little explicit help from staff members. Failure will result in a negative label of bad patient or "rubbish." A negative label reduces the probability of even average care. Patients are vulnerable to this social control because health, and possibly life, are at stake and there may be few alternatives for treatment.

Anxiety is further heightened by the difficulty of getting information about one's own health and condition. The more the patient is like the physician in social class of origin, the longer the patient and physician have been acquainted, and the higher the patient's education and social class, the more likely the patient is to receive desired information.[45] A patient without information has no basis on which to make informed decisions about the treatments available. The less the patient knows, the more control the staff has.

Issues of control and information access are directly tied to the impact of treatment on patient self-esteem. Lower-status patients report that medical personnel talk down to them. Caregivers assume that certain patients are incapable of understanding and following instructions and are unreliable sources of information. Such consumers may be treated more like pieces of furniture than like competent people. For example, pregnant women are sometimes refered to as "maternal environments," simply vessels to hold infants until a practitioner can bring it forth.[46] Patients who question staff perceptions or who fail to behave correctly may be referred for psychiatric evaluation and, thus, stigmatized. The consumer's future health and ability to function are also threatened by health care stratification. Some will receive only minimal care because they possess devalued traits. Bad patients may be released early to rid the staff of an irritant. Occasionally, lower-status and minority patients benefit from being somewhat disvalued. Miller,[47] in research on patients with head or neck cancer, found that physicians treated upper-class patients longer than middle- or lower-class patients before referring them to specialists. That might be because physicians identified more with upper-class patients. Such positive discrimination may result in a closer relationship between physician and patient, but those with cancer need specialized treatment more than they need a warm, personal relationship with the family physician. The longer referral was postponed, the less likely the patient was to recover.

Finally, at the top of the status differential are those whose high social value may earn them extraordinary lifesaving efforts. This can be a blessing if it returns the patient to health, or it can be a curse if the patient is kept alive, but at a low level of quality. Clearly the inequalities in health care have serious implications for consumers.

SOCIETY

Stratification in the health care sector reinforces and perpetuates inequality in the larger society. It also operates as a form of social control. Treatment of various categories of patients tends to follow patterns of inequality in other areas of society. This reinforces stereotypes and prejudices held by medical staffers who are, at the same time, members of the larger society. In some respects, medical theories and treatment even expand discrimination against particular categories. The social stereotype of women as highly emotional, irrational people whose function is reproduction and child care is strengthened and extended by medical practice. Texts used in medical schools often refer to females only in the gynecological and psychiatric sections. And medical students may be advised to concentrate on female patients' reproductive role and ignore their sexual needs. Full-time wives and mothers who report symptoms of depression, fatigue, and headaches are often treated as mental cases and advised to commit their lives to their families. Women suffering from stress-related disorders may be advised to marry and give up their career goals.[13,16] Poor, minority patients may be blamed for their own illnesses, if medical personnel judge their lifestyles to be immoral or inferior.[1,3]

Perpetuation of inequality wastes talent and productivity that could otherwise benefit the entire society. Those with little or no access to care die earlier and experience more health problems. Minority children have higher infant mortality rates and more frequent illness. This interferes with development and education. Later, minority workers, especially in lower-status jobs, miss more work days than others due to illness and temporary or permanent disabilities.

Perpetuation of social inequality also has a direct impact on those who deliver health care. Women and minorities are only found in significant numbers in the lower-status positions in the care structure. Women, especially white women, may be encouraged into nursing, while male nurses face prejudice, especially from male physicians. But male nurses tend to move more rapidly to the higher, administrative levels of nursing than females do.[13] (There is a parallel with public school teachers here.) Blacks and Hispanics are disproportionately represented in the lowest status medical jobs as nurses' aides, orderlies, attendants, and janitors. The highest status positions, physicians and administrators, are typically still held by white males. This not only has an impact on individuals, it also restricts the pool of capable people for decision-making positions. In addition, morale problems develop when people in lower-status jobs see their work devalued and their expertise ignored. (This frustration may be similar to that experienced by patients whose comments are ignored.)

It is easy to see how stratified health care reinforces inequality in the larger society, but more difficult to see how health care exerts social control, how it discourages nonconformity. Labeling a person "ill" has a tremendous coercive impact. It requires that the patient cooperate and accept medical treatment. Failure to comply may result in psychiatric intervention and court ordered treatment. Some have argued that the mental illness label, in particular, is a tool of the powerful used to prevent challenge and remove people who are in one way or another a problem for society.[48] Other institutions of society, such as the criminal justice system, have similar power, but medicine has added legitimacy by claiming scientific objectivity. Sick people are treated, chemically or surgically, and confined.

By turning authority to determine who is well and who is ill over to a relatively small and largely unchecked occupational group, society risks losing the individual's freedom to be different in favor of a kind of moral and behavioral uniformity.[49] In many respects, medicine has gradually taken over functions that were once reserved to other sectors of society.[1] Numerous types of deviance and criminality now carry a medical explanation, removing them from the justice system. Hyperactive children are medically treated with Ritalin. Aging, a natural process that took place alongside other roles and relationships in the family and community, has been medicalized and family members and friends have been all but shut off from offering aid and support. There are clearly cases in which medicine is vital to all these conditions, but many would argue that "medicalization" has gone too far. Reaction against this can be seen in such actions as the women's health movement, the home birth movement, and some hospice arrangements.

In summary, stratification of health care has a significant impact on nurses, consumers, and society. It perpetuates and legitimates prejudices and stereotypes within the society and deprives it of the full participation of some of its members. At the occupational level, stratified health care creates practical and ethical dilemmas for nursing professionalization—conflicts between advocacy and medical teamwork. And at the consumer level, stratification may mean that some patients experience personal degradation, suffer prolonged ill health and disability, or even die prematurely.

Future Considerations

Predicting the future is always risky, but there are four points related to health care stratification that are certain to be of importance. These future considerations involve the gap between social classes, the changing structure of health care, the changing age structure of society, and the social control power of the medical professions.

HEALTH CARE: RIGHT OR PRIVILEGE?

Residents of the United States generally assume that health care is a right guaranteed to them all.[50] Yet our previous discussion indicates that this is not the reality. In practice the United States is divided over whether care should be available to even the poorest or whether it is a big business. In many ways the patient today is becoming more knowledgeable about care and treatment procedures and options. And increasingly those with a consumer approach to medicine are seeking care from private, for-profit organizations, including the relatively new Health Maintenance Organizations (HMOs). This raises a number of important stratification issues for the future. Will the for-profit operations attract the affluent consumers and leave the nonprofit, public, and charity facilities to serve the poor? Will the profit-oriented facilities choose to offer services that have guaranteed income (eg, from Medicare), or those that generate large amounts of money because they are new or can attract research funds? Either choice will omit the less lucrative services, such as routine obstetrics and minor surgery. Will the trend toward for-profit hospitals draw certain kinds of medical personnel away from public and charity facilities? The private facilities can usually offer higher income and better working conditions. Even if the public facilities retain well-qualified staff members, will they eventually become demoralized by the large numbers they serve? Will these facilities become the ghettos of health care? Will the latest advances in procedures and technology be available only for affluent patients in private hospitals?[8,51]

For services and technology that are in limited supply, deciding which of several patients will benefit most from treatment adds another dimension.[52] If 20 patients need a heart transplant and only five organs are available, what will determine who gets another chance at life? Existing inequalities would indicate that older patients and those who are poor or from a minority group, or whose lifestyles are disapproved of by the surgeon in charge will have a low priority. Already there has been concern that patients who have access to the media or an influential sponsor, such as the President of the United States, may get preference over other patients who have waited longer and whose conditions are more serious.

Questions of right or privilege frequently involve government intervention. If health care is a right and a matter of social good, then the society must find a way to provide, and finance, equal access and adequate treatment for all citizens. If, on the other hand, it is a privilege—a consumer good—then those who can afford it will have care and others will do without. One in five people aged 50 to 54 in the United States is uninsured, and most of those aged 55 to 64 are probably underinsured. We have the most health insurance coverage, HMO membership, and other financial supports for health care when we are middle-aged and need it the least.[20] Federal programs such as Medicare and Medicaid do exist, but

> Federal policy since 1981 has simultaneously increased the number of citizens without means to pay for care, transferred responsibility for these citizens to state and local governments, and encouraged private sector competition for paying patients.[53]

Changes in Medicaid eligibility (aid to the poor) disqualified approximately one million people between 1981 and 1985. Most were the working poor and their children.[53] The question is what, if anything, will the federal government do to limit cost to consumers and direct policy for rationing limited resources such as organs, high-tech equipment, and research funds? Which disorders will receive substantial federal money for research? Will the funds benefit research on disorders of the elderly or the young, the well-to-do or the poor, those who conform to middle-class standards or those who have alternate lifestyles? The answers to these questions will have serious implications for such populations as AIDS and Alzheimer's patients.

CHANGES IN THE STRUCTURE OF HEALTH CARE

In addition to changes in the types of organizations offering health care, the emergence of new care specialties and the increasing use of technology in care will have implications for stratification. Clinical nurse specialist and nurse practitioner are two relatively recent alternatives in nursing. Patients express acceptance of expanded nursing roles, especially if it results in shorter waits for care, but it is not clear what the implications are for care stratification. Some express concern that nurse practitioners will become "physicians to the poor," while physicians treat the affluent. Others see these as promising signs that physicians are losing some of their supremacy and that new arrangements will allow patients a greater role. This is especially likely if these new caregivers are trained to be sensitive to ethnic and class differences in communication, attitudes, and norms.[17,24]

With regard to the increasing use of high tech to diagnose and treat patients, there is less agreement about the likely outcome. Concern is expressed that high tech leads to low levels of interaction between staff and patients—that it depersonalizes health care. Not long ago, caregivers could do little beyond holding the patient's hand and offering verbal comfort. Today miraculous cures are accomplished, but hand holding and comforting words are becoming scarce. Emotional support has a valid place in maintaining the well-being of patients and should not be discarded lightly. Some even worry that the combination of profit-motivated care facilities and high technology may end in a new "medical-industrial complex" in which both patients and caregivers are lost in the shuffle. Today technology can help people of all ages survive when they would not have only a few years ago. In many cases this is a blessing, but not in all. Humans must take into account one factor that the machines do not—what will be the quality of the life that survives? What impact will that have on society and the survivor's family? Will high-tech facilities make allowances for patient input and for differences among various subgroups, such as ethnic and racial minorities, or will all be expected to conform to the same procedures and be treated like inanimate parts on an assembly line?[9,46]

CHANGING AGE STRUCTURE

Societies are dynamic, just as are health structures. One of the most important changes already taking place in the social structure involves the age of potential consumers of health care. The United States, like most other developed nations, has an aging population. That means that an increasingly larger proportion of the population is in the older ages, rather than the younger. We have already seen that youth is valued in health care and that the elderly may receive less care and are more likely to be labeled bad patients. Consequently, the aging of our society is likely to have a major impact on health care. One factor is that as people get older they experience more chronic and less acute disorders. We noted earlier that physicians tend to prefer patients with acute disorders, which are more interesting and for which treatment has an immediate impact. What will happen to health care as more people live longer lives and spend more time in hospitals with chronic illnesses? Will medical specialties and priorities shift to provide this population with care, or will there be a critical shortage of beds and caregivers for that population? Will medical research shift to give more attention to the disorders accompanying old age? And again, who will pay the bills? Changes in Medicare guidelines have resulted in situations in which the elderly may become destitute from paying medical bills. According to Robert Butler of the American Public Health Association, Medicare was designed as if all the people on it were 40 years old instead of 65.[20] Will society experience a dramatic increase in elderly suicides as people try to avoid burdening their families with huge medical expenses, or will solutions be found?

MEDICINE AS A MECHANISM OF SOCIAL CONTROL

Not long ago many forms of physical and mental illness were attributed to demon possession, or viewed as divine punishment for sin. Gradually medical science redefined the situation and relieved the afflicted person of blame, placing it on germs and other factors largely beyond the patient's control. Recently, however, another shift has been evidenced, and it would appear that victims (patients) are again being blamed for their own health problems. Lung cancer patients smoke themselves to death; liver damage is caused by the patient's excesses with alcohol; AIDS victims seal their fate by being promiscuous; and heart conditions result from failure to get enough exercise or improper diet. Individual behaviors do contribute to various disorders, but this approach ignores society's role in shaping people's behavioral patterns. Earlier, we saw that health professionals take a dim view of patients who cause their own illnesses. A blame-the-victim attitude, therefore, does not bode well for those who may be perceived as causing their own ill health. It also threatens to increase the population of patients who fall into that category. As health care costs rise, will insurance companies force differential rates for self-inflicted and spontaneous illnesses? Will insurance policies cease to pay for illnesses that the patient could be supposed to have been able to prevent?[54] Would such distinctions benefit some in society at the expense of others?

> The important point here is which segments of society and whose interests are health workers serving, and what are the ideological consequences of their actions? Are we advocating the modification of behaviors for the *exclusive* purpose of improving health status, or are we using the question of health as a means of obtaining some kind of moral uniformity through the abolition of disapproved behaviors?[49]

In the long term this is an issue of freedom and could have enormous implications for the values and principles of society as a whole. If people do not voluntarily choose to follow health advice, will medical leaders seek to force their advice on the public? Medical experts once suggested that water supplies be fluoridated to improve health. The people voted and rejected the plan, but drinking water was fluoridated anyway. The medical experts convinced the government that this was a public health issue, and as such should be done "for the good of the population."[1] No one is suggesting that fluoridation was detrimental to the society, but the procedure used demonstrates how medicine's claim to scientific objectivity and the public interest can overcome the public will.

As of this writing, AIDS is an urgent medical issue for society. Current debate surrounds who should be required to have the blood test for the virus and what restrictions should be placed on those who test positive. The dangers of AIDS are appalling, but there is obvious reason to be concerned about the risks of damage from the testing. It risks creating a new deviant underclass that is subject to serious discrimination in social interaction, employment, *and* health care. The dangers involved with giving medical authorities broad social control powers are evident, and are likely to receive more, rather than less, attention in the future.

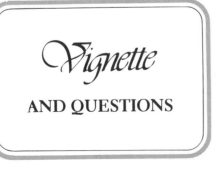

Vignette

AND QUESTIONS

Nurse Smith recently graduated from a baccalaureate program at a small college in the rural Midwest and has started working at Metropolitan Hospital. Mr. Goldman, a middle-aged Jewish salesman, has been one of Nurse Smith's patients for several days. This morning Nurse Smith requested a conference with Head Nurse Jergens to discuss Goldman's case. Smith explains that Goldman complains loudly about the pain from his hernia surgery, but refuses to take medication because it might slow his recovery. Smith is frustrated by Goldman's complaints and endless questions, and suggests that Goldman needs psychiatric counseling for mental instability.

Nurse Jergens is aware that Mr. Goldman's Jewish background and Nurse Smith's Protestant upbringing result in different definitions of the situation. Jergens wants to help Smith become a more effective nurse and, therefore, needs to address the following questions:

1. What information would help Smith to understand Goldman's behavior?

2. How does Smith's view of Goldman's medical situation differ from Goldman's view?

3. If Goldman is referred for psychiatric evaluation, what impact might it have on the care and treatment of his physical health now? in the future?

INFORMATION SOURCES

Harwood A (ed): *Ethnicity and Medical Care.* Cambridge, MA, Harvard University, 1981

Macklin R: Are we in the lifeboat yet? Allocation and rationing of medical resources, Social Research 52:607, 1985

Martinez RA (ed): *Hispanic Culture and Health Care: Fact, Fiction, Folklore.* St. Louis, CV Mosby, 1978

Strauss A (ed): *Where Medicine Fails.* Chicago, Aldine, 1979

Wolinsky FD, Marder, WD: *The Organization of Medical Practice and the Practice of Medicine.* Ann Arbor, Health Administration Press, 1985

REFERENCES

1. Zola IK: Medicine as an institution of social control. In Conrad P, Kem R (eds): *The Sociology of Health and Illness.* New York, St. Martin's, 1981, p511

2. Zborowski M: Cultural components in response to pain. Journal of Social Issues 8:16,

3. Millman M: *The Unkindest Cut: Life in the Backrooms of Medicine.* New York, William Morrow, 1977

4. Mechanic D: The concept of illness behavior. In Mechanic D (ed): *Handbook of Health, Health Care, and the Health Professions.* New York, Free Press, 1983

5. Madsen W: *The Mexican-Americans of South Texas,* 2d ed. New York, Holt, Rinehart, and Winston, 1973

6. Cockerham WC: *Medical Sociology,* 3d ed. Englewood Cliffs, NJ, Prentice-Hall, 1986

7. Kub JP: Ethnicity-An important factor for nurses to consider in caring for hypertensive individuals. West J Nurs Res 8, 4:445, 1986

8. Reinhardt UE: Economics, ethics and the American health care system. *New Physician,* October 20, 1985

9. Strauss A: Medical ghettos. In Strauss, A (ed): *Where Medicine Fails.* Chicago, Aldine, 1979, p11

10. Kurtz ME, et al: Teaching medical students the effects of values and stereotyping on the doctor/patient relationship. Soc Sci Med 21:1043, 1985

11. Reed WL: Suffer the children: Some effects of racism on the health of black infants. In Conrad P, Rochelle K (ed): *The Sociology of Health and Illness.* New York, St. Martin's, 1981, p314

12. Waldron I: Why do women live longer than men? In Conrad P, Rochelle K (eds): *The Sociology of Health and Illness.* New York, St. Martin's, 1981, p45

13. Weaver JL, Garrett SD: Sexism and racism in the American health care industry: A comparative analysis. Int J Health Serv 8:677, 1978

14. Macintyre S, Oldman D: Coping with migraine. In Davis A, Horobin, G (eds): *Medical Encounters: The Experience of Illness and Treatment.* New York, St. Martin's, 1977, p55

15. Armitage K, Schneiderman L, Bass R: Responses of physicians to medical complaints in men and women. JAMA 241:2186, 1979

16. Scully D, Bart P: A funny thing happened on the way to the orifice: Women in gynecology textbooks. American Journal of Sociology 78:1045, 1973

17. Fitton, F, Acheson HW: *The Doctor/Patient Relationship: A Study in General Practice.* London, Department of Health and Social Security, 1979

18. Quadagno J: Occupational sex-typing and internal labor market distributions: An assessment of medical specialties. Social Problems 23:442, 1976

19. Dodge S: Factors related to patients' perceptions of their cognitive needs. Nurs Res 18:502, 1969

20. Friedman E: The all-frills yuppie health care boutique. Society 23:42, 1986

21. Starr P: *The Social Transformation of American Medicine*. New York, Basic Books, 1982

22. Mullner R, Anderson O, Anderson R: Upheaval and adaptation. Society 23:37, 1986

23. Culler S, Ohsfeldt, R: The determinants of the provision of charity medical care by physicians. Journal of Human Resources 21:138, 1986

24. Sidel V, Sidel R: *A Healthy State: An International Perspective on the Crisis in United States' Medical Care*. New York, Pantheon Books, 1977

25. Nanry C, Nanry J: Professionalization and Poverty in a Community Hospital. In Strauss A (ed): *Where Medicine Fails*. Chicago, Aldine, 1979, p71

26. Roth J: Some Contingencies of the Moral Evaluation and Control of Clientele: The Case of the Hospital Emergency Service. In Conrad P, Kern R (eds): *The Sociology of Health and Illness*. New York, St. Martin's, 1981, p377

27. Cockerham W, Kunz G, Leusher G, Spaeth J: Symptoms, social stratification and self-responsibility for health in the United States and West Germany. *Soc Sci Med*. 22:1263, 1986

28. Duff R, Hollingshead A: *Sickness and Society*. New York, Harper & Row, 1968

29. Glaser B, Strauss A: The social loss of dying patients. Am J Nurs 64:119, 1964

30. Sudnow D: *Passing On: The Social Organization of Dying*. Englewood Cliffs, NJ, Prentice-Hall, 1967

31. Strauss A, Fagerhaugh S, Suczek B, Wiener C: *Social Organization of Medical Work*. Chicago, University of Chicago, 1985

32. Becker H, Geer B, Hughes E, Strauss A: *Boys in White*. Chicago, University of Chicago, 1961

33. Suczek B: Chronic medicine. In Strauss A (ed): *Where Medicine Fails*. Chicago, Aldine, 1979, p203

34. Smith D, Luce J, Dernberg E: The health of Haight-Ashbury. In Strauss A (ed): *Where Medicine Fails*. Chicago, Aldine, 1979, p38

35. Davis A, Horobin G (eds): *Medical Encounters: The Experience of Illness and Treatment*. New York, St. Martin's, 1977, p212

36. Jeffery R: Normal rubbish: Deviant patients in casualty departments. In Kelly D (ed): *Deviant Behavior*. New York, St. Martin's, 1984, p357

37. Lorber J: Good patients and problem patients: Conformity and deviance in the general hospital. In Conrad P, Kern R (eds): *The Sociology of Health and Illness*. New York, St. Martin's, 1981, p395

38. Holohan A: Diagnosis: The end of transition. In Davis A, Horobin G (eds): *Medical Encounters*. New York, St. Martin's, 1977, p87

39. Leininger M: *Transcultural Nursing*. New York, Wiley, 1978

40. Copp L: The nurse as an advocate for vulnerable persons. Journal of Advanced Nursing 11:255, 1986

41. Keddy B, Gillis M, Jacobs P, et al: The doctor-nurse relationship: An historical perspective. J Adv Nurs 11:745, 1986

42. Turnipseed L: Female patients and male nursing students. J Obstet Gynecol Neonatal Nurs 15:345, 1986

43. Stein L: The doctor/nurse game. Arch Gen Psychiatry 16:699, 1967

44. Reverby S: Re-forming the hospital nurse: The management of American nursing, in Conrad P, Kern R (eds): *The Sociology of Health and Illness.* New York, St. Martin's, 1981, p220

45. Waitzkin H: *Information giving in medical care.* J Health Soc Behav 26:81, 1985

46. Guillemin J, Holmstrom L: The business of childbirth. Society 23:48, 1986

47. Miller M: *Who receives optimal health care?* J Health Soc Behav 14:176, 1973

48. Szasz T: *Ideology and Insanity.* Garden City, New York, Doubleday, 1970

49. McKinlay J: A case for refocusing upstream: The political economy of illness. In Conrad P, Kern R (eds): *The Sociology of Health and Illness.* New York, St. Martin's, 1981, p613

50. Doob C: *Sociology: An Introduction.* New York, Holt, Rinehart, and Winston, 1985

51. Geraldine Dallek, *Hospital care for profit.* Society 23:54, 1986

52. Menzel P: *Medical Costs, Moral Choices.* New Haven, Yale University Press, 1983

53. Hughes R, Lee P: Public prospects. Society 23:63, 1986

54. Crawford R: Individual responsibility and health politics in Conrad P, Kern R (eds): *The Sociology of Health and Illness.* New York, St. Martin's, 1981, p468

ARLENE LOWENSTEIN, RN, PhD

CHAPTER 18 — *Diagnosis Related Groups: Controlling Health Care Costs*

Background and Overview

The implementation of **diagnosis related groups (DRGs)** as a basis for governmental funding of hospitals for care of Medicare patients has had a major impact on the delivery of health care services and on the practice of nursing. Although the law that began the widespread use of DRGs was designed for payment to hospitals and limited in scope to the Medicare population, the **DRG concept,** which is a method of classifying patients, has been picked up by many other groups and become widespread in the health care industry. Hospital and nursing administrators and non-governmental third-party reimbursers, such as Blue Cross, Blue Shield, and private insurers, are beginning to use DRG classifications for many purposes. DRGs are being used for quality assurance, by state governments for hospital payment for Medicaid patients, and for special payment programs of Blue Cross and private insurers. An important use of DRGs is in defining "product lines" for hospital and nursing management. Certain DRGs are considered as product or service lines, and hospitals are restructuring management to provide product-line managers responsible for seeing that care for specific groups of patients is efficient and cost effective. Those managers may or may not be nurses. DRGs are also being used to assist in identifying nursing costs and to provide new nursing care delivery methods.

333

Prior to 1983 hospitals were reimbursed for patient care in what was known as a **retrospective cost-based method.** It was believed that the total cost of a patient's care could not be determined before the patient left the hospital. After discharge the cost of services provided to the patient could be calculated, and a bill submitted to Medicare. The more costs incurred, the more money the hospital received, so the incentive was for hospitals to provide more costly services and keep the patient in the hospital. The DRG system, which was implemented in October of 1983 after the Social Security Amendments of 1983 (PL 98–21) were signed into federal law, provided a different reimbursement method for hospitals. The DRG system was based on a **prospective payment system (PPS),** in which fixed payment rates could be determined in advance of the provision of hospital services for Medicare patients. It was hoped that the use of a fixed rate system would provide better incentives to hospitals to reduce the cost of care and the patient's **length of stay (LOS),** which would subsequently reduce government expenditures for hospital payments.

Medicare came into existence in 1965 and government expenditures to hospitals began climbing quickly. The 1972 Social Security Amendments (PL 92–603) made provision for some limits on Medicare reimbursement. Under the provisions of that law the Department of Health and Human Services (HHS) also began funding projects to explore prospective reimbursement systems. Even though some limits were set on reimbursable costs, Medicare hospital expenditures continued to rise at an alarming rate during the 1970s and early 1980s. There was a real fear that the Medicare insurance system would be out of funds by the 1990s if no action were taken.

The **Tax Equity and Fiscal Responsibility Act of 1982 (TEFRA)** was an important first step in cost containment. TEFRA placed a ceiling on certain cost increases that could be reimbursed per case (patient) for hospital inpatient services over a three-year period, reducing the allowable costs each year. TEFRA established **peer review organizations (PROs)** to provide safeguards on utilization of health care services and quality control. The TEFRA legislation also required Health and Human Services (HHS) to develop legislative proposals for prospective reimbursement by the end of 1982. That was done and Congress approved the prospective reimbursement proposals in April 1983 and the prospective payment bill, known as Title VI of PL 98–21, the Social Security Amendments of 1983, was signed into law on April 20, with implementation effective October 1, 1983. The **Health Care Financing Administration (HCFA)** developed regulations to interpret and implement the law. Several modifications of the law and regulations have been made since passage and implementation in 1983.

Although the legislation was developed and implemented quickly, the process that brought about the change occurred over 15 years of experimentation and testing. The DRG system that was eventually chosen for use evolved primarily from a research project carried out in the 1960s and 1970s at Yale University, by Drs. Robert Fetter and John Thompson. They were interested in classification of patients by medical diagnosis for utilization review purposes, and they looked at hospital length of stay for patients in certain diagnostic categories. The diagnosis related groupings that were developed at Yale were used with further modifications in an experiment in New Jersey to relate DRGs to hospital costs and to develop a prospective pricing system that was implemented in New Jersey hospitals in 1980.[1] The use of DRGs is not the only method of classifying patient cases, but it was the system selected by HCFA. The original projects were modified to develop a system for national use.

DIAGNOSTIC CODING

DRGs are based on the diagnostic and surgical procedure codes from the **International Classification of Diseases—Ninth Revision—Clinical Modification (ICD-9-CM).** The ICD-9 is a classification system developed by the World Health Organization to permit more uniform data collection. The clinical modification (CM) of the ICD-9 codes was developed by the National Center for Health Statistics to provide a mechanism to present a clinical picture of a patient and to adapt the ICD-9 classification system to the needs of hospitals in the United States. The ICD-9-CM codes are more precise than ICD-9 codes. The ICD-9-CM classification system was implemented in 1979 and has become the single classification system used by United States hospitals. The system requires periodic changes and updating to reflect technologic procedure changes and new diseases. The revisions are carried out by the ICD-9-CM Coordination and Maintenance Committee, an interdepartmental committee of the federal government.

The DRG system also needs periodic updating. The **Prospective Payment Assessment Commission (ProPac)** was set up by Congress to monitor the DRG system and make recommendations for updating, taking into account changes in the ICD codes, along with technological and scientific advances, the quality of health care provided in hospitals, and long-term cost effectiveness in the provision of inpatient hospital services. Nursing, medicine, and other health care professions are represented on ProPac. ProPac is advisory and makes recommendations for regulation and legislative changes to HCFA and HHS.[2]

CLASSIFICATION

To classify a patient into a DRG for payment, the ICD-9-CM diagnosis and procedure codes are recorded on the chart and discharge summary by the patient's physician, with help from medical records personnel who are the experts in coding. The patient's principal diagnosis is used for classification into **major diagnostic categories (MDCs).** The principal diagnosis is not necessarily the admitting diagnosis, but the diagnosis that, after discharge, is considered to be chiefly responsible for the patient being in the hospital. There are currently 473 specific DRGs, and all but three are categorized into MDCs. Most MDCs are based on a particular organ system (Table 18-1). Once the MDC is established, a computer program, known as Grouper, uses the MDC and factors in secondary diagnoses, certain medical or surgical procedures, complications, and demographics (age, sex, and discharge status), to come up with a DRG for that patient and to assign certain weights that will determine average LOS for a patient in that DRG and the amount the government will pay. Table 18-2 lists the ten most common DRGs according to claims for Medicare payment nationwide.

The original legislation allowed age over 69 to be factored into the DRG determination. Studies by HCFA and ProPac have shown that **complications** and **comorbidity (CC)**, rather than age, are the major cause of increasing hospital services for Medicare patients.[3] A complication for DRG purposes is described as a condition that arises during the hospital stay and prolongs LOS by at least one day in approximately 75 percent of patients with that complication. Comorbidity is a preexisting condition that, when combined with a specific principal diagnosis, increases LOS by at least one day in approximately 75 percent of patients. The 1987 revisions of the Medicare DRG system are expected to eliminate age over 69 as a factor in assigning a DRG, but will retain complications and comorbidity.

HOSPITAL PAYMENT

Payments to hospitals for care of Medicare patients are now made according to DRG, at predetermined, fixed rates that represent average costs of treating those patients (See Figure 18-1). If a hospital can provide services at a lower cost than the DRG payment, it may keep the savings. Hospital services costing more than the payment rate will not be reimbursed, leaving the hospital to absorb the loss. There are limited provisions for payment for patients who have unusual needs that create a longer than average stay and higher costs. These patients are called **outliers,** and justification for the increased stay must be acceptable for the funding agency for reimbursement over and above the DRG rate. There is a ceiling on the amount of funds that may be used for outlier payments so that many hospitals have not been reimbursed for care, even though patients may meet the basic criteria.[4] Some increases in outlier payments were included in the regulatory changes planned by HCFA for 1988.[3]

Certain types of hospitals have received special treatment in the law and are exempt from the prospective pricing system, although there are plans to eventually include some of them. These hospitals continue to be paid on the basis of reasonable costs, but fall under the TEFRA limits for the allowable rate of cost increases. The hospitals currently excluded from

TABLE 18.1

Diagnostic Related Groups: 23 Major Diagnostic Categories

MDC 1:	Diseases and Disorders of the Nervous System
MDC 2:	Diseases and Disorders of the Eye
MDC 3:	Diseases and Disorders of the Ear, Nose, and Throat
MDC 4:	Diseases and Disorders of the Respiratory System
MDC 5:	Diseases and Disorders of the Circulatory System
MDC 6:	Diseases and Disorders of the Digestive System
MDC 7:	Diseases and Disorders of the Hepatobiliary System and Pancreas
MDC 8:	Diseases of the Musculoskeletal System and Connective Tissue
MDC 9:	Diseases of the Skin, Subcutaneous Tissue, and Breast
MDC 10:	Endocrine, Nutritional, and Metabolic Diseases and Disorders
MDC 11:	Diseases and Disorders of the Kidney and Urinary Tract
MDC 12:	Diseases and Disorders of the Male Reproductive System
MDC 13:	Diseases and Disorders of the Female Reproductive System
MDC 14:	Pregnancy, Childbirth, and Puerperium
MDC 15:	Normal Newborns and Other Neonates with Certain Conditions Originating in the Perinatal Period
MDC 16:	Diseases and Disorders of the Blood and Blood-forming Organs and Immunological Disorders
MDC 17:	Myeloproliferative Diseases and Disorders and Poorly Differentiated Neoplasms
MDC 18:	Infections and Parasitic Diseases (Systemic and Unspecified Sites)
MDC 19:	Mental Diseases and Disorders
MDC 20:	Alcohol/Drug Use and Alcohol/Drug Induced Organic Mental Disorders
MDC 21:	Injuries, Poisonings, and Toxic Effects of Drugs
MDC 22:	Burns
MDC 23:	Factors Influencing Health Status and Other Contacts with Health Services

Source: Health Care Financing Administration, US Department of Health and Human Services, Baltimore, MD

the prospective payment system are psychiatric, rehabilitation, and children's hospitals, designated psychiatric or rehabilitation units that are distinct parts of a general hospital, long-term hospitals with an average inpatient length of stay greater than 25 days, certain designated cancer hospitals, and hospitals outside the 50 states and the District of Columbia.

Psychiatric hospitals and designated psychiatric units in general hospi-

TABLE 18.2

DRGs Representing the Most Frequent Causes of Hospital
Admission of Medical Patients

DRG NO.		Fiscal Year 1986* RANK	Fiscal Year 1985 RANK	Fiscal Year 1984 RANK
127	Heart failure and shock	1	1	1
089	Simple pneumonia and pleurisy, age > 69 and/or complication or comorbidity	2	2	6
140	Angina pectoris	3	3	5
014	Specific cerebrovascular disorders except TIA	4	5	4
182	Esophagitis, gastroenteritis, miscellaneous digestive disorders, age > 69 and/or complication or comorbidity	5	4	2
296	Nutritional and miscellaneous metabolic disorders, age > 69 and/or complication or comorbidity	6	8	10
138	Cardiac arrhythmia and conduction disorders, age > 69 and/or complication or comorbidity	7	7	8
096	Bronchitis and asthma, age > 69 and/or complication or comorbidity	8	6	12
209	Major joint procedures	9	13	14
336	Transurethral prostatectomy, age >69 and/or complication or comorbidity	10	14	13

* Bills received through September 1986.
Source: Bureau of Data Management and Strategy, Health Care Financing Administration, US Department of Health and Human Services, Baltimore, MD

FIGURE 18.1

Computation of DRG Reimbursement

Diagnosis	Codes		DRG		DRG Relative Weight
Acute Cholecystitis with Cholelithiasis	574.00	→	206	→	.7735**
Operative Procedure					
Cholecystectomy	51.22	→	198*	→	1.1399**

Reimbursement Determination:

$$\left[\begin{array}{cc} \text{Labor-Related Portion} & \text{Wage Index} \\ \text{of} & \text{for} \\ \text{Standard Average Cost} & \text{"X" Area} \\ \$2{,}287.78 \quad \times & 1.2253 \end{array} \right] = \$2{,}803.21 + \$873.57 =$$

(Non-Labor Related Portion of Standardized Average Cost)

DRG Relative Weight*

$3,676.78 × 1.1399 = $4,191.16 (TOTAL HOSPITAL REIMBURSEMENT)

If No Surgery Performed:

DRG Relative Weight**

$3,676.78 × .7735 = $2,843.98 (TOTAL HOSPITAL REIMBURSEMENT)

---

* Operative procedure determines DRG in this category.
** Weights published Federal Register, 9/3/86.

tals were excluded because it was believed that, due to the wide variation in treatment plans within a psychiatric diagnosis, DRGs would not accurately predict the hospital services and resources that would be needed for psychiatric patients. Although HCFA is sponsoring studies in this area, no common agreement has been reached and the exemption is being continued. Alcohol and substance abuse units have also been exempt, but existing units are expected to be moved under PPS shortly, and PPS already applies to new units. Hospitals in Puerto Rico are also being brought in under PPS.

In addition to complete exemption, certain groups of hospitals have different payment rates. Rural hospitals are paid at a lower rate than urban hospitals, and sole community hospitals, those hospitals that are the only source of inpatient services for a specific geographic area because of isolated location, weather conditions, etc., have a special payment formula. When PPS was first enacted, four states were permitted exemptions because they already had cost containment or prospective payment systems in effect. Two of the original four, New York and Massachusetts, are now under PPS Medicare regulation except for a few demonstration projects in upstate New York. Maryland and New Jersey, where the original studies originated, have developed their own systems, and HCFA has accepted those systems for Medicare payments.

Patients in long-term care hospitals and rehabilitation hospitals do not fall easily into the established DRGs. HCFA is sponsoring classification studies for these patients. One such project in New York State is exploring the use of a long-term care prospective payment system that employs case mix measures and classifies use of resources into **Resource Utilization Groups (RUGs)** for determining payment.[5] RUGs are based on categories of activities of daily living, rather than diagnosis. Some long-term care, or skilled nursing facilities, have been included on an optional basis in programs that provide prospective per diem (or daily) payment rate, rather than a diagnosis at discharge rate.[6]

The prospective payment system and DRG categorizations do not apply to ambulatory care at this point in time. Many hospitals have begun to develop or increase outpatient services not covered by DRGs, such as day surgery units, in an attempt to provide revenue not under prospective payment. Studies are going on to establish classification systems for ambulatory patients. Other methods of reimbursement are used for ambulatory settings, such as capitation and preferred provider agreements, which provide set fees for care for certain groups of patients. These studies and systems are significant for future consideration as alterations are made to the current DRG system.

Impacts on the Nurse, the Consumer, and Society

THE NURSE

DRG based payments to hospitals have important implications for nursing in both hospitals and community settings. The incentives in this system are to reduce hospital costs and patient length of stay. O'Connor stresses that nursing is "the production department of any hospital enterprise, and must be at the heart of any hospital responses to prospective payment."[7] Nurses assess patient needs and plan and coordinate patient care. Nurses monitor patient goal achievement and response to therapy and use this information to evaluate and restructure care in coordination with physicians and other health care disciplines. Nurses assist patients and families in planning for care after discharge from the hospital. Nurses provide appropriate health education for patients and their families so that the need for future hospitalizations may be reduced. All of these activities impact and are impacted by the increased emphasis on cost and length of stay.

The assessment, monitoring, and coordination activities of nursing care provide information about the patient and family that is needed by the health care team to assess progress, to assess the need for additional tests and changes in therapies, and to evaluate patient and family readiness for discharge. The change to the prospective payment system has emphasized the value of nursing information in patient care. Communication and collaboration with physicians and other members of the health care team can make a difference in the course of a patient's hospital stay. This was demonstrated in a study that in some hospitals fewer patients died than a severity of illness index predicted would die, while the opposite was true in other hospitals. The difference in patient outcome was attributed to better communication and collaboration between nursing and physicians in those hospitals that had fewer deaths than predicted and poor communication and collaboration in hospitals where more patients died than were predicted.[8]

Prevention of complications during hospitalization must also be a major goal of nursing care. Noscomial infections are prime examples of complications that can increase length of stay, as well as being uncomfortable and dangerous for patients. Haley found that 32 percent of noscomial infections were preventable and over 95 percent of cost-savings obtained from preventing infection meant financial gains to the hospitals he studied.[9] Upgrading a DRG to include the infection as a complication did not increase the allowable amount enough to compensate for the additional cost. The study estimated that reasonable control of noscomial infections could mean a $350,000 saving for a 250-bed hospital. Nursing plays a key role in realizing those savings.

The impetus to discharge patients early has led to increased patient acuity in the hospital and concern that patients not be discharged before they can maintain their health. In his keynote speech at the National Invitational Conference on Costing Hospital Nursing Services, Edward Halloran made the point that conditions nurses treat are what keep patients in the hospital. He believes that while physicians may admit patients, nurses should be the ones to discharge them.[10] Nurses are in a crucial position to begin discharge planning early in the patient's stay, to assist in the determination of when a patient is ready for discharge, to provide health education to patient and family so that the patient can manage his care at home, to identify patient needs for community resources and home care services, and to coordinate available services.

Nursing and Cost Containment.   DRGs have brought about an increased awareness of hospital expenses and the recognition that hospitals are vulnerable to closure if revenues do not meet those expenses. In response to this awareness, nurses at all levels in the institutions have become involved in cost reduction. A major challenge has been to reduce costs without reducing quality of care. Hobson and Blaney demonstrated that nurses can make a difference in cost savings to the hospital in at least three areas: cost effective use of supplies, by increasing patient motivation and effective patient teaching, and by providing input into improving the scheduling of diagnostic tests and patient procedures.[11]

The adoption of DRGs and prospective payment meant that hospital management and financial information systems had to be upgraded. It was crucial that institutions become interested in identifying and modifying costs. Nursing has traditionally been considered part of room and board for reimbursement purposes. The advent of DRGs and prospective payment focused new attention on determining the actual nursing costs. Once costs are identified, specific nursing interventions and strategies for cost containment can be instituted.

The **relative intensity measures** (**RIMs**) study in New Jersey was one of the first programs to identify nursing costs. The study was initiated by the New Jersey State Health Department as part of the DRG prospective payment system trials in the state, prior to national adoption of the system. Mathematical equations were used to calculate nursing minutes of patient care according to DRG category.[12] Many other methods for determining nursing costs have evolved since the inception of PPS. Edwardson and Giovannetti's analysis of 33 methods of cost-accounting for nursing showed only three of the projects were published earlier than 1983. Twenty-two methods were based on DRGs, either alone or in combination with other methods.[13]

In reaction to the need to reduce costs, many hospitals went through a period of layoffs of personnel in preparation for prospective payment and as occupancy rates began to fall. Support services and nonprofessional personnel are primary targets when layoffs are considered, and this, in turn, has an impact on nursing practice. Direct patient care activities formerly assigned to other disciplines were returned to nursing.[14] The staffing mix changed as LPNs and nursing assistants took the brunt of the layoffs, although many hospitals did not fill RN vacancies and reduced the number of RN positions. The ratio of RNs to patients increased.[15] Nursing administrators preferred RNs over the lower costing LPNs and nursing assistants. RNs were educationally better prepared to cope with the increased patient acuity that appeared as emphasis on reducing length of stay began to be felt, and RNs were able to provide the flexibility that was needed as support services were reduced. In addition, many hospitals were moving to primary nursing, and that method of care delivery focused on the RN as primary nurse. Adequate numbers of RNs were needed to insure effectiveness of primary nursing.

Nursing Delivery Systems. As the staffing mix changed and the push for cost containment continued, new forms of patient care delivery systems were explored. DRGs required new hospital information systems, and nursing administrators have been challenged to use the information to examine nursing costs and seek more efficient and less expensive methods of care delivery. Halloran's research showed that nursing diagnoses were better predictors of patient's length of stay than DRGs, and could be used to manage staffing.[16] In his institution nursing information systems have been developed to use nursing diagnosis to assist with DRG management.

DRGs are based on medical diagnosis, and this is not always compatible with determining nursing resources needed or certain nursing care delivery systems, such as primary nursing. Some proponents of primary nursing as a delivery system emphasize the advantages of the system to effect cost savings. There is evidence that primary nursing with a high proportion of RNs can reduce nursing hours. Primary nursing has been associated with shorter hospital stays along with higher quality care, fewer omissions in care, and fewer postoperative complications.[17]

The New England Medical Center Department of Nursing developed the primary nursing system they were using into a system they call nursing case management. They found primary nursing was the best model for professional practice until the health care industry began to use DRGs. They noted that the increased percentage of acutely ill patients, decreased lengths of stay, and the development of case-based management information and accounting systems created stress even in the most progressive primary nursing departments.[18] Their nursing department developed a **case management system** that included primary nursing but carried it further. A case manager is assigned who may serve as a patient's primary nurse when the patient is on the nurse's unit, but if a transfer occurs, the case manager continues contact with the new primary nurse. Traditional care plans were changed and reflect projected timelines and critical paths to outline key nursing and physician processes needed to reach outcomes during a patient's entire episode of illness. This increased continuity and nursing impact by moving primary nursing away from a unit-based system to a patient-based system that considers the total hospitalization.

Nursing and Documentation. Appropriate payment to the hospital may depend on DRG classification. The admitting diagnosis is only a predictor of the final DRG. Staff nurses can take an active role in ensuring the correct classification by documenting changes in health status and being aware of incomplete documentation that may impact on the coding system or delay payment to the institution. Many hospitals have established DRG coordinating committees and created a DRG coordinator position. A committee or coordinator can provide necessary updates to the system, keeping physician and nursing personnel aware of system changes and providing a forum for problem solving that can increase nursing's ability to have input into the system.

Nursing and Revenue Production.   Shortening the length of stay of a patient has an impact on hospital occupancy and requires hospitals to bring in more patients to make up for the shorter stays. The competitive stance of both for-profit and not-for-profit hospitals has increased dramatically since the advent of the prospective payment system. Hospital and nursing administrators are establishing marketing programs and marketing services to physicians, who are the main source of patients for hospital admission, as well as to consumers. Studies of southern hospitals by Byrd and Watford both showed nursing administrators, from head nurses to directors of nursing, actively involved in marketing activities.[19,20]

Besides decreasing expenses, nursing administrators have been challenged to seek ways of increasing revenue-producing activities of nursing departments. Hospital nursing departments have established consulting services, continuing education programs, and special patient care programs to bring in additional funds to their hospital. The New England Medical Center nursing department established a Center for Nursing Case Management to develop and market their activities in the case management delivery system. Good Samaritan Medical Center in Phoenix developed a consultation service utilizing all levels of nursing staff.[21] Nurses have begun to recognize the importance of promoting the value of nursing activities to the health care system.

THE CONSUMER

With the emphasis of PPS on shortening the length of stay, widespread concern has been raised that quality of care may be compromised. Congressional hearings have been held to address quality issues from the consumer viewpoint.[22] HCFA has been required by law to report to Congress each year for the first four years following implementation on the broad impacts of PPS, including quality of care issues. PROs, external review boards set up by Congress to monitor utilization and quality of care, are administered by HCFA and differ from state to state. **Peer review organizations (PROs)** review hospital admissions and use of invasive procedures, but they are also charged with developing and meeting specific objectives in five general areas relating to quality of care.

- reducing unnecessary hospital readmissions due to previously substandard care
- reducing the risk of mortality associated with selected procedures and/or conditions requiring hospitalization
- lowering unnecessary surgery
- curtailing avoidable postoperative or other complications
- assuring provision of medical services which, if not given, would have significant potential for causing serious patient complications[23]

PROs are limited in what they can accomplish. HCFA is responsible for funding PROs and may have cost-containment objectives that may or may not be compatible with quality of care issues. In addition, although PROs have a substantial budget, the amount available for quality of care issues is relatively small and their responsibility stops at the hospital door.[23] The debate on how much quality the system can afford goes on. Quality care is difficult to measure and has different meanings for different people. Nursing is in an important position to provide input about patient care and define and monitor quality of care issues.

It is difficult to balance the cost issues against the quality issues. Consumer groups, such as the American Association of Retired Persons (AARP), have supported PPS because of their concern about rising health care costs, but are also concerned about barriers to access to care and quality issues. AARP has been concerned about "DRG creep," a by-product of the DRG system that occurs when providers manipulate the system by pushing patients into higher-paying DRGs, or encourage certain DRG categories of patients while discouraging others. The Grey Panthers, an activist elderly group, have shared their concern with Congress that DRGs provided hospitals with economic incentives to provide only the minimum care required to earn a specific DRG payment.[22]

SOCIETY

Early discharge of patients has meant increased need for home health services and a higher acuity level for community based nursing services. Patients may leave the hospital before nursing care goals can be met or before they can benefit from patient teaching activities. The impact of DRGs does not stop at the hospital door. Floyd and Buckle documented the changing population in their practice at Johns Hopkins as showing an increase in frail elderly.[24] These patients experience problems that require increased nursing contact hours and complex discharge planning. They reported that many of the elderly patients in their facility suffered some cognitive impairment. Malnutrition was a major health problem and unsteady gait, decreased mobility, and incontinence were problems exacerbated by complete bed rest during hospitalization. These patients require supervision and assistance when discharged to home. Joint planning between inpatient and home care services was important to address the patient care issues. They also found a need for education of both inpatient and home health nurses to address content specific to age-related health changes, communication styles, and teaching-learning skills.

Nurses in the community are well aware of the impact of prospective payment. One nursing director of a home health care agency developed a guide for care planning for home care that combines DRGs with functional health patterns adapted from work done on nursing diagnosis.[25] Classified by DRG for easy reference, the method calls for continuity between hospital and community to assist in planning for home health services and demonstrates how DRG information can be used in providing nursing care in the community setting.

Increased acuity and potentially increased physical decrements in the population being discharged from the hospital can create problems for families who need to care for these patients in the home setting. As societal demographics change and the aged population increases, primary caregivers for patients discharged to home may also be elderly and frail, with as many needs as the patients themselves. Women have traditionally been the group to care for their own and their husbands' parents, but many women are now working and cannot stay home to provide the needed care. Day care services for the elderly are limited and need improvement. Because of the increased acuity, changes in the traditional home care service hours may also be required, with service available in the evening as well as during the day. Communication between hospital and community nurses is crucial to provide continuity of care, identification of quality of care issues, and identification of barriers to access for health care services.

Despite the dire predictions when PPS was introduced, studies by the American Hospital Association and HCFA data show that the vast majority of hospitals have succeeded in streamlining their operations and improving efficiency. According to HCFA, those hospitals are experiencing substantial operating margins on their Medicare patients. HCFA's statistics show that hospitals reported 12 to 16 percent profit margins for Medicare patients in 1984 to 1985.[3] This poses an interesting problem, in that the purpose of the legislation was to reduce costs by providing an incentive for hospitals to profit, but when hospitals do show a profit there is concern that costs could be cut further if profits were lower. Punishing hospitals that have been most cost efficient by lowering their profit margins can remove incentives to reduce costs.

Future Considerations

The use of DRGs and prospective payment systems has both its supporters and detractors. The jury is still out on the long-term effects of the system, but there is agreement that health care costs will continue to be a major concern and need to be dealt with. Medicare expenditures include more than monies spent for inpatient care, and it is difficult to measure how changes in the system will impact expenditures. New regulations for the system come out each year and changes are made in reimbursement rates and costs eligible for payment. Changes in rates based on regional differences across the country, current amounts allowed for capital costs, and medical education expenditures are all undergoing revision and will be reduced. These changes will affect individual hospitals differently; some will benefit, and some teaching hospitals in particular will need to find other sources of revenue or cut back programs or capital expenditures. The potential for National Health Insurance rises and falls with political administrations, and the latest concerns deal with catastrophic illness insurance. All of these financing methods and system revisions have the potential for influencing the direction and use of DRGs and prospective payment systems.

The implementation of DRGs has made the health care industry more aware of the need for education for health care providers. Physicians and nurses can no longer focus on clinical issues alone. The emphasis on DRGs as product or service lines brings a business vocabulary into play. Knowledge of economics and marketing concepts is becoming important as competition increases and cost containment effects begin to be felt within institutions. The need for education is not limited to health care managers. Nurses at all levels are beginning to become aware of the concepts and their effects.

The use of DRGs has been spreading to other areas of the health care sector. Blue Cross is using DRGs to develop reimbursement levels for prudent buyer programs, special programs that can be contracted with hospitals. There is also potential for private insurers to utilize DRGs for reimbursement, and much work is being done in the ambulatory care sector to adapt DRGs for reimbursement purposes. Prospective payment is now being implemented for selected ambulatory surgical procedures. The use of **product line management,** a system of hospital operations and management that focuses the organization's activities on the delivery of a defined group of services to a specific patient, based on DRGs has been on the increase. This impacts nursing directly when changes in the structure of organizations are made so that nurses are responsible to physicians or other nonnursing management personnel. Although this is not all bad and can provide a better organized program for certain types of patients, care needs to be taken that nursing's input in the system is not fragmented and that nursing's responsibility to patients is not sacrificed in the name of efficiency. The use of matrix organizations that have nurses responsible to the nursing department, but also to a clinical program director, is one method that may appear more frequently in the future and has the potential to provide safeguards and standards for nursing care. Nursing managers can also serve as **product line managers,** the individuals responsible for the marketing and financial responsibilities of the defined-group of services constituting the product line. Therefore, they need to be willing to acquire needed skills to serve in that role, to accept that level of responsibility, and to educate others that there are advantages in having nursing provide that management rather than nonnurse managers.

Other methods have been suggested by health care researchers and policy makers to replace DRGs in the future. **Capitation,** the payment of a uniform fee or amount of money for each person, is being used in ambulatory care settings and pays a negotiated amount of money for a package of services. It has been talked about as an eventual replacement for DRGs and prospective payment. Replacing DRGs with other case-mix methods such as the severity of illness index and disease staging has also received attention. Researchers studying those methods have attempted to demonstrate a stronger relationship between other case-mix methods and costs of care than DRGs provide. Nursing researchers have also been looking at those cost-mix methods and comparing them with nursing classification systems and DRGs.

Severity of illness attempts to reflect the *overall* severity of illness of the patient, and not just the severity of the diagnosis. Severity of illness has a functional component as well as a diagnostic and procedural one. Nursing had input into the original classifications developed at Johns Hopkins by Dr. Susan Horn. Other researchers have made modifications and are developing the concept further. It is still a medical classification, however, and will not in itself classify patients for nursing cost purposes.[26] Although one nursing study of critical care units found a very high correlation between the nursing intensity measure used and the severity of illness index, the researchers also found that the addition of nursing intensity measures together with severity of illness improved the prediction of overall resource utilization.[27]

Disease staging (DSM) is a case-based classification method developed by Systemetrics, Inc. and Dr. J. Gonnella of Jefferson Medical College. DSM utilizes four levels of illness for each diagnosis, based on concepts similar to the stages currently used in classifying oncology patients: stage 1, minimal; stage 2, limited problems but significantly increased risk of complications over stage 1; stage 3, multiple-site involvement, generalized system involvement, poor prognosis; and stage 4, death. Sublevels are used for finer definition. A study sponsored by the nursing administrators of the Appalachian Council of University Teaching Hospitals was unable to correlate DSM with nursing care hours or hospital charges, but they recommended that additional studies with larger samples be developed.[28]

Regardless of the direction the prospective payment system takes, nursing needs to continue to be involved in identifying and documenting the cost and benefits of nursing care. At first the layoffs and cutbacks that occurred as PPS was implemented helped end the nursing shortage that had occurred a few years earlier. Over time that changed, however, and shortage conditions have begun to emerge again. This is a major issue today as enrollments into nursing programs have continued to decline, but the need continues for RNs in the health care system, in both hospitals and community settings. As the impact of PPS continues and patients are discharged earlier and at a more acute level, more RNs are needed and being used in community settings, further reducing the number of nurses available for hospitals. Changes in staff mix and patient care assignments in hospitals, as vacancies occur and positions cannot be filled, may impact on the successful implementation of developing nursing care delivery systems, unless other strategies are developed to increase professional satisfaction and reduce turnover.

Nursing care is an important and expensive resource in the health care system, and the impact of DRGs and new payment systems has challenged the nursing profession to demonstrate that professional nursing standards of care lead to efficient and cost-effective practice that can provide quality health care for consumers. It is crucial to the society that benefits from nursing care that nurses be involved in governmental policy decisions that have the potential to affect nursing practice. As citizens, nurses have political power that can be used effectively to promote a positive direction for future legislation and the provision of nursing care in the health care system. Individual nurses, as well as nursing leaders, need to harness that power by staying informed through research and education, actively participating in the political process, and communicating their views and experiences to the decision makers in our society.

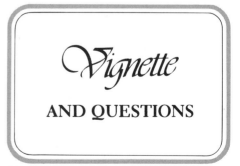

Mrs. W., a 66-year-old widow, was admitted to an academic health center with an admitting diagnosis of malignant neoplasm of the vulva. She was also a mild diabetic, noninsulin dependent, was somewhat obese, and had mild hypertension. She lived by herself, in a suburban community near her son and daughter. She was scheduled for a radical vulvectomy with the potential for pelvic evisceration, including bladder removal. Because of the primary diagnosis, Mrs. W. was assigned into the MDC 13 category, diseases and disorders of the female reproductive system. The ICD-9-CM codes were established for each secondary diagnosis and each procedure during her hospitalization. Four ICD-9-CM codes were used for the surgery itself, codes for the pelvic evisceration, the vulvectomy, the excision of lymph nodes, and the excision of peritoneal tissue. Additional codes for blood transfusion, other parenteral infusions, and a CAT scan were added. During hospitalization she acquired an infection of the urinary tract. The procedure codes plus the codes for the secondary diagnosis, including the diabetes, obesity, hypertension, and infection, were classified by the Grouper computer program into DRG 353, pelvic evisceration, radical hysterectomy, radical vulvectomy, and given a weight of 2.3887. The weight assigned represents the assumed resource use relative to other DRGs. The higher the weight, the higher the DRG payment. In this case the assigned weight assumes 2.4 times the average resource use of most DRGs. The LOS was computed based on geographic and average figures to a range of 14.8–17.3, with an outlier LOS of 32. The hospital was paid a total of $9677 for her stay. Mrs. W.'s actual stay was 18 days. She was discharged to home with home health assistance.

The weighting for this DRG showed that Mrs. W. would require a significant number of resources. Resources translate into cost for the hospital. Mrs. W.'s actual stay of 18 days was slightly higher than the average stay for this DRG. Had her length of stay been 16 days, the hospital would save the cost of two days. Computing an average daily rate for her stay, the hospital could save $1075, although in reality costs may be higher earlier in her stay than at the end. Despite that fact, the hospital would still benefit from reducing the length of stay as much as possible.

The goals for Mrs. W.'s nursing care need to take both cost and quality issues into account. Mrs. W.'s ability to resume self-care and take responsibility for maintenance of her health and prevention of complications from the diabetes, obesity, and hypertension need to be primary concerns in deciding when she is ready for discharge. Nursing assessment and nursing interventions can provide information and strategies to meet those concerns. Discharge planning needs to begin immediately to identify resources to be utilized in the community, so that appropriate treatments and teaching can be carried out or followed up in the home situation, rather than keeping her in the hospital. Avoiding infection and other complications during hospitalization will contribute to earlier discharge. Infection was not prevented for Mrs. W., but it was controlled early. Nursing's role in monitoring response to illness and therapy provides important information that permits early recognition and treatment, keeping further problems at a minimum. Nursing also has a major role in assisting Mrs. W. to resume self-care and to assess when she can safely accomplish that or when appropriate resources can be used to support her in her home environment until she can achieve that goal. The nurses assigned to Mrs. W. have a responsibility to her to avoid an early discharge if they have concerns that she is not ready. In that instance those nurses all need to be able to validate their concerns through documentation of problems and efforts to resolve them, and by developing an appropriate plan of care with time frames and alternative strategies.

1. How can nursing and/or hospital quality assurance be utilized in evaluation of this patient's care?

2. Who should be involved in discharge planning for Mrs. W.?

3. What mechanisms can be set up for communication between the unit staff and community resources utilized for Mrs. W.?

4. How can feedback regarding Mrs. W.'s course at home be provided to the unit staff? Why is that important in looking at prospective payment issues?

5. What information needs to be available to nursing management to promote cost containment and cost-effective care?

6. What information needs to be available to staff nurses to promote cost containment and cost-effective care?

7. What strategies can nurses use to balance cost containment with the provision of quality care?

8. What strategies can nurses use to promote involvement in policy making decisions that impact the provision of nursing care?

INFORMATION SOURCES

National League for Nursing supplies books and other publications on DRGs and nursing.

National League for Nursing
10 Columbus Circle
New York, NY 10019

Shaffer FA (ed): *Patients and Purse Strings: Patient Classification and Cost Management.* New York, National League for Nursing, 1986

Shaffer FA (ed): *DRGs: Changes and Challenges.* New York, National League for Nursing, 1984

A New Era for Nursing. Videocassette. New York, National League for Nursing, 1984

American Nurses' Association provides publications and research reports on DRGs and nursing.

American Nurses' Association
2420 Pershing Road
Kansas City, MO 64108

For an in-depth report on DRGs see:

Caterinicchio RP: *DRGs: What they are and how to survive them.* Thorofare, NJ, Slack, 1984
Office of Technology Assessment, Congress of the United States: *Medicare's Prospective Payment System.* New York, Springer, 1986
Spiegel A, Kavaler F: *Cost containment and DRGs: A guide to prospective payment.* Owings Mills, MD, National Health Publishing, 1986

The US Government provides publications, research reports and agency and congressional reports. HCFA, a division of HHS, publishes proposed regulation changes and impact statements in the *Federal Register.*

Superintendent of Documents
US Government Printing Office
Washington, DC 20402

Health Care Financing Administration (HCFA)
200 Independence Ave, SW
Washington, DC 20201

Nursing journals oriented to management, professional, and clinical issues frequently include articles on DRGs. Medical journals and the following journals outside of nursing may also be helpful.

Healthcare Financial Management
Hospitals
Health Care Financing Review

REFERENCES

1. Bentley J, Butler P: Case mix reimbursement: Measures, applications, experiments. Healthcare Financial Management 34:27, 1980

2. Prospective Payment Assessment Commission: Third Annual Report. Federal Register 52:22169, June 10, 1987

3. Health Care Financing Administration. Medicare program: Changes to the inpatient hospital prospective payment system. Federal Register, 52:22080, June 10, 1987

4. Spiegel A, Kavaler F: *Cost containment and DRGs: A guide to prospective payment.* Owings Mills, MD, National Health Publishing, 1986

5. Mitty E: Prospective payment and long-term care: Linking payments to resource use. Nsg Health Care 8:14, 1987

6. Grimaldi P: Prospective payment begins for medicare SNF care. Nsg Mgmt 18:17, 1987

7. O'Connor P: Health care financing policy: Impact on nursing. Nsg Admin Quar 8:19, 1984

8. Knaus WA, Draper EA, Wagner DF, Zimmerman JE: An Evaluation of outcome from intensive care in major medical centers. Ann Inter Med 104:410, 1986

9. Haley RW, White JW, Culver DH, Hughes JM: The financial incentive for hospitals to prevent noscomial infections under the prospective payment system. JAMA 257:1611, 1987

10. Nurses identify reasonable costs of care. Amer Nurse, June, 1987

11. Hobson CJ, Blaney DR: Techniques that cut costs, not care. AJN 87:185, 1987

12. Grimaldi P: DRGs and nursing administration. Nsg Mgmt 13:30, 1982

13. Edwardson SR, Giovannetti, PB: A review of cost-accounting methods for nursing services. Nsg Econ 5:107, 1987

14. Sovie MD: Managing nursing resources in a constrained economic environment. Nsg Econ 3:85, 1985

15. Booth RZ: Financing mechanism for health care: Impact on nursing services. J Prof Nsg 1:34, 1985

16. Halloran EJ, Patterson C, Kiley, ML: Case-mix: Matching patient need with nursing resources. Nsg Mgmt 18:27, 1987

17. van Servellen GM, Mowry MM: DRGs and primary nursing: Are they compatible? JONA 15:32, 1985

18. Zander K: Nursing case management: A classic. *Definition: The Center for Nursing Case Management.* Newsletter of the New England Medical Center Department of Nursing 2:1, 1987

19. Byrd LA: *Marketing emergency services: The degree of involvement among nurse executives.* Master's Thesis, Med Col of GA, 1986.

20. Watford D: *Marketing hospital based obstetrical services: The degree of involvement among nurse executives.* Master's Thesis, Med Col of GA, 1987

21. Anderson R: Alternative revenue sources for nursing departments. JONA 15:9, 1985

22. US Congress, House of Representatives, Select Committee on Aging, *Hearing* on *Sustaining quality health care under cost containment*, H.R. 499, Feb. 26, 1985 (Washington, DC:US Government Printing Office, 1985)

23. Office of Technology Assessment, Congress of the United States. *Medicare's Prospective Payment System.* New York, Springer, 1986

24. Floyd J, Buckle J: Nursing care of the elderly: The DRG influence. J. Gerontological Nsg 13:20, 1987

25. Birmingham JJ: *Home Care Planning Based on DRGs: Functional Health Pattern Model.* Bethany, MD, Fleschner, Philadelphia, Lippincott, 1986

26. Giovannetti P: Where do we go from here? In Schaffer FA (ed): *Patients and Purse Strings: Patient Classification and Cost Management.* New York, National League for Nursing, Pub No. 20-2155, 1986, p349

27. Lucke K, Lucke J: Severity of illness and nursing intensity as predictors of treatment costs. In Schaffer FA(ed): *Patients and Purse Strings: Patient Classification and Cost Management.* New York, National League for Nursing, Pub No. 20-2155, 1986, p181

28. Sherman J: DRG 001: A multihospital comparison. Nsg Mgmt 17:11, 1986

CONNIE R. CURRAN, RN, EdD, FAAN

CHAPTER 19 *Systems of Health Care Delivery: Their Diversification and Decentralization*

Background and Overview

In the past five years, the American public has witnessed more changes in the health care system than in the previous 50 years. There has been heightened awareness among health professionals and consumers alike to critically examine the nature and distribution of health resources in this country, as well as the methods of delivery and reimbursement for health care. Lacking in a comprehensive, coordinated approach to the delivery of health services, many health care providers and consumers have questioned the actual existence of a health care delivery "system" in this country. Thus it is imperative for nurses to develop an understanding of salient issues that surround the various health care delivery systems and of the social forces that influence the nurse's role in those systems.

It is the purpose of this chapter to provide a brief overview of some of the major types of health care delivery systems presently operating in the United States, including: hospitals, nursing homes, home health care institutions, health maintenance organizations (HMOs), and ambulatory care settings. Following the presentation of these health care delivery systems, the impact that the "corporatization" of health care has had on the nurse, the consumer, and society will be examined. The chapter will conclude with speculations about the future of health care delivery systems and provide a vignette for analysis and discussion.

TYPES OF HEALTH CARE DELIVERY SYSTEMS

Hospitals.   The first hospitals in Europe were religious and charitable in nature and served as a refuge for the sick who sought care for their ailments. The church provided shelter and supplies needed to care for the sick, while the actual patient care was provided by members of the congregation. The term "angels of mercy" was coined by the recipients of that care to describe the women of the church who gave so freely of their time to meet the needs of the ill.

The religious influence of the early European hospitals was felt by the first hospitals in America. This influence was noted in the provision of care, food, and shelter, not only for the ill, but also for the poor. However, in 1751, the first voluntary hospital, Pennsylvania Hospital, was founded in Philadelphia and marked the first separation of the caring for the sick from the caring for the poor.

In the late 1800s advances in asepsis, surgical anesthesia, and the training of nurses began to influence the effectiveness of care provided by hospitals. Medical care was becoming increasingly complex and physicians were finding that they no longer could independently handle patient care demands and thus turned to hospitals for the new technology and the provision of care provided by trained nurses. As a result, hospitals increased from 178 in 1873 to more than 4300 in 1909[1] with the average patient's bill being less than $10.00 a day.[2]

In an effort to provide for a more equal distribution of hospitals across the nation, the Hill-Burton Act of 1946 was passed and federal funds became available for hospital construction. Thousands of hospitals were built in small towns and rural communities throughout the country. Hospital insurance became an employee benefit; and it was during this time that the Blue Cross system was developed to assist with inpatient hospital care. In an attempt to meet the financial demands of health care for the poor and the elderly, Medicare and Medicaid programs were developed in 1965. As more and more Americans utilized either private insurance or Medicare and Medicaid coverage, hospitals continued to expand.

As a result of hospital expansion, hospital care has become big business. In 1985 there were 5732 hospitals; of these, 45 percent had fewer than 100 beds, 45 percent had between 100 and 400 beds, and only 10 percent had more than 400 beds.[3] In that same year the total hospital revenues reached $138 billion with outpatient revenue alone comprising $26.3 billion. These high outpatient revenues reflect the rapid growth in ambulatory care services. The average cost of hospital care by this time was $460.19 a day, a 12 percent increase from 1983.

A revolutionary change in the way hospitals were paid occurred in 1982, with the Tax Equity Fiscal Responsibility Act (TEFRA). Until 1982, hospitals were reimbursed for the costs of their services retrospectively. This system resulted in annual increases in health care expenditures until they accounted for 11.6 percent of the country's gross national product. In an attempt to control costs, a prospective reimbursement system was developed, diagnostic related groups (DRGs). The DRGs are based upon average lengths of hospitalization for various illnesses and procedures and, based upon these estimates, the hospital is paid a prospective fee. If the hospital can provide care for less than the fee, it is permitted to keep the excess. However, if the hospital charges exceed the fee, it must absorb the financial loss. The prospective reimbursement system has caused many hospital financial officers to examine the efficiency of their hospital's rendered services.

In the first three years of prospective reimbursement, inpatient days dropped by nearly one-third. This decrease in patient days, combined with the 1950s increase in the number of hospitals, resulted in large increases in hospital bed vacancies. Consequently, about ten percent of the country's hospitals closed. In an attempt to keep economically solvent and competitive in the marketplace, many other hospitals joined together to form **multihospital systems.** Today, one out of three of the nation's hospitals belongs to such a system.

Two methods of organizing a multihospital system exist and these include horizontal and vertical integration. **Horizontal integration** is one that involves sharing, cooperation, or merger of *like* institutions, whereas **vertical integration** includes the linkage of *unlike* institutions. Vertical integration is a complex system that combines resource development, manufacturing, distribution, and consumption.[4] In health care, a system of vertically integrated services might include primary, secondary, tertiary, rehabilitative, and custodial care. One provider is capable of delivering potentially all of the services a patient might require during an illness, or perhaps in a lifetime. Proponents of such a concept agree that this is an economical and efficient method of delivering high quality, accessible health care.

Why are multihospital systems such an attractive solution to hospital management problems? It has become advantageous for hospitals in close physical proximity to collaborate rather than compete. Analysis of community needs often reveals that the volume of patients justifies one service in an area, rather than two. Additionally, large chains of hospitals can save millions of dollars through group purchasing arrangements. By joining together and purchasing large quantities of supplies, hospitals are able to negotiate lower costs. Furthermore, entering a joint venture might facilitate sharing of highly specialized personnel, often in short supply. Whatever the motive, it is likely that multihospital systems will continue to emerge and dominate the marketplace by 1995.

Nursing Homes.   Nursing homes are the dominant long-term care institutions in the United States. Approximately 2.4 million Americans use this service annually.[5] Roughly five percent of all persons aged 65 and over currently reside in some type of nursing home. It is estimated that 20 percent of all elderly will spend some time in a nursing home before they die. As the population ages and the incidence of chronic diseases increases, the number and proportion of elderly seeking admission to nursing homes also will rise. With the advent of a prospective payment system, new demands are being placed on nursing homes. Hospital stays have been reduced and, thus, patients are being transferred to nursing homes in more acute states of illness.

The passage of Medicare and Medicaid in 1965 provided public monies for nursing home care, which resulted in accelerated growth in the nursing home industry. In the early 1960s there were just over 8000 nursing homes and 300,000 beds, whereas by 1969 there were 11,465 nursing homes and over 800,000 beds.[6] In 1980 there were close to 23,000 nursing and related care homes with just under 1.5 million beds and 1.4 million residents.[7] Despite these increases, there continues to be a shortage of nursing home beds in many regions of the country. Although less of a concern for private paying patients, many patients dependent on Medicare and Medicaid have faced serious nursing home placement problems.

Another consequence of Medicare and Medicaid has been the establishment of definitions as to the types of institutions providing nursing home care in order to determine eligibility for federal reimbursement. Additionally, guidelines were needed to govern and assure quality of patient care within these homes. Nursing homes became classified according to the complexity of care they provided. **Skilled nursing facilities** (**SNFs**) provide 24-hour nursing services under the supervision of a physician. This type of setting generally cares for convalescent patients and those with long-term illnesses. **Intermediate care facilities** (**ICFs**) provide for patients who require less intensive care. Nursing services are available, but not around the clock. Residents of ICFs are typically not capable of living independently, but do not require 24-hour nursing care. Both facilities are certified and meet federal standards within the meaning of the Social Security Act. Medicare will reimburse only SNFs, but Medicaid will reimburse both SNFs and ICFs. The average length of stay in a nursing home is 75 days, which reflects the large number of short, SNF stays. These short stays are posthospitalization for recuperation and rehabilitation.

The majority of nursing home staff consist of nurses' aides, not registered nurses. Hospitals are staffed at a rate of 3 staff per patient, while nursing homes are staffed at a 0.5 staff to patient ratio. Thus the factors of a low staff to patient ratio and a largely nonprofessional staff make nursing home costs much less than hospital costs. However, from 1960 to 1980, nursing home expenditures in this country soared from $500 million[8] to $24 billion.[9] Over half of these funds (57 percent) came from public sources, primarily Medicaid. In 1977 over three-quarters of all nursing homes were proprietary (for profit). In recent years there has been significant growth in multihome proprietary chains, with over one-third of all nursing homes being a part of such a chain.

As a result of lower costs and therefore improved profitability for long-term care facilities, many hospitals are converting their excess unoccupied beds to SNF beds. Converting these unoccupied hospital beds to SNF beds assists with patient placement as well as hospital census problems. Affiliation between hospitals and nursing homes is another approach to placement and census issues. Merger and affiliations between nursing homes and hospitals can facilitate transfers between settings and provide continuity of care.

Home Care. Home care is not a new concept. As early as 1776 the Boston Dispensary made home nursing services available. In 1877 the New York City Mission began hiring graduate nurses to provide home care and the concept eventually led to the formation of the Visiting Nurses Association.

In 1909 the Metropolitan Life Insurance Company became the first insurance company to offer home nursing benefits to its policy holders. The services became so popular and in demand that by 1928 Metropolitan Life was affiliated with 953 organizations that provided visiting nurse services.[10]

In 1947 Montefiore Medical Center in New York developed its "Hospital Without Walls." Their services were comprehensive and included medical care, pharmaceutical services, social work services, occupational therapy, physical therapy, and nursing services. Housekeeping, hospital equipment, and transportation services also were made available. The Montefiore home care program average cost was $3.00 per patient day compared to $12 to $15 per day for hospital care. Thus home care provided the opportunity for low cost, individualized, comprehensive care.

Several government programs were developed to finance home care. In 1961 the Community Health Services and Facilities Act authorized grants for the development of home health care services. In 1966 Medicare and Medicaid funds became available for home care, with the Social Security Act also covering such services. Even though these funds assisted with the costs of home care, most patients continued to receive all of their treatments as hospital inpatients.

In 1982, however, the change in hospital reimbursement motivated many hospitals to develop home care services as a way to reduce a patient's length of hospital stay. By 1984, 42 percent of all hospitals offered some type of home health care services.[11] Hospitals were learning that they could provide home care at significantly less cost than inpatient hospital care. Thus Medicare certified hospital-based home care programs saw a 60 percent increase between 1984 and 1985.[12]

The home care market is now growing at about 20 percent per year. Visiting nursing associations, community health associations, and hospital-based home care services are some of the nonprofit organizations providing home health care. The growth in technologically oriented proprietary corporations into home care services has also been seen in recent years. In fact, for-profit agencies now make up the largest segment of the market. This followed the 1980 removal of the former Medicare ban on reimbursement of for-profit home health services. Home infusion therapy is currently one of the fastest growing segments of the home care market, totaling $227 million in 1985.[13] Total revenues for home care services and products have skyrocketed. In 1983 expenditures in this area were close to $6.3 billion.[13] It has been projected that the total home care market could reach $24.8 billion by 1995.[14]

Hospices.   Hospices provide a unique blend of home care, long-term care, and hospital care. Modern hospices began in England in 1967 and were founded because of the belief that the dying have special needs that cannot be met by hospitals focused on caring. The first US hospice was founded in New Haven, Connecticut, in 1971, and by 1985 there were a total of 1345. Over half (53 percent) of the hospices are independent organizations, 27 percent are based in hospitals, 19 percent in home care agencies, and one percent in nursing homes. Hospices serve approximately 19,000 patients and their families daily.[15]

Health Maintenance Organizations. Although the term **health maintenance organization** (**HMO**) did not appear before the early 1970s, the concept of prepaid health plans was developed in the 1920s. In 1929 two physicians contracted with the city of Los Angeles to provide health care to city employees for a predetermined fee. In the early 1930s Dr. Sidney Garfield provided prepaid health care to construction workers. The success of Garfield's plan led to the development of a similar plan for Kaiser construction workers, which was the precursor of the Kaiser-Permanente's plan, one of the oldest and largest HMOs in the United States.

In 1973 the first HMO Act was passed, authorizing $325 million for the provision of a demonstration program for the development of HMOs. This particular act mandated such comprehensive benefits that it resulted in HMOs that were more expensive than traditional health insurance plans. In 1976 amendments were made that reduced the restrictions of the original act and resulted in more competitive prices for HMOs.

Three types of HMOs exist and include:

- **Staff/Group Plan.** In this type of plan physicians are employed by the HMO to provide services to HMO enrollees. Salary or capitation are the usual payment mechanisms.
- **Close Panel.** In this type of plan, HMO enrollees may constitute only a small portion of the total patients. Physicians contract to provide services to enrollees.
- **Individual (or Independent) Practice Association (IPA).** In this plan physicians work in their own settings, providing care to both their prepaid patients and their fee-for-service patients. The physician bills the IPA plan.

By 1985, 18 million Americans, approximately eight percent of the insured population, were enrolled in prepaid group plans.[16] Results of a recent study revealed that 94 percent of the companies surveyed were providing alternative delivery systems to employees and their dependents.[17] Estimates suggest that 20 percent of the population will be members of HMOs by 1993. HMOs combine traditional insurance and the health care delivery function within one organization. Participants of such a program are voluntary and pay a fixed amount, independent of the cost of services. HMOs are now enrolling Medicare and Medicaid populations.

A recent bill developed by representative Richard Gephardt from Missouri proposes the development of Community Nursing Organizations (CNOs). CNOs are similar to HMO for Medicare patients.

Ambulatory Care.   Ambulatory care covers all health care given to a person who is not a bed patient. A large amount of ambulatory care is given by private physicians on a fee-for-service basis; however, ambulatory care also is provided within organized settings. These include hospital-based ambulatory services, clinics, emergency care, surgery centers, and neighborhood health centers. The number of freestanding ambulatory care centers (FACCs) in operation in 1984 was 2300.[18]

Utilization of ambulatory services varies with age, sex, region, and income. In 1981 the frequency of physician visits increased with patient age. Children under 17 years of age averaged 4.1 visits per year, while persons over 65 years of age had 6.3 visits per year. Females had one visit more per year than males, and blacks had about the same number of visits as whites. Geographically speaking, the highest number of visits were in the West, and the lowest in the North Central and South regions. Physician visit rates for families earning less than $7000 in 1981 was 5.6, in contrast to 4.4 for the over $25,000 groups.[19]

In recent years hospitals have expanded their ambulatory care services. The latter half of 1985 reflected rapid increases in the use of hospital outpatient services, particularly in the area of ambulatory surgery. It is estimated that by 1988, 571 freestanding outpatient surgery centers will exist, performing 1.2 million procedures.[20] The expansion of these services has been an attempt to reduce costs associated with hospitalization, as well as an attempt at illness prevention.

Impacts on the Nurse, the Consumer, and Society

THE NURSE

Diversification and decentralization of the health care system have had numerous impacts on the nursing profession. As hospitals have expanded, so too have career opportunities for nurses. While there is a greater demand for nurses in health settings outside of the hospital environment, employment opportunities within the hospital have also increased. This expansion in employment opportunities has contributed to a shortage of registered nurses.

In 1970 there was one nurse for every four patients; in 1987 the nurse-to-patient ratio was one to ten. Decreased length of hospital stay has resulted in increased patient acuity and increased needs for specialized nursing care. More highly specialized nurses are needed to assess, plan, implement and evaluate care given to the acutely ill. The increased patient acuity level has led to an increase in the cognitive, affective, and psychomotor skills needed by nurses. However, to adjust to decreasing patient days and decreasing census, many hospitals reduced their number of employees. When downsizing occurred, it was usually the nonprofessional staff that was terminated. Because of the increases in patient acuity and technology, the number of registered nurses employed by hospitals actually increased. In attempting to meet the nursing care needs of the changing patient population, many hospitals developed "primary nursing." This system of care further increased the demand for registered nurses.

Hospital mergers and vertical integration have resulted in expanded career patterns for nurses. These diversified hospital organizations have created personnel systems directed at employee development and retention. Nurses are able to choose from a variety of work settings and roles within those settings, or create new roles and responsibilities based on their expertise and the needs of the institution. Several proprietary systems have career development programs that assist employees to move up career ladders within and across sites. These systems develop many of their leaders from within. Managers move from smaller to larger institutions. A nurse could work in a variety of clinical areas, sites, and roles, yet spend an entire career with one employer.

Prospective reimbursement and increased regulation by insurers have created greater financial pressures for health care delivery systems. Because nursing is usually one of the largest expenses within the hospital, nurse managers and executives must have sophisticated financial management skills. The increased emphasis on business skills has led many nurses to pursue a graduate degree in nursing, which is supplemented by courses or degrees in business administration.

In many hospitals the nurse executive responsibilities have increased. Titles have changed from "director of nursing" to "vice-president for nursing" and today, many nurse executives hold the title "associate administrator of patient services." These titles reflect an increased status for nurse executives as they assume greater responsibility for total patient care services. Clearly, the changing climate of the health care industry has created greater demands and rewards for nurse executives. Professional nursing practice has become a highly visible force within various health care organizations.

THE CONSUMER

The numerous, rapid changes within the health care delivery system have frequently caused great confusion among health care consumers. It is not an unusual occurrence for an obstetrical patient who spent five days in the hospital when delivering a baby six years ago, to be discharged two days post-delivery in 1989. The consumer/patient wonders what has happened. Many patients and their families are fearful about early discharges. Without adequate communication from all health care workers, confused consumers soon become dissatisfied customers.

Pressure to limit health care costs has extended to employers. Many employers have changed the health insurance benefits provided to the employee. The total insurance package provided in the 1970s has frequently been replaced by co-payment insurance in which the employee pays a portion of their insurance costs. The 100 percent insurance package of the 1970s is likely to have been replaced by limited coverage, requiring the patient to pay a portion of the costs for the care received. These insurance changes have resulted in confusion and additional expense for consumers.

Many employers are offering a variety of health insurance plans to employees. The employee often has to choose between HMOs, preferred payment organizations (PPOs), and traditional hospital insurance programs. The employee has more autonomy in choosing health care coverage, and more responsibility in paying for it. Many of the program choices are new and untested. Frequently, the consumer does not realize the limitations of a particular program until already involved in the plan. The variety of choices has resulted in "program shopping" by both employers and employees. This shopping has led to frequent changes in benefit programs, and, once again, added more uncertainty to an already confused consumer.

Hospital advertising was unheard of prior to 1980. With decreases in patient days and increases in financial pressure, hospitals developed marketing programs. Magazine and newspaper ads, television and radio commercials, billboards, and direct marketing have all been designed to reach new patient populations. American consumers are actively making some real choices about the nature of their health care services. Health care professionals have in turn developed more egalitarian relationships with patient/consumers. The common claims of high quality care have encouraged consumers to question the definition of "quality care."

Furthermore, greater visibility of militant consumers has emerged with the increase in medical and nursing specialization, and "bureaucratization" in health care delivery.[21] One might reasonably ask, "How will the consumer/patient of tomorrow tolerate receiving health care from an increasingly large bureaucracy?"

SOCIETY

The concept of health is evolving along with the changes in the types of health care delivery models discussed in this chapter. Society's view of health has shifted from a traditional paradigm in which disease was the central focus, toward a more positive, holistic approach with emphasis on health promotion. This conceptual change in health from a unidimensional to a multidimensional perspective has perhaps had the greatest single impact on the health care delivery system in this country. What health means to a society dictates how that society will respond to the health needs of its members—economically, politically, socially, and ethically.

In 1958 the World Health Organization defined health as "a state of complete physical, mental, and social well-being, and not merely the absence of disease and infirmity." Following this definition, various models of health emerged, including the psychosocial framework, in which health is viewed as the interaction of mind, body, and society. Perhaps the most influential concept of health shaping the current health care delivery system is that which equates health care with a positive lifestyle. Society's recent attention to "quality of life" and "high-level wellness"[22] reflects a change from the traditional medical model of cure to a more social model of care and health promotion.

Future Considerations

In the fifteen years from 1970 to 1985, the number of people aged 65 and older increased 42 percent. In the over-85 category, there was an 89 percent increase during the same years. By the year 2000, the 65-and-older age group will rise from 12 to 13 percent of the total population. People over the age of 85 will produce an even greater effect, increasing from 1.1 to 1.8 percent of this country's population.[23]

What are the implications of these demographic trends? Chronic conditions, such as hypertension and arthritis, exist in four out of five persons aged 65 or older. This population segment, especially those over the age of 85, use proportionately more health services than the younger population. Although chronic illnesses are not usually life-threatening per se, they often require ongoing health care treatment and frequently cause limitations of daily activities. Chronic disease will continue to be the major challenge in health care as professionals work together to preserve or restore the functional ability of the patient/consumer. As the need for assistance with personal care rises with age, so too does the possibility of institutionalization. As the nursing home bed crisis escalates, more patients will be cared for by family members, creating even greater demands on home care support services. It is likely that additional responsibilities will be placed on families, given the restrictive fiscal support by Medicare for recuperation and rehabilitation from acute and chronic illnesses.[24]

Although the 1980s have revealed fundamental changes in the health care delivery system, setting the climate for new alliances and the building of vertical systems, it is unlikely that total integration, vertical or horizontal, will ever exist in this pluralistic society. The 1990s will bring greater competition and more joint ventures as consumers continue to voice their health needs and preferences. The ultimate success of health delivery models will depend on the ability of those models to deliver high quality, cost-effective services.

Ms. Smith is a senior in a baccalaureate program. As an honor student, she will have numerous employment opportunities. Since her junior year, her primary clinical interest has been the gerontology client. Her immediate career goal is to find a position that will enable her to increase her clinical skills with the aged population. Her long-range goal is to enroll in a graduate program and move into a clinical speciality

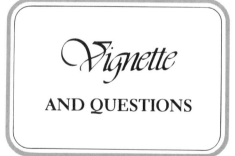

Vignette

AND QUESTIONS

role. She wants to begin her career in an extended care setting, but is curious about eventually moving into an acute care or ambulatory care setting.

Due to the variety of health care delivery services for the elderly, Ms. Smith is considering employment in a multiple hospital system. She could begin her employment in their extended-care setting. As her career interests unfold, Ms. Smith will be able to transfer to other sites within the multihospital system, including ambulatory and acute care. The tuition reimbursement benefits will enable her to begin part-time graduate study. She will retain seniority, rank, and collegial relationships while changing her work. Multihospital systems allow the nurse to change her work without changing her employer.

1. What type of integrated system is Ms. Smith considering as her first employer? What are the differences between vertically and horizontally integrated hospital systems?

2. What are some advantages and disadvantages of multihospital systems for the new graduate nurse? the consumer?

3. What is the difference between a proprietary and nonproprietary hospital?

INFORMATION SOURCES

Multihospital Systems: Perspectives and Trends. Chicago, American Hospital Association and Arthur Andersen & Co., 1987

Jonass J. (ed): *Health Care Delivery in the United States*, ed 3. New York, Springer, 1986

West Maine: Nursing and the Corporate World. Journal of Nursing Administration 17(3):22, 1987

REFERENCES

1. Weinstein MR: The illness process, psychosocial hazards of disability programs. JAMA 204:209, 1968

2. Johnson EA, Johnson RL: *Hospitals in Transition.* Rockville, MD, Aspens Systems Corporation, 1982

3. American Hospital Association: *Hospital Statistics.* Chicago, American Hospital Association, 1986

4. Brown M, McCool BP: *Vertical Integration: Exploration of a Popular Strategic Concept.* Rockville, MD, Aspens Systems Corporation, 1986

5. Liu K, Palesch Y: The nursing home population: Different perspectives and implications for policy. Health Care Finan Rev 3:15, 1981

6. Department of Health, Education and Welfare, National Center for Health Statistics, The National Nursing Home Survey: 1977 Summary for the United States, DHEW No. (PHS) 79-1794, Hyattsville, MD, 1979

7. Sirrocco A: National Center for Health Statistics: An Overview of the 1980 National Master Facility Inventory Survey of Nursing and Related Care Homes. Advance Data from Vital and Health Statistics, No. 91, DHHS Pub. No. (PHS) 83-1256, Hyattsville, MD, 1983

8. Freeland M, Schendler CE: National health expenditure growth in the 1980s: An aging population, new technologies, and increasing competition. Health Care Finan Rev 4:18, 1983

9. Gibson RM, Waldo DR: National health expenditures, 1980. Health Care Finan Rev 3:1, 1981

10. Stewart, JE: *Home Health Care*. St. Louis, CV Mosby, 1979

11. Home Care Agencies Up 25 Percent Since 1984. Hospitals 59:64, 1985

12. ABT Associates: *Home Health Services: An Industry in Transition*. Cambridge, MA, ABT Assoc-Publ, 1984. Prepared under contract for the Health Care Financing Administration, Office of Demonstrations and Evaluations

13. Jackson B, Jensen J: Home Care Leads Rising Trend of New Services. Mod Healthcare, 14:214, 1984

14. National Association for Home Care: Home Health Market Trends. Caring 3:16, 1984

15. Moga D: The Hospice Equation, Business and Health 2:7, 1985

16. National HMO Census, Excelsion, MN: Interstudy, 1985

17. The business roundtable task force on health, corporate health care cost management and private sector initiatives. In American Hospital Association: *Digest of National Health Care Use and Expense Indicators*. Chicago, American Hospital Association, Dunlop Group of Six, 1986, p16

18. Survey of Freestanding Centers, SMG Marketing Group, Inc., Chicago, IL, March 1984 and 1985

19. US Department of Health and Human Services, *Health United States, 1984*, USDHHS Pub. No. (PHS)85-1232: US Government Printing Office, 1984

20. Survey of Freestanding Centers, SMG Marketing Group, Inc., Chicago, IL, March 1984 and 1985

21. Salloway JC: *Health Care Delivery Systems*. Colorado, Westview Press, 1982

22. Dunn HL: High-level wellness for man and society. Am J Public Health 49:786, 1959

23. Division of Hospital Planning and Environmental Assessment of the American Hospital Association: *The Environmental Assessment Overview 1987*. Chicago, American Hospital Association, 1987

24. Detmer SS: The future of health care delivery systems and settings. J Profess Nurs 2:20, 1986

MARY GRANEY TRAINOR, RN, PhD

NANCY WIEDERHORN, RN, DNSc

Financial Equity for Services Rendered

CHAPTER 20

Background and Overview

For the past several years, state and federal legislation have been concerned with the issues involved in whether or not insurers must reimburse all licensed health care practitioners for services acknowledged to be independent legal functions of their various professions. Recognized as health care professionals, this group, which includes such health professionals as nurse practitioners, physicians' assistants, chiropractors, podiatrists, and psychologists, has traditionally been denied access to the reimbursement system, even though they are licensed by the state to provide health services to individuals covered by health insurance plans. Recent legislative activity promulgated by individual nurses, state nurses' associations, and special interest groups has resulted in legislative changes mandating third-party reimbursement for nursing services.

Over 85 percent of the American population has some form of private health insurance coverage and more than 23 million people, half of whom also carry private insurance, participate in the federal Medicare program.[1] Since patients are most likely to seek care rendered by professionals whose services are paid for by health insurance, the ability to obtain direct reimbursement for nursing services from private and government third-party payers has a direct bearing on the role of the nurse in the health care system.

Concurrent with the rise of public interest in private health insurance, **third party reimbursement,** direct insurance payment to nurses for services rendered, was identified by the American Nurses' Association in 1948 when it was included as a platform issue at the convention.[2] However, since nursing services were specifically excluded as reimbursable when the health insurance laws were originally written, physicians and health facilities had already gained control of the reimbursement system, thus limiting competition among providers and inhibiting the growth of nursing autonomy.

It was not until the 1960s that health care providers and planners began to recognize that a potential pool of physician extenders existed within the health care system, a group that could be quickly trained and utilized to perform some of the physicians' routine tasks at a time when a physician shortage was becoming apparent. By adopting the Nurse Training Act of 1971, the federal government indicated awareness of the necessity for enhancing the scope of nursing's role in the health care system by providing funding for specialized nursing programs to educate pediatric nurse practitioners, family nurse practitioners, maternity nurse practitioners, midwives, adult care practitioners, primary care practitioners, and others. The first program designed to educate nurse practitioners was developed in 1965 at the University of Colorado. To date, more than 140 programs exist in the United States.[3]

The development of specialization in nursing practice necessitated changes in many of the state nurse practice acts, amending them to allow nurse practitioners to perform acts under "special medical protocols" that would otherwise be outside the scope of nursing practice. With the emergence of more autonomous nursing roles, a movement toward independent practice developed, with nurses providing services through such nontraditional practice arrangements as private and group nursing practice, consultation with industry as well as other health care providers, and nurse-managed health centers. But who would pay for the services of the new nurse entrepreneurs?

STATUS OF REIMBURSEMENT

Legislation. It is a matter of state law whether or not insurance companies must reimburse health care providers for services rendered to their health care policy holders. Under state law, insurers may reimburse groups of health care providers unless a specific prohibition exists and, since no state specifically prohibits nurse reimbursement, many private insurers have chosen voluntarily to reimburse some nurses for the services they provide. However, in some states it has been necessary for the legislature to pass statutes mandating insurers to reimburse for nursing services.

Despite the opposition of some medical groups and insurance companies, to date, 25 state legislatures have passed laws concerning direct reimbursement for nurses. The provisions in the laws vary considerably, with some states requiring reimbursement for the services of only one type of nurse practitioner, most commonly nurse midwives, nurse anesthetists, and psychiatric/mental health nurses, and others contain broader statutory language that mandates benefits for many kinds of nursing services. While some statutes require reimbursement through a mandatory benefit law, others have a mandatory option law that only requires an insurer to offer nurse reimbursement as an option in policies it sells.[4] As of June 1986, of the 25 states presently permitting direct reimbursement for nursing services, 14 permit reimbursement for nurse practitioners.[5]

Payers. The third-party payers affected by reimbursement legislation include nonprofit private health insurance companies such as Blue Cross and Blue Shield, and for profit insurance companies such as Aetna, Hartford, and Travelers. Other private health insurance plans affected by nursing reimbursement legislation include self-insured employer plans, union plans, health maintenance organizations, and preferred provider organizations.

As is the case in state law, it is a matter of federal law whether or not federal health care policies such as Medicare, Medicaid, the Civilian Health and Medical Program of the Uniformed Services (CHAMPUS), and the Federal Employees Health Benefits Program (FEHBP) must reimburse nurses for services rendered. Unlike state law, however, under federal law specific authorization must exist before a health care provider may be reimbursed. As a result, changes in federal law are necessary before nurse practitioners can be reimbursed for their services.

Medicare and Medicaid are the two largest government sponsored health insurance programs in the United States. A federal health insurance program, **Medicare,** was created in 1965 as Title XVIII of the Social Security Act in order to provide for the health needs of people over 65 and for the disabled. Established in the same year, **Medicaid,** Title XIX of the Social Security Act, was established as a joint federal-state program to provide medical assistance to specified categories of low-income people. While current Medicare law provides that nursing services will be reimbursed only if they are rendered under the immediate supervision of a physician, Medicaid programs allow for reimbursement for services provided by nurse midwives, and in some instances for selected nursing groups such as nurse anesthetists, psychiatric nurse specialists, and nurse practitioners.[2]

CHAMPUS, the Civilian Health and Medical Program of the Uniformed Services, provides for direct reimbursement for services of certified nurse practitioners and certified psychiatric nurses, while federal direct reimbursement was denied to nurse practitioners under the Federal Employee Health Benefits Program as of the closing session of the 1986 Congress.[6] This was so, despite a presidentially authorized Office of Personnel Management (OPM) study, which concluded that neither cost nor utilization of services would necessarily increase if other health care providers were reimbursed directly.[6]

Services.   Whenever reimbursement legislation is enacted, an important issue is whether reimbursement services will include only those services currently being reimbursed when provided by another practitioner, or whether all services under the lawful scope of practice of the nurse will be included. To the present, every piece of nursing reimbursement legislation includes language that provides for reimbursement for nurses only when the policies currently reimburse for those services. Thus nursing is prevented from receiving reimbursement for services provided that are unique to nursing and are the essence of nursing practice.[2] The one exception is the Maryland 1979 reimbursement law, which in very general language requires that ". . . whenever a policy . . . provides for reimbursement for any service within the lawful scope of a duly licensed health care provider, the insured shall be entitled to reimbursement for such services. . . ."[2]

Impacts on the Nurse, the Consumer, and Society

Third-party reimbursement gives nurses the autonomy stipulated by state regulatory boards of nursing. Denying such reimbursement violates the nurse's right to independent practice and deprives society access to alternative modes of health care. The prevalent practice of requiring a physician's signature or "close supervision" is incompatible with professional independence[1] and undermines nursing's credibility with consumers. Currently, the specialty groups most affected by denial of third-party reimbursement are psychiatric clinical nurse specialists, nurse midwives, and nurse practitioners. Certified registered nurse anesthetists (CRNAs) will not be considered in this discussion because of the special nature of their problem. Generally CRNAs are considered adjuncts to medicine rather than nursing[1]; thus health insurance plans usually cover their services.[7] Although the move toward independent practice may be considered embryonic at this time,[3] its impact on nurses, consumers, and society poses serious challenges for the profession.

THE NURSE

Independent practice is impossible without third-party reimbursement. Consequently, economics in the currently competitive health care market becomes one of the most compelling nursing issues. Several events influenced this competition: increased supply of physicians, cost containment legislation, initiatives from the private sector to control health costs, and the enforcement of antitrust legislation to the health sector.[8] As a result, it has been predicted that the fee for service solo physician practice will become extinct within the next ten years,[9] to be replaced by group practices employing varying health care providers.

In response to the rapid growth of health maintenance organizations (HMOs), and preferred provider organizations (PPOs), independent practice associations (IPAs) are developing in which nurses play a vital role. Like physicians, nurses are employed by HMOs; with PPOs the provider is paid on a fee for service basis. The term **preferred provider** indicates that the insurance company or other purchaser contracted with the provider for services at an agreed upon usually discounted price. PPOs provided a challenging opportunity for a group of nurse practitioners in New Hampshire when they contracted with the state to become the PPO for the primary care of the developmentally disabled.[10]

Beginning efforts by nurses to compete with other health care providers illustrate a need to develop marketing strategies that not only clearly state their services in terms the public understands, but also identify the professionals and their credentials. Because businesses and individuals are uninformed about nursing services, nurses must "define, price, package, and market their services."[9] In addition to informing the public about cost containment and nursing effectiveness, nurses will need to use available legal and political channels to protect their interests.

Although they vary from state to state, reimbursement laws in general specify that the necessary qualifications for reimbursement of nurse practitioners and nurse midwives include certification of the nurse provider. California requires both a master's degree and two years of experience, but no certification for reimbursement of psychiatric nurse specialists; and Minnesota requires certification and post basic education for nurse midwives and nurse anesthetists. Provider categories also vary from state to state, with most provider states including legislation for reimbursement for midwives only, some including nurse anesthetists, three states including psychiatric/mental health nurse specialists, and a few states including the language "registered nurses" in their legislation.[2]

Legal aspects of third-party reimbursement continue to be defined in the courts and by state legislatures. Some obvious concerns relate to such issues as malpractice, legally accepted definitions of nursing, and the implications of the Sherman Antitrust laws.

The obvious need for malpractice insurance was dramatically illustrated with the recent experience of nurse midwives who lost their malpractice insurance when insurance providers refused to reissue their policies as they expired. The American College of Nurse Midwives (ACNM) appealed to the Association of Insurance Commissioners, who enabled the formation of a consortium of ten companies that agreed to provide professional liability insurance for certified nurse midwives.[11] Similarly, the American Nurses' Association (ANA) contracted for a new registered nurse liability program with self-employed nurses.[12] This action by the ACNM and the ANA provided an essential service to their membership, who could not have continued to function in expanded nursing roles without the protection of liability insurance.

Many states have not clarified what is meant by advanced nursing practice; consequently, the malpractice issue becomes obscured by the lack of legal definition of scope of practice and realistic standards for nurse specialists.[13] One principle applied to physicians for malpractice might be used for nurses. This principle states that "It is considered malpractice for a physician not to refer to a specialist when the patient's condition requires assistance or expertise beyond his skills or training."[13] By working with their state regulatory boards in defining the boundaries for advanced practice and establishing standards of care for various nurse specialists, nurses take the right of defining nursing practice out of the hands of third-party payers and physicians and put it into the hands of nursing, where it belongs.

A legal recourse for third-party reimbursement is the Sherman Antitrust law, which promotes competition in the workplace. For many years the "learned professions," which included health professionals, were thought to be exempt from federal antitrust laws.[1] Recently, however, several court cases have challenged that notion. Of particular interest to nurse practitioners is the case of the Virginia Academy of Clinical Psychologists vs. Blue Shield of Virginia, in which clinical psychologists sued Blue Shield of Virginia for refusing to pay for services of psychologists unless these services were billed through a physician.[1] The court ruled in favor of the psychologists, stipulating that it found no reason to believe that there was any therapeutic justification for recognizing the MD as superior to a board-certified psychologist in the provision of psychotherapy. The court ruling went on to state that it was "not inclined to condone anticompetitive conduct on an incantation of good medical practice."[14] If nurses can establish that a market exists for their services and that physicians and nurses compete in that market, then the Sherman Antitrust laws can be used in the courts to correct current abuses.[1] Whether nurse practitioners will successfully challenge third-party reimbursement obstacles in the courts will depend upon judicial willingness to apply antitrust doctrines to condemn restrictive practices perpetrated against them. The same safeguards of the Sherman Antitrust Act that have been used to condemn restrictive practices against other allied health care providers should apply with equal force to nurse practitioners.

Learning the art of politics allows nurses to develop effective strategies to create change. Nurses must see to it that state regulatory boards rather than legal statutes define nursing practice and thus reimbursement.[4] Statutes requiring that nurses function under the direction and supervision of physicians are no longer acceptable in this age of advanced specialty nursing education and practice. By combining the resources of specialty groups, greater support can be mobilized for broad statutes that will reimburse nurses in a variety of expanded roles. The American Nurses' Association has written comprehensive guidelines compiled from state associations that have achieved successful reimbursement legislation, and makes them available upon request.[15]

THE CONSUMER

Opposition to third-party reimbursement by physicians and private insurers is frequently couched in terms of concerns about quality of care and cost containment for the consumer. Nurses function beyond the medical model and its treatment of pathology as they assist clients to develop their capabilities for self-care. Research studies have consistently pointed out that care by nurses has beneficial consequences.

Recent research studies have concluded that when compared to care by obstetrical residents, patients cared for by nurse midwives had fewer low-birthweight babies and a greater number of infants born symptom free.[16] In another study, nurse midwives achieved major reductions in prematurity and neonatal mortality.[15] Similarly, another study indicated that pregnant adolescents cared for by nurse midwives were less likely to be anemic and had more spontaneous vaginal deliveries and larger babies than similar groups of adolescents cared for by obstetricians.[17] When nurse practitioners were compared to physicians in comparable clinical service areas, patient outcomes were similar.[18]

Insurance companies and physicians claim that increasing the number of health care providers will also increase the cost of care. Although no substantial data exist to support this claim, a number of reports suggest that nurse specialists can reduce costs and thereby provide direct cost benefits to the consumer.[15] In their guide to third-party reimbursement,[15] the ANA cites a report by Karoff and Kramer, who found that psychiatric nurses charged less per visit than did psychiatric social workers, clinical psychologists, psychiatrists, and other physicians.

Many nursing clinical specialists use a sliding scale to determine their fees, basing charges on family income and number of family members, thus providing the consumer with a direct monetary benefit of reduced co-payment costs. In other studies, costs for perinatal care decreased following the establishment of a nurse midwifery program in a rural area;[21] and costs at a childbearing center were 37.6 percent of the usual cost of in-hospital care.[22] In a study describing the use of nurse practitioners in an obstetrical-gynecological practice, savings were passed on to all patients by not increasing office fees for a period of three years.[23] In another practice studied, the nurse practitioners' fees were found to be 44 percent less than those charged for identical services by physicians.[23]

Limited research has been done to definitively demonstrate the cost-effectiveness of nurses. Studies need to be done to measure the effect of midwives on health care costs and on the health of mothers, babies, and families. Similarly, research is required involving nurse practitioners and clinical nurse specialists in order to answer questions about quality and costs. Large-scale studies need to be done that would consider "national outcome data, basic safety in all settings, quality of care, consumer satisfaction, service to the under-served, and cost effectiveness."[24]

SOCIETY

Containing health care costs will continue to be a major issue as we move into the 1990s. Although direct third-party reimbursement to nurses in expanded roles could contribute to such containment, we currently lack the necessary information to support this claim. Too frequently a physician's signature and medical diagnosis are required on health forms, without which insurance companies refuse reimbursement to nurses. Consequently, the economics of health care continue to be controlled in large part by physicians, with other health care providers such as nurses having little impact over policies.

Feldstein[8] claims that perpetuating a system whereby the physician is the primary caregiver and fee collector will no longer be tolerated in the competitive marketplace. He believes that the current competition gives the public a greater choice of delivery systems. Feldstein envisions future health corporations offering a spectrum of care, ranging from health maintenance and the provision of acute care to various levels of care in retirement settings. Clearly, nurses can provide important contract services within this framework. However, in order to successfully compete in the health care marketplace, nurses will need to recognize common goals, mobilize their forces, and unite to create a strong organization that can mount effective marketing strategies to sell their services.

Future Considerations

As nurses identify their unique services in "diagnosing and treating human responses to actual or potential health problems," one of the major obstacles that impedes their ability to function at their optimum capacity is denial or restriction of third-party reimbursement. Reimbursement policies that require physician supervision hamper nursing practice and deny the unique contribution that nursing offers. Once nurse practitioners have established that there is a market for their services, and that physicians and nurse practitioners compete in that market, then the denial of third-party reimbursement to nurses can be judicially challenged.

Whether nurse practitioners will successfully challenge third-party reimbursement obstacles in the courts will depend upon judicial willingness to apply antitrust doctrines to condemn restrictive practices perpetrated against them. The same safeguards of the Sherman Antitrust Act that have been used to condemn restrictive practices against other allied health care providers should apply with equal force to nurse practitioners.

Collaboration between state nursing associations and nursing specialty groups, other allied health professionals, and consumer groups should help to achieve passage of third-party reimbursement legislation in those states in which none has so far been enacted. Nurses must also lobby for passage of federal direct reimbursement of nurse specialists; educate insurance carriers about services for which nurse practitioners seek reimbursement; identify new alternatives for financing health care services; and develop tools to document the cost effectiveness of nursing practice.[5] As LeBar has stated, "Only when all nurses' services are reimbursable and only when all nurses are affected by health insurance laws, will nurses truly be an equal provider in the health financing system and significantly increase access to their services."[2]

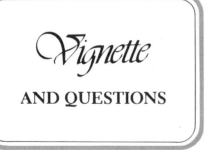

Vignette

AND QUESTIONS

Ms. Trayhorn, a certified clinical specialist in adult psychiatric mental health nursing, recently established an independent practice with another nurse in a state that has legislated direct reimbursement to clinical nurse specialists. She contacted various insurance companies to obtain the necessary information for third-party reimbursement. While most insurance providers cooperated with her request, a major company consistently thwarted her efforts by giving her inaccurate or misleading claim information. During her latest contact with this company, she was told that the name of a supervisory physician was necessary before she could be given a provider number to use on clients' insurance claims.

In this situation, the nurse needs to consider the following issues:

1. What are the reasons that insurance companies refuse third-party reimbursement?

2. What resources within the profession can the nurse call upon for help at this time?

3. What arguments can the nurse formulate that will justify third-party reimbursement without a physician's signature?

4. What strategy can the nurse use if the insurance company continues to refuse reimbursement?

INFORMATION SOURCES

American Journal of Nursing; News Section published in each issue: PO Box 1063, New York, NY 10102-0008

Capital Update; provides information on national legislation: American Nurses' Association, 1101 14 Street NW, Washington, DC 20005

Obtaining Third-Party Reimbursement: A Nurses' Guide to Methods and Strategies. Council of Primary Health Nurse Practitioners, 1984. American Nurses' Association, 2420 Pershing Road. Kansas City, MO 64108

The American Nurse; Official newspaper of the American Nurses' Association, 2400 Pershing Road, Kansas City, MO 64108

Nurse Practice Act individual state boards of nurse examiners

REFERENCES

1. Kelley K: Nurse practitioner challenges to the orthodox structure of health care delivery: Regulations and restraints in trade. Amer J Law and Med 11:195, 1985

2. LaBar C: Third-party reimbursement: Status of legislation. Oncology Nurs Forum 12:53, 1985

3. Studner JM, Hirsh HL: Nurse practitioner: Functions, legal status and legislative control. Medicine and Law 5:61, 1986

4. Cohn SD: Survey of legislation on third-party reimbursement for nurses. Law, Medicine and Health Care 11:260, 1983

5. Stallmeyer J: Direct reimbursement for NPs under FEHBP. Nurse Practitioner 11:14, 1986

6. *Capital Update*, American Nurses' Association, Washington Office, 4, Oct. 20, 1986

7. Hershey N: Entrepreneurial practice for nurses: An assessment of the issues. Law, Medicine, and Health Care 11:253, 1983

8. Feldstein PJ: The emergence of market competition in the US health care system: Its causes, likely structure and implications. Health Policy 6:1, 1986

9. Griffith H: Who will become the preferred providers? American J Nurs 85:538, 1985

10. Diehl DH: Private practice—out on a limb and loving it. Amer J Nurs 86:907, 1986

11. Amer Nurse, Sept. 1986, p3, 11

12. Amer Nurse, Nov.–Dec. 1986, p1, 11

13. Phillips RS: Nurse practitioners: their scope of practice and theories of liability. J Legal Medicine 6:391, 1985

14. Professional Briefs. Medical Economics, Nov. 13, 1980, p13

15. *Obtaining Third-Party Reimbursement: A Nurse's Guide to Methods and Strategies.* American Nurses' Association: Kansas City, MO, 1985

16. Slome C, Wetherbee H, Daly M, et al: Effectiveness of certified nurse midwives. Amer J Obst Gynec 124:177, 1976

17. Corbett MA, Burst WV: Nurse midwives and adolescents: The South Carolina experience. J Nurse Midwifery 21:13, 1976

18. Ramsay JS, McKenzie JK, Fish DG: Physicians and nurse practitioners: Do they provide equivalent health care? Amer J Public Health 72:55, 1982

19. Merenstein JH, Rogers KD: Streptococcal pharyngitis: Early treatment and management by nurse practitioners. JAMA 226:1278, 1974

20. Hardin SG, Durham JD: First rate. J Psychosocial Nursing 23:9, 1985

21. Reid ML, Morris JB: Perenatal care and cost effectiveness: Changes in health expenditures and birth outcome following the establishment of a nurse midwife program. Medical Care 17:491, 1979

22. Lubic R: Evaluation of an out of hospital maternity center for low risk patients. In Aiken L (ed): *Health Policy and Nursing Practice.* New York, McGraw-Hill, 1981, p90

23. Briggs RM, Heckock DE, Rassie DS, Brickell NJ, Kakar SR: Medlevel personnel in obstetrics and gynecology practice. Western J Med 132:466, 1980

24. Baxter LM: Documenting nurse midwifery outcomes: The need for a national database. J Nurse Midwifery 31:169, 1986

A N N   H.   C A R Y, RN, MPH, PhD

CHAPTER 21 *Home Health Care*

Background and Overview

The home health care industry is a potent force in the health care marketplace. Demographic, socioeconomic, and technological developments have contributed to the shifting of health care delivery from the home (1880s) to the hospital (1900s) and now to the home once again (later 1900s). As history begins to unfold toward the year 2000, consumers and providers alike will experience accelerated yet often contradictory trends in the development of the home health industry. These trends should become more stable as the health policy agenda becomes congruent in solving the cost-containment, continuity, and quality of care dilemma for the escalating numbers of health care consumers. Meanwhile, the current unprecedented rush for change has created both opportunities and pitfalls for providers and consumers of home health services.

The role of nurses in the development and delivery of home health care has historically been paramount in the industry. Agencies traditionally have appointed nurses in both administration and formal caregiver positions. Home care agencies are dominated by nurse professionals and have pulled heavily from community health nurse professionals. These patterns may be increasingly subjected to challenge as highly technical care is required by acute home care clients and as other professional administrators (health care, MBA) seek career opportunities in the expanding industry. Nurse administrators and managers must strengthen their fiscal, research, marketing, and personnel knowledge, while community health nurses are being increasingly challenged to update their technical procedural skills to augment their teaching, counselling, advocacy, and case management activi-

379

ties. Consumer demands driven by fiscal reimbursement and self-care values are rapidly requiring functional changes in nurses' roles in the home care industry.

The historical portrait of health care reflects the delivery of services primarily in the home throughout the centuries. In 1796 the first home care program was established at the Boston Dispensary, with services being administered by lay persons and financed by philanthropists, charity, or private payer sources.[1,2] Visiting nurse agencies in Boston, New York, and Philadelphia expanded in the 1880s and 1890s so that by 1890 there were 21 VNAs in the US, with most employing only one nurse.[3] Graduate nurses were hired to replace lay personnel in the late 1800s to provide home care to the sick.[4] Dock (1922) asserts that by 1910 there were over 1900 agencies providing home nursing services.[5] County health departments, VNAs, the American Red Cross, and the Metropolitan Life Insurance Company were the major providers of home care until the end of World War II. It was in 1947 that a model program for hospital-sponsored home health services utilizing inhouse medical and social service personnel as well as contracted community nursing services was initiated at the Montefiore Hospital in New York City. In addition to the Medicare reimbursed services available today, Montefiore also provided transportation, housekeeping, medication, and appliances.[6] The comprehensive nature of the service on a 24-hour basis is enviable to consumers, even in contemporary times. From the end of World War II to the passage of the Social Security Amendments (Titles XVIII, XIX) in 1965, the delivery of health care shifted from the home to the hospital setting. This shift was predominantly driven by the Hill-Burton construction policies that financed the building of hospitals and nursing homes, as well as limited the public funding of health care to those in institutions.[7] Additionally, the postwar advances in surgical treatment and medical management protocols encouraged the utilization of institutional settings for care and cure. Parallel to this, hospitalization insurance plans became common employee benefits, so that the middle class could now afford hospital care, which became the center of the health care system.

As the costs of health care in institutional settings began to rise rapidly in the 1950s and 1960s, and health care accessibility and equality became a social progress concern, the legislative climate originally produced in the Social Security Act of 1935 signalled the debut of government funding for the health care of the elderly and poor 30 years later. The Social Security Amendments (SSA) of 1965—Medicare (Title XVIII) and Medicaid (Title XIX)—sanctioned both institutional and home care as reimbursable services for the underserved groups. This legislation legitimized home care as a government regulated, reimbursable form of health care service for Medicare and Medicaid recipients.

The impact of this legislation was to create forces that drove both the supply and demand for an initially insignificant industry. This was accomplished in a number of ways:

- It shaped the uniformity of requirements for agencies seeking Medicare certification (conditions of participation).
- It broadened the type of formal caregiver (RN, LPN, OT, ST, SW, PT, HHH) for which reimbursement would be allowed.
- It established a source of reimbursement for covered services.
- It established the physician as the gatekeeper of services.
- It changed the mix of agency types delivering home care services, as well as the reimbursement services.
- It increased the number of agencies.
- It increased the number of categories of providers eligible for reimbursed services by the government funding sources.

The composite thrust of these implications was to change the delivery of home health services from organizations and "mom and pop" enterprises to a market-driven, full-scale industry. Even though the home health expenditure barely exceeds three percent of the Medicare budget, the service delivery is growing annually at a rate of 20 percent. Expenditures are expected to rise to five percent by 1990 and to 10 percent by the year 2000.[8]

The growth of the home care industry had been significant from 1965 to 1979. The number of Medicare-certified agencies in 1966 was 1275 and more than doubled to 3000 in 1979.[9,10] But the most rapid growth trends have been seen in the first half-decade of the 1980s and can be characterized as prolific. **The Omnibus Reconciliation Act of 1980 (PL 96-499)** and subsequent annual amendments drafted changes in the home care benefit that reduced some restrictions on agency growth statistics while attempting to promote cost-effective delivery. In light of striking previous restrictions—the limitation in number of visits, prior hospitalization and state licensure requirement for proprietary types of agencies—the number of Medicare-certified agencies in 1985 swelled to 5964.[11]

Table 21-1 indicates the growth of home care from a service to an industry in less than 20 years.

The percentage increase between 1983 and 1985 in home health care agencies was 40 percent. In addition to the official tabulation by HCFA of the numbers of home health agencies in 1985, the National Association for Home Care estimates that there may be as many as 6,000 *additional* agencies that do not choose to participate in the delivery of home health services as a Medicare-certified agency.[12]

Arthur Anderson (1984) and *Business Intelligence Report* have predicted an annual growth rate in the number of home health agencies of 20 to 22 percent during each of the next five years.[13,14] The largest market agency segment of growth in the types of agencies have been the proprietary (for profit) and hospital-based agencies at 60 percent each from 1984 to 1985.[9]

An additional factor reflecting the current trend in industry growth is the utilization pattern of home health services. These patterns belie the

TABLE 21-1

Medicare-Certified Agencies by Type 1966–1985[10,11]

Type	1966	1983	1985
Proprietary	–	997	1927
Official/County	579	1288	1274
Hospital-based	81	579	1260
Private, nonprofit	–	674	831
VNA	506	520	518
Skilled nursing home-based	–	136	129
Combined	83	–	–
Other	26	64	25
	1275	4258	5964

increasing number of clients served and the trend in visits for home health clients. Note in Table 21-2 the annual increase for the year 1983–84 alone.

FACTORS INFLUENCING UTILIZATION

Factors that are promoting the intensified utilization patterns include:

- The growing prevalence of the Medicare eligible population. In 1983 persons 65 or older numbered 27.4 million or 11.7 percent of the US population. By the year 2000, persons 65+ will represent 13 percent of the population. The year 2030 anticipates the elderly force in the US as 21.2 percent of the population. This reflects the elderly population in 2030 as two and one-half (2.5) times the 1980 population. If current fertility, immigration, and mortality statistics remain stable in the next century, the only age groups to experience significant growth will be those over 55.[12]
- The growth in the numbers of agencies available to provide access to the home health benefit (Table 21.1).
- The intensity and numbers of visits required by the home health population. Since the inception of the DRGs, home care agencies have reported a 38 percent increase in referrals.[15] The "quicker" and "sicker" institutionally discharged clients are requiring more skilled visits by agencies.
- The relatively inexpensive cost of home care compared to nursing home and hospital care. In 1984 the average Medicare home visit

TABLE 21-2

Medicare: Utilization of Home Health Services for Selected Calendar Years 1975–1984

Calendar Year	Persons Served (in thousands)	Home Health Visits (in millions)	Visits Per 1000 Enrollees	Visits Per Person Served	Average Charge Per Visit
1975	500	10.8	431	21.6	$ 20
1977	700	15.8	597	22.5	25
1979	870	20.0	717	22.9	30
1980	960	22.6	792	23.4	33
1981	1080	26.2	902	24.3	36
1982	1190	31.3	1060	26.3	40
1983	1380	37.6	1252	27.3	43
1984 (E)	1450	40.5	1330	28.0	46
Annual Percentage Increase					
1975–1983	13.5	16.9	14.3	3.0	10.0
1983–1984	5.1	7.7	6.2	2.6	7.0

E=estimate
Source: Health Care Spending Bulletin, 85-04[12]

cost $46, as compared to $62 per day for a nursing home and $300 per day in a hospital.[12]

It is estimated that over 1.3 million individuals receive home health care services every year.[12] This number is expected to escalate as the pool of Medicare and Medicaid eligible clients grows and actually reflects an underutilization of the home health care benefit due to a lack of knowledge of the viability of the service by consumers, referring physicians, and other health care professionals.

HOME HEALTH CARE—DEFINITION AND MODELS

In 1965 the Medicare law mandated home health care as a Social Security health care benefit package. The conditions of participation were the regulations that guided agencies applying to be Medicare-certified agencies. Since the reimbursement structure was not in place for Medicare clients receiving home care services, these regulations have promulgated more consistency in the types of services being offered to Medicare recipients.

Home health care is defined as comprehensive health care services provided to clients and families in their residences for the purpose of promoting, maintaining, and restoring health or maximizing independence.[3] Services covered by Medicare reimbursement currently include the following:

- Intermittent, skilled nursing care
- Physical, occupational, and speech therapy
- Medical social services
- Intermittent home health aides
- Medical services or interns and residents under an approved hospital teaching program
- The forementioned services furnished on an outpatient basis under arrangements made by a home health agency involving equipment not available at the clients' home

In order for Medicare coverage to be obtained for clients, they must have met the following requirements.[12]

- Clients must be in need of services that are reasonable and necessary for the treatment of illness or injury.
- Clients must be considered homebound (to leave the home would be considered taxing and of considerable effort).
- The service for the clients must be part-time or intermittent rather than continuous.
- The clients must be in need of "skilled" nursing services.

The most frequently delivered type of professional service is nursing delivered as "skilled" nursing care and for home health aide supervision. Nursing professionals have the most frequent contact with clients among any other type of home health professional and constitute the largest component of the labor force.

The most common diagnoses for which home care clients are now admitted are circulatory diseases, diabetes, and cancer.[15] The major problems of the home care population reflect mobility limitations, functional status limitations, and mental conditions.

The largest number of home health visits are made to clients over 65 years of age, although there appear to be emerging aggregates of service developing for the pediatric and disabled populations.[12,16]

Medicare and Medicaid programs are the primary reimbursers of home health services. Private health insurers have been increasing their coverage of home health services at rapid rates since 1980. Blue Cross and Blue Shield report that 90 percent of their plans include a home health benefit.[10] Additionally, HMOs have been recently allowed to provide the home health benefit as a package provision to Medicare clients.

Table 21-1 indicates the classification scheme of home health delivery systems. Agencies may be classified as follows:

- **Official**—Agencies on the state and local levels that are given their powers through legislation and their revenue sources primarily through state and local tax bases. An example would be the home health department or section of a local health department.
- **Voluntary**—Agencies governed by a community board of directors, having been organized through no legislative authority and whose sources of income are not based on tax revenues. A voluntary agency utilizes nontax funds, such as United Way, cancer and heart societies and association contributions, third-party payments, and private donations, grants, and payments. Visiting Nurse Associations or services constitute the majority of this type of home health organization. These agencies are typically nonprofit and tax exempt under Section 501C of the Internal Revenue Code.
- **Combination Agencies**—In some communities, the official and voluntary agencies merge as a cost-effective strategy in delivering home health services. These may be administered jointly by a board of directors and governmental authorities. These types of agencies appear to be on the decrease as official agencies are tending toward a focus on programs other than home health care services.
- **Hospital and Skilled Nursing Facility-based**—Agencies that are housed within another service delivery system where the established institutional board of directors is responsible for agency governance may fit this category. The hospital or nursing home structure determines whether the home care agency is official, voluntary, private, nonprofit, or proprietary.
- **Proprietary**—Profit-making agencies are ineligible for tax exemption. Before 1982 these agencies could not participate in the federal health insurance programs in the absence of state licensure laws. This legislative change has encouraged the prolific growth of this segment of the industry. Proprietary agencies can receive revenues from Medicare if they are certified agencies. The majority of revenue comes from private pay insurance. Ownership of the agency can be by individual or corporation, and franchising is an additional option. Owners/investors may or may not choose to manage the agency. An example would be Upjohn Home Health Care Services, Inc.
- **Private Agencies**—Home care agencies can be nonprofit, private (tax exempt), or proprietary private (nontax exempt) structures. Either type may be owned by an individual or a corporation.
- **Other**—Agencies that may not fit the aforementioned categories due to the uniqueness of organization and administration are classified

as "other." Examples include prepaid health plan home care agencies (HMOs), an American Indian Nation agency, or a skilled nursing facility-based official.

In addition to the above classifications, agencies may be categorized as **freestanding** (not contained within another service delivery system) or **institutionally housed** (housed within another system). Therefore, possible combinations may include:

- freestanding voluntary
- freestanding official
- freestanding proprietary or nonprofit
- hospital-based nonprofit or proprietary
- SNF-based proprietary, or voluntary, or nonprofit
- freestanding chain-based proprietary
- other

REIMBURSEMENT SOURCES

Reimbursement for home health care services is a key issue for the industry's growth and survival. Before the passage of the Social Security Amendments (Titles XVIII and XIX) in 1965, most home health services were paid through subsidized donations and contributions, as well as self-pay by clients. Today the industry boasts of an array of payer sources for home health care as consumer demands and third-party reimbursers deliver the cost-benefit of home health care.

Medicare (Title XVIII).   Those eligible for this entitlement form of health care benefit may include:

1. Those over 65 who have paid into the Social Security or Railroad Retirement systems
2. Individuals disabled at least 24 months
3. End-stage renal disease clients
4. Spouses of 1, 2, and 3
5. Dependent children of 2 and/or 3

Part A of Medicare (Hospital Insurance) is the entitled service. **Part B** is an optional enrollment service for a monthly premium fee. Both parts A and B provide for home health services. If at least one of these services (currently identified as skilled nursing, physical therapy, or speech therapy) is needed, additional covered services can be added (home health aid, occupational therapy, medical social work, medical supplies and equipment). Custodial care and homemaker/chore services are not covered in this benefit. Medicare provides the major source of reimbursement in the home health industry. Medicare reimbursement is available only to agencies that meet the federal Conditions of Participation and are currently Medicare-certified.

Medicaid (Title XIX).   Home health care is a federally mandated service for every *state* Medicaid plan. Medicaid is administered by each state and receives a percentage (50–83 percent) of its program funding from matching federal funds. Eligibility requirements are by each state and include categorical and income factors. All states must avail the home health Medicaid benefits of nursing care (not necessarily skilled), home health aid, medical equipment, and supplies. States may also elect to provide through their home health program physical, occupational, and speech therapy. No matching federal funds are available for medical social work.[17] Medicaid reimbursement can be made only to the home health agencies that are Medicare-certified. The Medicaid regulations governing home health care services are more liberal in requirements (no homebound need), thus encouraging utilization.

Title XX (SSA).   The impact of this program on home health beneficiaries is to provide homemaker/chore services to those in financial need. The eligibility requirements vary from state to state and funds for these services may no longer be available if states have failed to replace the federal, time-limited funding.

Titles III & VII (Older Americans Act—1965).   Limited funding for home health agencies has been available through these sources for services to the elderly, including senior centers, information referral, home repair, meals delivered to the home, and transportation. Currently it assists state and local agencies to develop coordinated comprehensive systems to respond to those over 60.

Veterans Administration.   A source of home health reimbursement for a limited population (veterans) is available for veterans' post-hospitalization. Eligibility may be limited to veterans who are indigent and/or who have service-connected disabilities. Many of the home care services utilized by the veteran population are administered through Veterans Administration hospital-based home care departments.

Private Insurance.   There have been noticeable trends in the increasing coverage of some types of home health services by nonfederal insurance plans.[12] Most notably, Blue Cross/Blue Shield reports that over 90 percent of its plans contain a home health care benefit.[10] As consumers, labor management contracts, and insurance companies demand the most cost-effective options for individual health care coverage, the home health industry may see large proportions of its reimbursement evolving from the private insurance carriers.

Self-Pay Donations.   The remaining source of reimbursement for home health care was originally the major source of payment until 1966. It is now estimated that 20 percent of the reimbursement for home health care comes from self-paying clients.[18] A much smaller amount comes from donations, philanthropists, and charitable groups.

The role of the reimbursement players in designing the destiny of the home health industry cannot be understated. Due to the interpretative inconsistencies of the HHS regulations governing eligibility and conditions for clients receiving home care services, home health agencies are scurrying to court alternate sources of reimbursement and to reduce their financial reliance on Medicare funds as major sources. In an era of competition, cost cutting strategies, and hazy health policy, the home care industry is striving to maintain an equilibrium in the area of stable reimbursement revenue. Both the concepts of prospective payment and capitation are likely to influence the reimbursement mechanisms in the near future.

Impact on the Nurse, the Consumer, and Society

THE NURSE

The ebb and flow of the home health care industry has not gone without unduly influencing and being influenced by the profession of nursing. Very early in the history of home care in the US, nurses functioned independently. Perhaps Florence Nightingale's teachings of a visiting nurses' work, paraphrased below, captures the essence of the nurse's role.[19]

> The nurse needs special training beyond the hospital nurse, since she must work with no hospital appliances on-site, must report to the doctor who receives only her report and is his staff of clerks, dressers, and nurses. She must be able to "nurse the room," teach the patient and family to do the same, and to advocate and supervise the cleanliness and care performed there. Where there are sanitary defects, these must be brought to the attention of the proper authority. Dustbins, the water supply, and drainage deficits must be remedied.

The nurses in home health care agencies are often continuing to operate with minimal medical supervision, are autonomous in their authority to diagnose and treat human responses, and are responsible for implementing creative techniques in assisting clients to adhere to their treatment plans. Because of the responsibility this freedom creates, the home care nurse must possess strong biopsychosocial assessment diagnoses, planning, implementation, and evaluation skills. The nurse's communication with other professionals for information and consultation is more often by phone rather than being conveniently on-site as in the institutional setting. Verbal discussions and orders must be clearly communicated and delivered in a timely manner. Family members, who may constitute the majority of informal caregivers and deliver about 80 percent of the care in the home, must receive current and correct teaching of content, procedures, and problem-solving mechanisms.[20] Their knowledge base and ability to perform critical activities in the absence of a professional must be expertly assessed, reinforced, and evaluated. The nurse must possess skills in supervising the care delivered by home health aides, who remain a critical component of the service delivery package to home care clients. The nurse or appropriate professional staff member, if other services are provided, are required to make a supervisory visit to the client's residence every 14 days in Medicare-certified agencies.

Current industry dynamics portray the impact on the nursing professional in a number of ways.

Reduction in Length of Stay.   Since the inception of the Social Security Amendments of 1983 instituting a prospective payment system (PPS) for hospitalized Medicare clients, the average length of stay has decreased from 9.5 days to 7.5 days (1984)[21] to 6.4 days in 1985.[22] This reduction has shortened the length of planning, evaluation, and contact that nurses have with the institutionalized clients. Nurses must accomplish more activities (teaching, coordinating services, performing treatments) with clients and families in shorter periods of time. It demands an economy of planning and intervention from the initial minutes of institutional admission. Additionally it requires earlier detection of discharge needs and timely coordination with the targeted referral resources. The fact that clients are maintaining a smaller proportion of the acute state of their illness in the hospital means that nurses with acute care skills are in demand, albeit the acute contact with the client may be of shorter duration.

Marketplace Demand in Home Health.   The growing labor force in the home care industry will be composed of more institutionally based providers who seek the increasing job opportunities in home care agencies.[23] The community health nursing managers of these providers will be called upon to orient, educate, and supervise the new community-centered caregiver. Advanced practice community health and management concepts for administrators and managers can facilitate the smooth transition of the nurse force from the acute to the community-based settings while anticipating and incorporating the emerging clients' needs for an appropriate service delivery package by the agency.

The need for nuse managers in agencies has intensified as the growth in home care agencies has escalated. Betweeen 1982 and 1985 there was a 54 percent increase in the number of agencies.[11] This increase posed a demand for nurse managers in new agencies.

The majority of professional providers and services in the home health industry are nurses, delivering skilled and supervisory services on behalf of clients. In extrapolating from the National Association for Home Care data revealing that there are an average of 7.1 nurses employed in an agency, the number of nurses working in the 5964 Medicare-certified agencies alone constitutes a nurse labor force of over 40,000 nurses. This number is a gross understatement of the entire nurse labor force in the industry, since it does not include the non-Medicare-certified agency labor force. The number of nurse positions will continue to increase as beneficiary and agency numbers escalate.

Skill and Role Functions.   The practice of nursing in the field of home health care is more than transferring hospital-acquired skills to a home setting. An important initial difference is the psychological expectations of both the client and nurse. The nurse must operate in the clients' familiar territory and power base (their home)—just the opposite of the institutional environment. Routines and treatments must be more carefully blended with the client/family's home routine to be succcessful. Adaptations in equipment, rearrangement of the living environment, adjustments in schedules, and coordination of contributing resources all require flexible and creative strategies on the part of the home health nurse. Engaging the client and family in supportive and self-care activities that may require more effort in the home in the absence of the array of institutional supportive services (ie, meals delivered according to dietary regime and bed linens changed) is the result of clear communication, common therapeutic values, motivation, and adequate social support. Because the client and family are required to form a psychological contract with the home care professsionals, the techniques required to engage, motivate, collaborate, and advocate for the clients' recovery are paramount.

Another skill that has become exceedingly necessary to update and polish has been the skill of delivering highly technical care in the home. For nurses who have been out of the mainstream of technological devices, procedures, and rehabilitative techniques, the more acutely ill client being admitted to home care agencies will present a challenge in updating knowledge. It behooves the nurses and the agencies to establish formal, informal, and practical sessions to arm these professionals with current technical skills. Clients requiring IV and monitoring blood lines, advanced wound care treatment and debridement routines, ventilator equipment, and medication perfusion pumps, and chemotherapy and antibiotic regimens need professional and technically proficient formal caregivers.

Case management activities must be skillfully and economically enhanced in order to keep home care efficient and appropriate. As techniques administered in the home become more complex, require additional team members, and become successfully predicated on the critical coordination of community support services (transportation, durable medical equipment, pharmaceuticals, biochemical disposition), the nurses' time spent in the case management activities may become as critical as the on-site care. This is a skill that requires clear communication, documentation, a thorough knowledge of community contacts and resources, and a professional organization. As the name implies, it requires more than a physical nursing skill. Rather, it requires the management functions of directing, controlling, planning, and evaluating the service delivery for the clients.

Implications in the marketplace for the role of nurses are that their functions of advocacy, coordination, care provider, case finding, transitioner, researcher, teacher, consultant, marketer, manager, and administrator must be clearly understood, strengthened, and reinforced to other professionals and consumers. Experienced community health nurse managers of the newly migrating institutional nurses will be called upon to orient, educate, and supervise the new community-centered caregiver. Advanced practice community health and management concepts for administrators and managers can facilitate the smooth transition of the nurse force from the acute to the community settings, while anticipating and incorporating the emergency clients' needs for an appropriate service delivery package by the agency. As the number of agencies continue to escalate, the number of management and staff positions for nurses may rise dramatically. For some nurse professionals, the transition to this entrepreneurial market will be smooth, and for others it may require a retooling of skills.

Specialized education.   Home health care can be considered a subspecialization of community health nursing. As such, it requires advanced preparation in a specific area so that the skills can be identified, assimilated, and applied. Many home care leaders today have emerged through the process of on-the-job training. After many years in a number of positions, they have used their practical, current experiences to advance their leadership objectives.

It has only been since 1983 that the formal educational preparation for nurses in the field of home health care was begun at the University of Michigan School of Nursing. Gradually nurses around the country are beginning to pursue master's degree preparation in the first few programs in home health care. Several schools of nursing have begun to refine their programs—among them the Catholic University School of Nursing, Washington, DC—and to provide consultation to others seeking to initiate the advanced nurse specialization.

Administrators of graduate nursing education programs (84 percent response rate, n=98) view the demand for home care nursing increasing both regionally and nationally (93 percent). Most of these administrators (80 percent) believe that nursing schools will give increasing priority to home health care in their curricula.[24]

Educational institutions have the unique mission of predicting, preparing, and evaluating the needs of society and nurses for tomorrow's emerging health care advances. While the demand has been clearly established in home health care, the supply of formally prepared advanced practitioners to navigate the helm of the home care industry has not kept pace to date.

Avenues for Research. There remains a dearth of nursing research in the field of home health care. Now that the health care community is viewing this delivery system with more enthusiasm and scrutiny, perhaps the interest in research will materialize. Many factors may contribute to the stagnation of research in this area:

- Lack of advanced practitioners and experienced researchers employed in agencies
- Limited fiscal resources within agencies to support research
- Limited existence of institutional review boards to encourage, screen, and monitor research activities

The need for research opportunities and the expansion of the field of knowledge in the home care arena is paramount to the continued definition of the nursing practice specialization in the field. Historical descriptive, correlational, quasi-experimental, and experimental studies on clients, interventions, informal caregivers, sick role dynamics, cost and quality of care, formal providers, predictors of client outcomes, and health services implications need to be initiated to glean a more reliable picture of the industry and its impact. The ground is as fertile for research in this area as in any other area of nursing practice.

Quality Control—Myth or Reality? The home health industry came under Congressional scrutiny in the form of committee hearings in the summers of 1986 and 1987. These hearings focused on quality of care issues concerning the clients being served. Although there are current mechanisms in place to provide for the judgment of minimum structural and procedural standards in state Medicare-certified agencies, agencies governed by state licensure laws and/or in agencies seeking accreditation from either the National League for Nursing (NLN), or the Joint Commission on Accreditation of Hospitals (JCAH), there are questions being raised about the implications of the quality controls, the lack of consistency in standards, enforcement of standards, and the lack of outcome quality assurance mechanisms operational in agencies. Nursing as a profession has consistently supported quality assurance, both within its professional ranks (educational standards, licensure, certification, continuing education) and in industries in which health care is provided by nurse professionals. There is no question that there are presently quality control mechanisms; however, there is much more that nursing can do to impact the development of standardized, reliable, valid, and critical indicators of the value of the home health service to clients. As in its own professional evolution, nurses can take the lead in creating, testing, monitoring, and evaluating additional quality indicators for their agencies and the industry. Nurses are employed or utilized by insurance companies, fiscal intermediaries, state licensing agencies, the NLN, and JCAH to monitor agency compliance. The move to strengthen the quality controls presently in the industry will create the need for more nurses to take leadership positions in implementing the oversight of industry standards. Clearly, nursing representation on a peer review organization whose function is to monitor a system predominantly composed of nursing services is a critical need for the industry.

THE CONSUMER

One of the most obvious implications for consumers of the burgeoning home health industry is that there are many more agencies supplying services in communities than ever before. With the industry multiplying at a rate of 20 percent during the mid-1980s and with these predictions continuing through the 1990s, it is conceivable the choices may become overwhelming. Agencies in the community vying for increasing market shares will be listening closely to the voices of consumers as they attempt to package services in high demand. Since the purchasing power of the consumer (federal and state government, private insurance, and self-pay individuals) is the strongest force driving the market, the industry may develop more entrepreneurial services to augment the traditional home health delivery package. Agency administrators sensitive to the pulse of community dynamics can capitalize on the emerging demands of consumers by integrating these new programs into their agency.

Because of the trends developing in the general health care industry, consumers now have more choices about where they receive health care services. Clients can now have many surgical procedures performed in outpatient surgical centers with follow-up monitoring of their condition in the home by nurse professionals. Chemotherapy, antibiotic intravenous therapy, and blood transfusions may become predominantly home administered procedures in the near future. The implications for consumers entail their having greater access to teaching about the procedures, complications, and recovery, and that they assume additional responsibility for self-care activities.

Consumers of home health services report that they prefer receiving health services in their homes, as opposed to institutionalization.[25] This often requires out-of-pocket expenses by clients and additional participation of family members as informal caregivers in the delivery of care. Expenses to caregivers can be in the form of hiring auxiliary help, lost wages from missed days of employment, and the full or partial payment for items/ equipment used in the home. Gaps in federal and private insurance coverage of components of the home care service can create a financial strain on clients. One example is HCFA's current prohibition of payment for home IV antibiotic therapy supplies, equipment, or services, but the provision for allowance of payment for home IV chemotherapy supplies, equipment, and services on a limited basis.[18] When reimbursement becomes more congruent in fostering the consistent use of the home care service as a more cost-effective delivery mode, the impact on consumption of services will be profound. Much legislative support and lobbying by consumers is needed to quell the inconsistent reimbursement decisions for current home care consumers. Consumer demands must be heard by legislators and insurers in order to facilitate the logical, cost-effective evaluation of the industry.

Consumers must compare the quality of services and agencies. As in any industry experiencing rapid growth, it is conceivable that there are agencies in the community attempting to capitalize on profits to the detriment of quality and client safety. Agencies that are not financially stable may cut corners on services or discontinue services, creating a dumping of clients in the community. Consumers in hospitals, nursing homes, and the community must request information about the variety of agencies available to them and seek the opinion of respectable health care professionals and other consumers in searching for an agency to meet their needs. Disputes with agencies from which services are received can be corrected through ombudsmen at the agency, the insurer, the intermediary, or the local or state level consumer agency. Consumers have both the right and responsibility to expect the services for which they have contracted, in a reasonable time period and with the highest attention to quality and discharge planning. Consumer feedback is critical in promoting a healthy home care industry and is the strongest deterrent to fraud and abuse. Nurses have the professional obligation not only to contribute to the clients' quality of care, but to inform the consumers of their rights and obligations, while receiving home health services and in advocating on behalf of clients for needed services in the community.

SOCIETY

The proliferation and increasing utilization of home health services by the US population, especially in the last five years, have sanctioned the value of competent, restorative, and progressive health care outside the institutional setting. These trends reflect an ebbing of the notion that the hospital is the only viable center of technology and acute care, a thought that prevailed in the 1950s through the 1970s. The rapid adaptation of medical technology resulting in smaller, more simplified, and reliable equipment for use in the home by clients has facilitated the perception that the home will become the new center of technology. Although the home health benefit lacks sufficient coverage by many insurers, is underutilized as a referral option by physicians, and is meeting only 25 percent of the aggregate need for service, it remains a potent player in the array of health care services for clients.[1] With continued consumer demand, broader and comprehensive reimbursement plans, and continued delivery of quality care in home health services, the industry should supply a larger component of the spectrum of health care services and progress in fulfilling the consumer capacity that is apt to approach saturation.

A very important influence of the home care industry is the cost-savings alternative it provides to insurers and clients. Cost-effectiveness and affordable health care are highly regarded values. The double digit inflationary increases in health care costs have been slowed by government legislation supplying limitations in coverage, higher deductibles, and higher premiums. It was only in 1985 that the almost 20-year cycle of runaway, double digit health care costs was broken in this country.[26] The utilization of home health services offers a cost savings for consumers when compared to other forms of health care delivery. The average hospital cost in 1985 was $600 per day, while length of stay fell to 6.4 days.[22] Although society could expect to keep its members in the hospital for less time, it paid more in doing it. A startling example of cost comparisons is the Katie Beckett case. Katie Beckett, now a school-age child, spent her first three years hospitalized, due to being on a ventilator. Her hospital care costs ran $15,000 monthly, compared to $2,000–$3,000 monthly costs for home care. Similar studies reveal that cost savings can range from one-half to two-thirds of institutional bills.[12,27] While the cost savings cannot be as dramatic in all cases of home health care, they represent a significant societal factor in deciding access and reimbursement for components of the health care system.

Indirectly, the ethical consideration facing society in the health care arena is the responsibility to provide members with health care resources in a cost-effective manner so that health care is economically accessible to all. While the home health option may not be appropriate for all clients, it contributes to solving the concern of spending large amounts of health care dollars in institutions for a limited number of catastrophic clients.

Industrial growth of home health care contributes to the employment opportunities for the health care labor force and related product industries. Healthy businesses contribute to the country's economic stability and encourage additional investment opportunities. Clients spending less time in institutions may be able to return to the work force earlier, thereby shortening their nonproductive time.

When consumers enjoy a service, when industry standards promote a high quality product, and when health care resources may be more cost-effectively managed in utilizing home health services, society benefits. With health care expenditures representing ten percent of the gross national product, health care delivery decisions can significantly impact on the growth of the country.[26]

Future Considerations

There are many avenues of possible changes in the field of home health care. These will be principally navigated through health policy and subsequent legislation.

The most important clarification to be made is a clear indication of the content of the health policy agenda for this country. **The Health Policy Agenda for the American People Summary** is a document that provides a description of policy areas, principles, and implementation recommendations for responding to issues as they affect the health care system.[28] The increasing proportion of our population reaching advanced age is demanding answers to the provision of care problem. Home care is primarily provided to those over 65 on a short-term, intermittent, acute episode basis. The notion of long-term in-home care services has not been legislated. This sends a confused message to elderly consumers about where competent long-term care can be provided (reimbursed). This same confusion is experienced by many Medicaid clients (all ages) who can petition long-term home care only on waiver through bureaucratic channels of many months duration. Meanwhile, health care dollars, subsidized by tax bases, are being spent on more costly services than needed by individuals. The health policy stance must become consistent, sharpened, and clarified in a timely manner so that economic and emotional waste does not continue for potential home care clients.

Regulation of the industry needs to be consistent, enforceable, and effective. It is possible to operate a health agency without a licensure requirement, certificate of need (CON) application, or certification by Medicare regulations. In 1986 only 36 states (and now the District of

Columbia) had licensure laws, 34 states required CONs, and only agencies volunteered for Medicare certification.[18] With the rapid growth in agencies, it is possible that consumer needs and interests are not well understood nor protected. Outcome oriented quality control measures must be constructed, applied, and evaluated to discern a focused picture of services to consumers. Nurses, as the major professional service represented in home health care, need to participate in all phases of the industry regulation. The contribution of the nursing profession in this area cannot be understated.

Closely aligned with regulation is the professional credentialing needed for professionals in the home health field. Certification of nurses in the subspecialty of home health needs to be developed, implemented, and evaluated. Whether the nurse occupies the position of administrator, supervisor, field nurse, or quality assurance specialist, boards of directors, consumers, and referring services need to have an indicator of the type of distinction earned by agency staff. All staff must be held accountable for their current and professional delivery of client services. The ANA has begun the process of developing standards of practice for home health nurses. These will be refined in the near future.

Uniform standards for the training of paraprofessionals (home health aides—HHA) in the home care industry are amiss. This is ironic in view of the fact that these individuals require greater training and subsequent supervision. While a model curriculum and teaching guide for homemaker home health aides was developed by the National Home Caring Council in 1978 (now absorbed by the Foundation for Hospice and Home Care), it is not being used in many federal and state programs. Basic training, supervision, and monitoring requirements need to be mandated and enforced for those personnel and could facilitate more individuals seeking entry into this labor segment.

Administrators of graduate nursing education programs view the demand for home care nursing as increasing and will give greater priority to home health care in their curricula.[24] Students must have practicum experiences with both clients and routines in home health agencies to augment the application of knowledge in diverse settings with other roles. Since the industry appears destined to assimilate an increasing proportion of the health care delivery system, new graduates must know how agencies deliver services and for what types of clients home care may be more successful. This knowledge can enhance their care of the clients in the institutional setting and assist them to accurately discharge clients to the correct service delivery option. Graduate programs in nursing must offer specialty preparation for administrators, educators, researchers, and clinical specialists utilized in the industry. These advanced practice graduates will be responsible for fashioning the care and advancement of knowledge and research of home health populations.

A consideration in the growth of any industry is that the services and products remain affordable to maintain the demand. Lest home health care be subjected to the same legislative ramifications imposed by radical reimbursement changes for hospitals, the agencies must continue to strive for cost-effective services. Since the industry is labor intensive, it behooves personnel to be efficient and productive to enhance cost containment. Alternately, reimbursement must be objectively offered, based on factors constituting costs. Pricing and reimbursement formulae are likely to change for home care services, but the exact nature and models have yet to be revealed.

The steady growth in the home health industry during the first 15 years of the Medicare/Medicaid amendments to the Social Security Act has been replaced by volatile growth in the industry since 1981. This growth is predicted to continue to be robust through the 1990s and represents the health care delivery system's response to the aging population's dynamics of growth, an emerging number of expanded services (pediatrics, chronic disabled), and a radical consumer, insurer, and federal mandate to deliver health care more cost effectively in the least restrictive environment. With the DRG process encouraging timely discharge from the institutional settings, caps being placed on one-fourth of the states' skilled nursing home beds, almost 31 million Americans eligible for Medicare services, and the underutilization of home health care services by the 1.3 million Medicare beneficiaries,[12] the growth of the home care industry in the next 15 years presents the most potent avenue of expansion for community health services and nursing among all other alternatives.

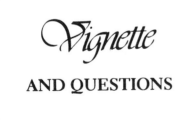

Vignette

AND QUESTIONS

Mrs. Olson is a 74-year-old widow who has been admitted to the hospital with a diagnosis of cerebrovascular accident (CVA) with bilateral hemiparesis and partial aphasia. She has lived alone for seven years in her own home and is adamant about returning to it to convalesce. Her needs upon discharge will be for medication regulation, monitoring and strengthening of mobility and muscle tone, continued progress in expressive communication, assistance in activities of daily living, maintenance of a catheter with subsequent bladder training, and the short-term administration of IV antibiotics for the remediation of a preexisting cellulitis condition in her left leg. As her primary nurse you are responsible for initiating and coordinating her discharge activities. After collaborating with Mrs. Olson and determining that she is insistent on receiving her treatment management at home, you convene a multidisciplinary meeting with professional staff to discuss the need for multidisciplinary services upon discharge and to review criteria in selecting home health agency options that can best serve Mrs. Olson's treatment needs. Factors that are important for this client include:

- The ability of the agency to deliver services on the same day of hospital discharge.
- Services provided by the agency:
   Skilled nursing care
   Physical therapy
   Speech therapy
   Occupational therapy
   Home health aides
   Social worker
- The availability of 24-hour, 7-day-a-week at-home coverage by nursing staff.
- The capacity of the agency to provide services in accordance with Mrs. Olson's reimbursement sources.
- The capacity of the agency to provide services that cannot be reimbursed by the clients nor their insurance sources.
- The agency's policy for clients whose coverage runs out.
- The ability of the agency to supply and/or coordinate supplies, pharmaceuticals, and equipment/device needs of the client.
- The skill levels of the staff members related to monitoring of her condition, IV therapy administration, and case management.
- The agency's reputation for client advocacy, ethical performance, fair pricing of service, appropriate referrals, and discharge planning.
- The accuracy the agency uses in following the plan of care and timely revisions and the communication feedback it provides with physicians and referral services.

The following questions may stimulate your consideration of additional aspects of carefully promoting continuity of care for Mrs. Olson:

1. What might be the role and responsibilities of family members of other informal caregivers in assisting the client to successfully manage at home?

2. In what activities might you involve family/informal caregivers on the unit as an adjunct to discharge planning?

3. What resources can you reference in educating Mrs. Olson about the list of agencies from which she may select to receive her home health services?

4. How can you encourage physicians and other staff members to increase their utilization of home care referrals for their clients?

5. For what client situations may a home care referral not be the most appropriate option at discharge?

INFORMATION SOURCES

National League for Nursing
Accreditation Program for Home Care and Community Health
10 Columbus Circle
New York, NY 10019-1350

National Association for Home Care
519 C Street, NE, Stanton Park
Washington, DC 20002

Joint Commission on Accreditation of Hospitals
840 N. Lake Shore Drive
Chicago, IL 60611

American Nurses' Association
2420 Pershing Road
Kansas City, MO 64108

National Center for Homecare Education and Research
Empire State Building
350 Fifth Avenue
New York, NY 10118

National Health Lawyer Association
522 21st Street, Suite 120
Washington, DC 20006

National Foundation for Hospice and Home Care
519 C Street, NE, Stanton Park
Washington, DC 20002

State Association for Home Care
(The National Association for Home Care will provide the name, address, and telephone number of the respective state home care association of inquiry.)

REFERENCES

1. Spiegel D: *Home Healthcare.* Owings Mills, MD, National Health Publishing Co., 1983

2. Hanlon JJ, Pickett E: *Public Health Administration & Practice.* St. Louis, Times Mirror/Mosby, 1984

3. Wiles E: Home health care nursing. In Stanhope M, Lancaster J (eds): *Community Health Nursing.* St. Louis, C.V. Mosby, 1984, p780

4. Jarvis L: *Community Health Nursing.* Philadelphia, F.A. Davis Co., 1981

5. Dock L: The history of public health nursing. Public Health Nurse 14:524, 1922

6. Cherkasky M: The Montifiore Hospital home care. Amer J Public Health 39:163, 1949

7. Mundinger MO: *Home Care Controversy.* Rockville, MD, Aspen Corporation, 1983

8. Halamandaris VJ: The future of home care. Caring 4:6, 1985

9. Home care agencies up 25 percent since '84. Hospitals 59:1985

10. HCFA Data: Medicare-certified home health agencies. Hospitals 60:49, 1986

11. NAHC Report 3. July 22, 1985

12. *The Attempted Dismantling of the Medicare Home Health Benefit - Report to Congress.* National Association for Home Care, 1986

13. Arthur Andersen and Co: *Health Care in the 1990s: Trends and Strategies.* Chicago: American College of Hospital Administrators, 1984

14. Mader TW: U.S. Health Service Businesses. *Business Intelligence Program*, No. 702, 1984

15. Mickel C: Premature-discharge allegations intensify. Hospitals. 59:31, 1985

16. Berk M, Bernstein A: Use of home health services: Some findings from the National Medical Care Expenditure Survey. Home Health Services Quarterly. 6:13, 1985

17. O'Malley ST: Reimbursement Issues. In Stuart-Siddall S (ed): *Home Health Care Nursing.* Rockville, MD, Aspen Corp., 1986, p23

18. Leader S: *Home Health Benefits Under Medicare.* Wash., DC, AARP, 1986, 17

19. Montiero LA: Florence Nightingale on Public Health Nursing. Amer J Public Health 75:181, 1985

20. *Technology and Aging in America.* Washington, DC, US Congress, Office of Technology Assessment (OTA-BA-264) 1985

21. Braunstein C, Schlenker R: The impact of change in Medicare payment for acute care. Geriatric Nurs, 6:266, 1985

22. Hospital Corporation of America and Equitable Group and Health Insurance Co, Dec. 1986

23. McCormick B: The current shortage of nurses may be a cost factor. Hospitals 60:51, 1986

24. Lawrence J, Ging T: *National Survey of Home Health Care Graduate Nursing Education.* University of Michigan, 1986

25. Cetron M: A public opinion of home care. Caring 4:13, 1985

26. Spencer R: US health care costs make smallest jump in two decades. *Washington Post*, August 1, 1985, p1

27. Home care for chronically ill children examined. *The New York Times*, Dec. 7, 1986, p32

28. *The Health Policy Agenda for the American People: Summary Report*, 1987

BARBARA C. GAINES, RN, EdD

CHAPTER 22   *Health/Illness Care:*
Who Pays?

Background and Overview

As Americans face rapidly increasing health care costs, we are forced to ask ourselves three questions. What kinds of health and illness care do we want available to all of our citizens? How do we want to pay for the available services? How much are we willing to pay? The following verbal picture, drawn from commonly cited statistics, provides a perspective for the discussion of the issues that will influence how we answer these questions.

Health care costs consistently increase at a faster rate than the consumer price index (CPI). Since 1984 Americans have spent over $1 billion per day on health. A substantial portion of these dollars is spent on personal health services, including physician's visits, insurance, hospitalization, and drugs and supplies. These familiar expenditures represent one month's wages for most Americans. However, Americans also spend indirectly but substantially on health care facilities construction research, and the education and training of health care professionals.

The billion-dollar-per-day figure represents approximately 11 percent of the country's gross national product (GNP). Under present financing mechanisms, health care expenditures can be expected to claim an increasing percentage of the GNP. Economists predict the amount will reach 14 percent of the GNP, or $1.9 trillion, by the year 2000. Several factors will contribute to this increase. Two of the more significant are aging of the population and the fact that health care is a big and profitable business.[1-6]

Former Secretary of Health, Education and Welfare, Joseph A.

Califano, Jr., reminds us that America will experience a four-generation society with two generations on Medicare and in need of nursing early in the 21st century. It is generally accepted that these elderly will require more nursing care services than the rest of the population, as well as more intensive medical services.[7] Currently, our Medicare-supported elderly pay from their own pockets for over 40 percent of the services they receive. We need only reflect on current legislative and administration debates on the solvency of the Medicare program and the need for catastrophic illness insurance to gain an understanding of the magnitude of the influence the aging population will have on health care delivery needs and costs.

With Medicare for the elderly, Medicaid for some categorically-defined needy groups, and employment related insurance for a majority of adult Americans, approximately 85 percent of us have access to health care. Because access is most often through fee-for-service group insurance, Americans are often unaware of the real cost of health care. However, for the unemployed as well as many persons who are employed, access is not uniform. Young adults, seasonal and part-time workers, and many persons working in small business settings are uninsured.[8,9] We are only beginning to realize that all of us face the potential of losing our access to health care each time we lose a job or change positions.

This brief scenario points out that health care is not evenly distributed in American society and that the potential for even greater inequities exists. Given that Americans spend 11 percent of the GNP on health, the largest expenditure of any industrialized nation in the world; that we continue to read about an oversupply of health care workers, especially physicians; and that we have too many empty hospital beds, the question of why we must have inequitable health care access and service is being asked with increasing frequency. The answer appears to be embedded in how we answer the questions posed at the beginning of this chapter. What kinds of health and illness care do we want to be available to all of our citizens? How do we want to pay for the available services? How much are we willing to pay?

HEALTH AND ILLNESS CARE

When authors talk about health care, and especially when that reference is in the context of **reimbursable care,** they are talking primarily about care provided to combat some disease process. This is partly the case because many of the services essential to health, such as clean drinking water, solid waste disposal, and other sanitary measures are provided by our communities through different funding mechanisms and, therefore, taken for granted. Additionally, some services, such as immunizations, are available either through health care or community programs and are also taken for granted.

The issue facing us as Americans when we try to decide whether a disease-oriented definition of reimbursable health care is adequate occurs when we consider the consequences of broadening it. Many people argue that our definition of health care is narrow because we allowed physicians, hospitals, and insurors to define health care.

Early in this century, when medical education was reformed, physicians became the undisputed arbiters of what health care services were needed and of how those services should be provided. Physicians' mastery of a rapidly increasing knowledge base and associated technology gave them a privileged status with their patients. The move to hospitals as the centers for care delivery was logical as the complexity of available services increased. Burke concludes that the result of the efforts of organized medicine hospitals and insurors was ". . . a delivery system and a payment model that were institutionally biased and physician controlled. Both private insurance and Medicare and Medicaid programs favored services provided by physicians, particularly those provided in hospitals."[10]

Objections to this sickness oriented, institutionally based fee-for-service system were countered with arguments that increasing government control would result in socialized medicine, a lesser quality of care, and an interruption of the free choice of citizens in the selection of their physicians and insurance coverage. As costs continued to rise, reforms to the system have been introduced in the legislature on numerous occasions. The proposals have met with limited success, however, as long as demanded services were generally available.[11] That is to say, as long as the majority of Americans found their health care satisfactory and reasonably priced, they valued freedom of choice over regulated services. Questions of waste, inefficiency, and inequity have become strident only as we face increasing personal costs for health care, an insurmountable national debt, and recognize that larger segments of our population have decreasing access in our present system. We are faced with the prospect of a **"two-tier" system,** a system in which everyone is entitled to some care regardless of ability to pay; or with a system that denies care for those who cannot pay. In economic terms Americans are being asked to consider whether health care should become a freely traded commodity or be treated as a social good.[12]

Currently, health care functions in the economy as a managed commodity. All services are available to people willing and able to pay the cost. Governmental regulation provides ceilings on selected costs, however, and funds selected services for groups defined as needy. As cost have escalated beyond what many are willing or able to pay, new cost management strategies have been imposed in both the private and public sectors. The ability of these cost management systems to influence what health care services are available ro each of us has caused us to rethink what services *should* be available and how we *should* pay for them.

It has been widely commented on in the literature that Americans believe that any medical service that might benefit an individual who is ill should be available.[12,13] With our burgeoning science and technology, this attitude has brought about a phenomenal increase in health care spending.

Reinhardt tells us coronary bypass surgery costs over $30,000 in California;[12] Florida residents are reported on television news and in newspapers trying to raise $300,000–$500,000 for a child's liver transplant; and person after person testified before Congress in 1987 about the exhorbitant costs of terminal and/or catastrophic illness. Of the incidents mentioned, it is likely that the bypass surgery was the only one where the individual's insurance made it possible for him/her to meet his/her share of the costs without undue hardship.

The uninsured, underinsured, and medically indigent, some 32 million people, cannot receive this sophisticated care without charitable contributions. They cannot, in fact, even receive low technology care in many instances. This has led many persons to suggest that care is rationed without acknowledging it. They argue further that a "two-tier" system with a defined set of services for all would be more honest and relevant at this point in our history. They often compare American services with those in other countries where national health insurance programs exist.[12,13] Califano points to the significant impact Medicaid has had on morbidity and mortality as an example of what guaranteed access to health care can do.[14]

Reinhardt, an advocate of health care as a social good, suggests that America can afford to make health care available to all and that it must. He argues that although the provision of health services to everyone would necessitate difficult choices about which services are essential, the rising sense of competition in the health care industry mandates that we resolve this issue. He goes on to remind us that the medically needy will only grow in a competitive system where cost-shifting does not occur to reimburse providers for indigent care.[9,12]

Most of the evidence in the literature suggests that Americans favor spending a larger percentage of the GNP on health care and would support a tax increase if necessary to maintain services to the poor, elderly, and disabled. They support some form of national health program and increasing control over physicians' fees and hospital costs, as well as prescription drugs. They would not, however, like their personal care arrangements disrupted—eg, their ability to choose their own physician, their access to technology, or their right to sue for malpractice challenged. Some argue that this apparent ambivalence has made the move to national health insurance impossible. Others argue that the data have been misinterpreted and that public comment is not incompatable with effective health care for all our citizens.[15,16] Along with the arguments supporting equity in access and services, many are arguing that a shift from illness care to preventive and health promotion activities would significantly increase the health of our citizens and save significant dollars.

While the arguments are intuitively appealing, Russell argues that prevention and health promotion, like curative-medical care, cost money. For example, she presents data showing that many preventive measures, such as blood pressure screening for hypertension, may actually increase health care expenditures. Although the costs of a single screening are small, persons diagnosed as hypertensive enter the health care system at an earlier time, require long-term management, and are forced to cope with a disease through treatment that is often more troublesome than the disease itself. Thus, she argues that these additional costs do not support prevention as the panacea to escalating health care expenditures.

Russell extends her cost argument in a discussion of lifestyle change. She suggests that sufficient data are not yet available to justify claims that lifestyle modification will reduce cost. While agreeing that lifestyle as a form of prevention is useful and effective, she reminds us that we do spend money in support of these changes. Many of the expenditures occur outside of the traditional medical sector and are not reflected in health care cost effectiveness analyses. Thus, the true costs of lifestyle modification are not known.[17] It is clear, however, that there are substantial costs. One need only walk through a department store or grocery store to see the increased variety of products available to promote spending for "health."

Despite considerable debate, it is now clear to policymakers that unlimited services cannot exist in a climate of cost containment, that broadening the scope of services to include health promotion will cause cost increases of unknown magnitude, and that Americans are not willing to abandon the poor, the elderly, or the disabled in the health care delivery system. What is not clear to policymakers, and that which will be the subject of continued debate, is whether governmental support should be extended beyond categorically defined groups. If that were to happen, some form of national health program would be necessary. Such a program has little if any support in the business community or in the current administration.

PAYING FOR HEALTH CARE

To better understand what decisions we want to make about health care delivery and its financing, a brief review of major financing mechanisms, their strengths, and shortcomings is provided.

Private Health Insurance.   Two major forms of private health insurance exist, nonprofit organizations such as Blue Cross and Blue Shield and commercial providers, such as Aetna. Unlike most forms of insurance that protect against the unusual or unexpected, health insurance was developed during the Great Depression to provide a stable means to pay for expected and needed care. Although insurance has always been available to individuals, the vast majority is purchased by employers in group plans.

Developed by the American Hospital Association and the American Medical Association, Blue Cross and Blue Shield are nonprofit organizations. They are predicated on a **cost-reimbursement model** in which the insuror reimburses the hospital and physician for reasonable costs for a given patient. Reasonable costs are determined by insurance commissions in most states, and thus rates are subject to regulation.

Commercial insurors are subject to monitoring by insurance commissions; however, rate regulation is excluded in these oversight activities. Rate regulation would be antithetical to the for-profit nature of these companies. Commercial insurors offer more alternative plans, many of which extend coverage beyond an individual's basic plan. These supplemental offerings may include catastrophic care and cash payments while a person is ill.[2]

The strengths of the **private insurance system** have been that it has provided hospital medical care to workers and their dependents at reasonable premium costs, allowed people to choose their own physician and type of coverage within groups, and supported indigent care in hospitals through a mechanism known as cost-shifting. In **cost-shifting,** paying patients pay higher rates to cover the costs of nonpaying patients.[12] The shortcomings have been that the cost-reimbursement model encourages increased use of services, especially costly services, and that hospitalization has been encouraged. The more services used and the longer the stay, the more money made. This mode of operation has allowed hospital costs to rise at rates of over 12 percent per year for many years.[4,10] Because of the nature of medical care delivered in hospitals, the cost-reimbursement model neglected health care services designed to promote health, such as nutrition counseling, exercise testing, and stress management. Given our inflationary economy, the increase in cost associated with service utilization has spawned new initiatives in the private sector.

Two additional types of private insurers are gaining prominence in the 1980s. **Independent prepayment plans** such as Kaiser-Permanente and Group Health in Seattle are capturing an increasing share of the market, having grown from six percent of the market in 1983 to over ten percent in 1987. These health maintenance organizations (HMOs) and other preferred provider organizations (PPOs) are either profit or nonprofit oriented. Their purpose is to obtain services and products from providers at reduced costs. This practice is known as "prudent purchasing."[5,12,14] HMOs offer clients comprehensive health services as opposed to hospitalization. PPOs offer services through selected physician groups.[2] Both regulate consumer use of services and confine physician choice to members of the prepaid group practice. The amount of regulation versus freedom within the organization is usually driven by its profit status, with nonprofits like Kaiser emphasizing freedom and the profit-oriented companies emphasizing regulation.[18]

Self-insurance is the second private insurance mechanism that is gaining importance in the private sector. Businesses are self-insuring their employees through a variety of means, including the purchase and operation of their own insurance companies.[2,4]

There can be no question that the growth in HMOs, PPOs, and self-insurance can be attributed in part to business's dissatisfaction with escalating health care costs. However, government dissatisfaction with the costs of Medicare and Medicaid has been an equally important force in determining changes in hospital financing.

Medicare and Medicaid.   **Medicaid** was developed to assist the nation's poor. The major recipients are persons who receive Aid to Families with Dependent Children (AFDC) and persons who qualify for Supplemental Security Income (SSI). AFDC families receive approximately 30 percent of the services and SSI persons 70 percent of the services. It is a joint federal and state program and covers a variety of inpatient and outpatient services. Because states determine eligibility for Medicaid, the programs vary widely in coverage and services. This diversity makes uniform regulation difficult. In the spirit of cost-containment HMOs became eligible to care for Medicaid patients, and some co-payments have been introduced.[2,14]

Medicare, which began in 1966, was developed to provide the elderly in the Social Security system with a variety of medical benefits, including hospitalization, nursing home and home care, and physician services. Amendments to the law in the 1970s extended the benefits to everyone aged 65 and over and to selected groups in need. Medicare does not provide comprehensive service or financial coverage. For example, most preventive services are not covered and hospital costs are paid to about 80 percent. Two proposals currently being debated in Congress, catastrophic care and a flat rate for physician reimbursement for Medicare services, will significantly reduce individual costs, if passed. From its inception in 1965 until 1983, Medicare reimbursed physicians and hospitals on a retrospective cost model patterned on the model used by Blue Cross and Blue Shield.[2,12,14]

In a major cost-containment effort in 1982 and 1983, the government initiated a **prospective payment system** for hospitals caring for patients on Medicare. The system, another example of prudent purchasing, reimburses hospitals on the basis of the patient's diagnosis instead of a services-rendered basis. Prospective payment is known by the acronym, DRGs.[2] (DRGs are discussed in detail in Chapter 18.) Since the advent of prospective payment, the federal government has succeeded in changing patterns of care with many services shifted to the less costly outpatient setting and length of stay in hospitals decreased.[14]

These private and public sector initiatives have brought about changes in the health care services available to those of us covered by insurance plans and to some extent modified what and how we pay for services. For example, if our employer self-insures and we choose to use a different health care option, our out-of-pocket costs will increase. These initiatives foster competition in health care service delivery and thus suggest that health care can and should be treated as a freely traded commodity. They do not address the health care needs of the uninsured, the underinsured, or the medically indigent. If Reinhardt and others are correct, a competitive approach will only increase the number of Americans who are medically indigent.[4,9] However, given the current climate, very few arguments appear in the literature in support of national health insurance.

National Health Insurance.   National Health Insurance (NHI) is by no means a new concept. It has a long and varied history, serving as a means to check the growth of socialist groups in Germany at the time of Bismarck and as a way to protect the health of merchant seamen during colonial times in America. From 1912 until 1965, when Medicare and Medicaid were enacted, numerous proposals for NHI had been introduced and defeated largely through the continued efforts of the American Medical Association (AMA). Early in the century the AMA was joined by business and labor in these efforts. However, since the mid-1960s, labor has become an active force shaping proposals for NHI. There seemed to be little doubt that NHI would become a reality under President Carter despite Republican opposition voiced as late as 1976.[19,20] In the third edition of his book, *Health Care Delivery in the United States*, Jonas has replaced the last chapter, which was titled "National Health Insurance," with a chapter titled "A Review of the Past; Visions of the Future." In this chapter he comments, "National Health Insurance (NHI) was indeed a major actor on the stage of the era in which those editions were written: the 1970s. In the 1980s NHI has all but disappeared from the stage."[21]

The failure of NHI proposals in the 1980s cannot be attributed to diminishing need. The failure appears to center once again on the balance between governmental and private control. Senator Kennedy's limited 1985 proposal to reduce the numbers of uninsured and constrain costs recognized this need. It used regulation requiring employers to insure former employees and less costly outpatient services.[21] However, it failed. Similar legislation may be reintroduced in 1989 or 1990.[22] As costs continue to rise and if the medically indigent grow, it is likely additional governmental initiatives will receive a new hearing.

Impacts on the Nurse, the Consumer, and Society

The impact of escalating health care costs in a national climate of cost containment has different implications for nursing, for consumers, and for society as a whole. Not only is cost containment experienced differently by varying segments of our population, it is also being experienced differently by various providers.

THE NURSE

Several responses to cost containment have specific ramifications for nurses. For example, many hospitals are moving to all registered nurse (RN) staffs, and increasing their emphasis on primary nursing. These hospitals believe that the flexibility achieved with all RN staffs is cost-effective. The staff nurses are being asked to function at high levels of efficiency, eg, by introducing discharge planning on admission and regulating unnecessary use of services and supplies. They are increasingly being asked to be aware of how they spend their time, since nursing salaries are a large part of hospital costs. Despite these increases in efficiency, nurses in small community hospitals are suffering some unemployment or at least a limitation on number of hours worked.[5,23,24]

Nursing administrators, on the other hand, have used cost containment as a new impetus to determine what nursing care actually costs. Initial studies await replication, but hold promise of demonstrating that nursing can be a revenue as well as a cost center.[23,24] For example, studies continue to demonstrate that patient teaching is cost-effective.[25] The ability to demonstrate excellence in nursing as well as efficiency is considered a plus in a competitive marketplace.

Nurses in community settings and nursing homes are seeing major changes in their clients' level of illness as a result of cost containment. People are sicker before they enter a hospital and less well when they leave. Financing for many supportive resources available in the past has been cut. Community health nurses are being asked to assume increasing responsibility for the assssessment and provision of services, as well as for the coordination of care.[5]

Many nurses are seeking new employment opportunities in the private sector. They are working in HMOs and providing services and consultation to surgicenters, urgent care centers, home birthing centers, and day care centers for seniors. Some are going into business for themselves. These entrepreneurs are nurses with advanced preparation, such as certified nurses, midwives, and nurse practitioners (NPs), many of whom are eligible for third-party reimbursement. They are faced not only with providing needed services but with issues of productivity and quality of care. There is substantial evidence to show that NPs can save the public health care dollars. They cost less to educate and train than physicians, make smaller salaries, and often charge less for services. How rapidly nurse practitioner services will grow will be influenced by how much resistance physicians offer to the expansion of NP care, and by the amount and type of regulation imposed by legislatures.[5,26]

Nurses, regardless of the practice setting, are experiencing substantial increases in the cost of malpractice insurance. These increases are a result of expanded practice roles and of an increasing desire of the public for error-free practice. Some nurses, eg, CNMs and NPs, like some physicians, have had difficulty obtaining coverage at any cost. The issues surrounding tort reform—of which malpractice is a part—promise to challenge the profession for the next several years.

One impact of cost containment common to all nurses has been resolved. Documentation of observations, findings, services provided, referrals, etc., has gained increasing importance. Documentation of the nursing care plan is critical to reimbursement and to the research that must be done to assist the profession to demonstrate the value of nursing in the health care delivery system.

THE CONSUMER

Increasing costs are a major concern for all of us as consumers. Insurance premiums continue to cost more with higher deductibles and co-payments common. The need to obtain second and third opinions before a nonemergency procedure can be performed requires lost time from work that is often costly as well.

Shorter hospitalization may mean fewer nosocomial infections, but it also means that patients discharged earlier or undergoing day surgery will require support upon return to their homes. Adding this group to those who are elderly or have incapacitating chronic illnesses has greatly increased the need for supportive nursing and homemaker services. Obtaining this support for those who live alone or who are members of families where all members work is proving costly. In New York, for example, the largest increase in Medicaid spending is for personal care services.[27]

In summary, higher utilization of health maintenance organizations, out-patient services, and intermediate care services will likely disrupt some patient/physician relationships. Early experience with nurse practitioners in many of these agencies has been extremely positive. It is impossible at this time, however, to provide all Americans with free choice of health care provider. Under the present reimbursement systems, federal employees, for example, may have only physicians as primary providers. Similar conditions exist under many private insurance plans. Increasing access to nurses as primary providers is another challenge for the profession for the 1980s and 1990s.[28]

SOCIETY

Societal concerns with regard to the costs of health care become very significant when we consider rationing. When we think of rationing we usually think of a rationing of services based on age, severity of disease, or some other illness-related variable. This is the basis on which care is rationed in many countries with national health programs. When we talk of rationing care in the United States, the critics assert we are talking about rationing based on the ability to pay. The rationale for their argument is that we are unwilling to deal with the ethical dilemmas posed by our current system. Jonas and others suggest our confusion is heightened when we are encouraged to see ability to pay as a problem itself instead of seeing it as a part of the larger problem of inequitable access. That is, health care continues to be viewed as a problem of individual right and responsibility as opposed to a problem of distributive justice. How we view it will of course influence what solutions we find useful in our future.

Future Considerations

There seems to be little question that competition is alive and well in the market place of health care. Hospitals are announcing profits. Multi-hospitals are becoming common. These corporate entities share services such as purchasing and laboratories and drop nonprofitable services such as obstetrical care. Many organizations are diversifying and entering the health care market for the first time. For example, IBM is number one in the hospital computer market, GE is developing highly sophisticated equipment such as CAT scanners, MRIs, etc., and Avon is now in the x-ray contrast media business. Pharmaceutical houses are opening new markets overseas and smaller companies of all kinds are merging or being purchased by larger companies. The net result according to Levitt is that power is being concentrated into fewer but larger corporate entities.[4]

Given the political tenor of the present time, it is impossible to say whether new NHI legislation will be introduced in the near future. It must be remembered that at this point much of this private sector activity is financed with public funds creating even more incentives for business and its competitive approach.[4] If NHI is introduced it will require the support of physicians, hospitals, and business. Given business's response to HMOs and PPOs, it is also impossible to predict what the scope of the NHI program would be. The legislation introduced by Senator Kennedy in 1985 stopped far short of care for everyone. It seems far more likely that categorically defined proposals extending care to already covered groups such as catastrophic illness coverage for Medicare recipients will occur in our present political climate. Additionally, physician reimbursement reforms are likely, as is the continued governmental support for HMOs.[29]

Despite what appear to be failures in the overall system, some progress is present. Change continues to be incremental in the health policy arena. There is a rising awareness of the hazards of sidestream smoke and sexually transmitted diseases, and of the benefits of seatbelts and other motor vehicular safety devices. While the influence of these policy activities on costs has not yet been determined, they are having a positive influence on the health of our population.

Thus it seems that although we are unable to decide what services should or must be available to all, Americans are continuing to raise the arguments in such a way that the issues are being actively debated at state and national legislative levels, in business and industry, in professional meetings and journals, and in the popular press. Nursing's voice is heard along with the others. Nurses are actively supporting candidates working for the health of the country through political action committees (PACs) and campaign work. Nurses are increasingly invited to sit on national health policy advisory groups. Nurses are actively seeking political office and producing research on significant health care delivery issues. Never before in our history have *all* the groups come together with the common goal of cost containment in health care spending. The attention of everyone holds promise that a clearer statement of health policy may be forthcoming. The continuing experimentation with new payment mechanisms both in the private and public sector suggests that efficient financing systems will be available to complement health policy as it unfolds. How much we will pay remains an unknown, but what that amount is and what it represents, both in services and proportion of the GNP, remains a conscious choice.

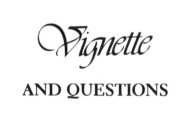

Vignette

AND QUESTIONS

You and three of your classmates in your "Issues" class are assigned to present an hour-long oral presentation titled "Health Care for the Uninsured, Underinsured, and Medically Indigent: Whose Responsibility Is It?" You are meeting with the faculty member, Dr. Leiber, to outline the elements of your presentation. Dr. Leiber reminds you that the major issues with regard to this question focus on the assignment of responsibility. She suggests that you consider the question in terms of legal and political responsibility, economic responsibility, and ethical orientations. Dr. Leiber then asks you to summarize your thinking by presenting a rational position for the nursing profession to espouse to legislators on this issue. As you and your classmates meet to prepare your presentation, you ask yourselves the following questions.

1. If, as Dr. Leiber suggests, the issues are the assignment and assumption of legal, economic, and ethical responsibility, what are the strengths and drawbacks to competitive versus governmental solutions?

2. Can the United States afford a national health program that would include comprehensive national health insurance, or should we consider rationing?

3. If nursing developed a public position supporting a "two-tiered" system of care, would you support it? If yes, what facts and principles would form the basis for your argument? If no, what arguments would you present?

INFORMATION SOURCES

National Center for Health Statistics
Superintendent of Documents
US Government Printing Office
Washington, DC 20402

Health Care Financing Administration (HCFA) publications:
  a. Health Care Financing Review
  b. National Health Expenditures
  c. Private Health Insurance
  d. Medicare and Medicaid Data Book
Superintendent of Documents
US Government Printing Office
Washington, DC 20402

American Nurses' Association (ANA) publications:
  a. Facts About Nursing
  b. Capital Update
  c. The American Nurse
ANA
2420 Pershing Road
Kansas City, MO 64108

National League for Nursing (NLN) publications:
a. Executive Director Wire
b. Nursing and Health Care
NLN
10 Columbus Circle
New York, NY 10019

State Boards of Nursing, Medical Examiners, and Health for Local Statistics

REFERENCES

1. NBC Nightly News, February 9, 1987

2. McCarthy CM, Thorpe KE: Financing for health care. In Jonas S: *Health Care Delivery in the United States*, ed 3: New York, Springer, 1986, p303

3. Munson R: The claim to health care. *Intervention and Reflection: Basic Issues in Medical Ethics*, ed 2: Belmont, CA, Wadsworth, 1983, p517

4. Levitt J: The corporatization of health care. In Jonas S: *Health Care Delivery in the United States*, ed 3: New York, Springer, 1986, p483

5. Davis CK: The federal role in changing health care financing. Nurs Economics 1:10, 1983

6. Starr P: *The Social Transformation of American Medicine*. New York, Basic Books, 1982

7. Califano JA Jr: A revolution looms in American health. *The New York Times*, March 25, 1986

8. Tallon JR: The case of mandatory employer health insurance coverage, in *National Debate on Health Care*. Dallas, TX, April 20–23, 1986

9. Reinhardt UE: The case for mandatory employer health insurance coverage. In *National Debate on Health Care*. Dallas, TX, April 20–23, 1986

10. Burke SP: The economics of nursing: Implications for clients, providers and educators. In Sorenson G (ed): *The Economics of Health Care and Nursing*. Kansas City, MO, ANA American Academy of Nursing, 1985, p33

11. Falk IS: Medical care in the USA: 1932–1972. Problems, proposals and programs from the committee on the costs of medical care to the committee for national health insurance. Health and Society 51:1, 1973

12. Reinhardt UE: Rationing the health-care surplus: An American tragedy. Nurs Economics 4:101, 1986

13. Aaron HJ, Schwartz WB: *The Painful Prescription: Rationing Health Care*. Washington, DC, The Brookings Institution, 1984

14. Califano JA Jr: *America's Health Care Revolution: Who Lives? Who Dies? Who Pays?* New York, Random House, 1986

15. Blendon RJ, Altman DE: Special report: Public attitudes about health-care costs, a lesson in national schizophrenia. N Engl J Med 311:613, 1984

16. Navarro V, Altman DE: Debate on popular opinion and U.S. Health policy: Are Americans schizophrenic? *Inter J Health Services* 15:511, 1985

17. Russell L: *Is Prevention Better Than Cure?* Washington, DC, The Brookings Institution, 1986

18. Adler S: Personal Communication, May 7, 1986

19. Falk IS: Proposals for national health insurance in the USA: Origins and evolution, and some perceptions for the future. Health and Society 55:161, 1977

20. Enthoven AC: Consumer-choice health plan (second of two parts): A national-health-insurance proposal based on regulated competition in the private sector. N Engl J Med 298:709, 1971

21. Jonas S: *Health Care Delivery in the United States*, 3d ed: New York, Springer, 1986, p504

22. Maraldo PJ: *Executive Director Wire*. New York, National League for Nursing, December 1986

23. Booth RZ: Financing mechanisms for health care: Impact on nursing services. J Profess Nurs 1:34, 1985

24. Hartley SS: Effects of prospective pricing on nursing. Nurs Economics 4:16, 1986

25. Karam JA, Sundre SM, Smith GL: A cost/benefit analysis of patient education. Hospital and Health Services Administration 31:82, 1986

26. Sweet JB: The cost-effectiveness of nurse practitioners. Nurs Economics 4:190, 1986

27. Schneider D: *Patient Classification Reimbursement: Quality Assurance in the Long Term Care System*. Portland, OR: February 19–20, 1987

28. Health Insurance Mandate Proposed. Capitol Update 5:5, May 25, 1987

29. Davis CK: Health care reforms: What can we expect? Nurs Economics 4:10, 1986

JANET NIEMI CHUBB, RN, MS

Deinstitutionalization of the Mentally Ill

CHAPTER 23

Background and Overview

During the past four decades the federal, state, and local governments, along with the private sector, have spent considerable time and money developing and reforming a system of treatment and care of the mentally ill. The result of this reform has been the development of the philosophy that community based treatment programs, rather than centralized institutional services, were the most effective and humane way of providing mental health services to the chronically mentally ill. Further, psychiatry has been altering its treatment approach from long-term institutional to short-term community-based psychiatry. It was the philosophy of the National Institute of Mental Health, along with the Joint Commission on Mental Illness and Health, that community-based psychiatric programs would prevent long-term disability. In keeping with the ethic of humane treatment, these federal commissions recommended reducing the size of state mental institutions by **deinstitutionalizing** or re-integrating the mentally ill client into the community.[1-3] While the intent of deinstitutionalization was to provide alternatives to institutional care, the sequelae of this movement has impacted the consumer, the provider, and society.

HISTORICAL EVOLUTION

In 1955 federal health policy was impacted by the international examination of mental health legislation and the development of mental health services by the World Health Organization.[3] The thesis of this committee was that effective mental health legislation should accurately reflect the current status of mental health needs and that legislation should advance the development of additional programs and services to meet these needs. In addition, the increase in the populations of state psychiatric hospitals, the increased financial burden of state governments to provide inpatient care, and the goal of the federal government of reducing state expenditures led to the development of the Mental Health Study Act and the establishment of the Joint Commission of Mental Illness.[4] Responding to these influences, federal mental health policy was developed that reflected a humane treatment focus as well as community based treatment programs. The Joint Commission on Mental Illness and Health called for improvements in mental health treatment, development of better short-term treatment modalities, the reduction in size of state hospital facilities, and the creation of aftercare and rehabilitation services.[5] In order to carry out these goals, the commission made very specific recommendations to President Kennedy and the Congress in 1960, which resulted in the passage of the Community Mental Health Centers Construction Act of 1963.[6-7]

The development of mental health policy is best understood when further examined from the perspective of the sociopolitical forces of the late 1950s. To elucidate, psychoactive drugs were being used throughout the country that allowed psychiatric patients to return to the community. In addition, there was increased public interest in the effects of poverty, racism, individual rights, and the care and treatment of the mentally ill. Legislation reflecting these concerns was evidenced in the **Draft Act,** which advocated the voluntary admission (as opposed to involuntary admission) of patients to mental hospitals in order to facilitate access of the mentally ill to treatment facilities.[8] President Kennedy's efforts drew public attention to the treatment of the mentally ill and mentally retarded. Community mental health programs aimed at combating mental illness and retardation and providing humane and ethical treatment through the use of community centered agencies were developed. In 1963 Congress passed one of the most enlightened pieces of legislation, the **Mental Health Centers Act.** This act provided seed money to help states develop new and expanded community-based mental health centers. The seed money was to encourage these centers to become self-sufficient and to aid in the "deinstitutionalization" of the mentally ill. This philosophy was congruent with the social and political tenor of the time and reflected Kennedy's "bold, new approach." [9-12]

The Mental Health Centers Act, along with the Medicare/Medicaid Bill of 1965, resulted in the reduction of the population of state institutions by 75 percent.[3,13-14] While the reduction achieved the desired goal, individuals in the state institutions were "dumped" into the community without systematic, comprehensive, or clearly defined strategies or plans to achieve the shift of care from the institutions to the communities. Deinstitutionalization was achieved in theory, but it did not achieve the intent of the policy: humanistic care and treatment of patients. Living facilities, treatment programs, and financial resources were unavailable or nonexistent for the deinstitutionalized patient. Therefore state institutions experienced a "revolving door" syndrome in which the chronically ill patients were readmitted.[1,15]

During this time the media sensationalized the need for mental health reforms by depicting numerous "true life" stories of patients who had been "dumped" into the community and who committed heinous crimes within hours or days of their discharge. Other stories recounted incidents of patients being hospitalized inappropriately for many years. For example, a woman committed in 1940 to a state institution for mental retardation was found in 1972 not to be retarded, but rather a genius. These incidents outraged the public, who demanded reform of commitment laws making it more difficult to involuntarily commit an individual to a state institution. Likewise, the public demanded stringent reforms in discharge laws. As a result, commitment and discharge statutes slowly began to change.

In 1970 the deinstitutionalization and the community mental health policies were a disaster. To rectify this situation, the federal government provided nominal fiscal support to communities to develop a system of support service among existing agencies for the deinstitutionalized patient. Concomitantly, lawsuits were filed by mental patients when the legislated programs failed to provide for the humane care and treatment of the mentally ill.

COURT CASES

Court cases regarding the implementation of the new mental health policy of deinstitutionalization were common during the 1960s and 1970s in spite of the numerous changes and approaches to the treatment of mental disorders. Until this time, the courts had maintained a "hands-off" policy toward the mentally disabled. However, between 1972 and 1977, a series of judicial decisions were made in response to society's request for tighter commitment and discharge laws and patient rights. The judicial decisions established a right to treatment in the least restrictive alternative, protection from harm, procedural and substantive safeguards in the civil commitment process, restrictions on forced administration of psychotropic drugs, electroconvulsive therapy (ECT), psychosurgery, and the right to educational programs for all handicapped children.[1,16,17] These changes reversed not only the legal aspects of reform in mental health treatment, but also the sociopolitical and ethical aspect related to reform in mental health treatment laws. Although the concept that the mentally ill are entitled to a full compliment of personal rights and civil liberties as they undergo treatment was embraced by the public, operationalizing the concept proved problematic. As mental health professionals attempted to establish community living facilities for the deinstitutionalized patient, they met public resistance to having mental patients in the community.

SUPREME COURT DECISIONS

In spite of state attempts via legislation to promote humane and ethical treatment while protecting patients and the public, suits continued to be filed in the Supreme Court by patients demanding treatment during hospitalization and community resources upon discharge.[18] O'Connor v. Donaldson was a landmark case in which a psychiatric patient held involuntarily in an institution for 15 years filed suit against the superintendent of the institution for denial of his civil liberties. The Supreme Court ruled in favor of Donaldson, stating that an individual who was not dangerous to him/herself or who could care for him/herself, or who could survive safely with responsible significant others, could not be confined against his/her will.[19-21]

Thus the court ruled that patients in public mental institutions who receive only custodial care be given treatment or be released.[2] When the Supreme Court ruled in favor of Donaldson, initially there was concern by the public that state institutions would release patients by the thousands. Some institutions released patients rather than provide treatment, but massive numbers of discharges did not occur. Instead, once again, as during the Kennedy era, the consciousness of the relevant publics was raised regarding the rights of the mentally disabled. The ethic of humane care and treatment gained momentum as evidenced by a small number of communities developing alternative resources. New York City developed Fountain House, a sheltered living and work environment, while communities such as St. Louis, Missouri, and Madison, Wisconsin, developed similar group programs in response to the Supreme Court decisions.

Other lawsuits continued to be filed in order to explore and secure the rights of the mentally disabled. For example, in the case of Wyatt v. Stickney, the court ruled that when an individual is denied his/her liberty because of confinement in an institution, the institution must provide something in return (treatment) for the deprivation of liberty. As a result of this court decision, states were forced to make changes in their institutional environment that included changes not only in the physical plant (ensuring the right to privacy), but also changes in the criteria for adequacy of treatment. Clearly, this mandated that institutions must provide for a humane psychological and physical environment by providing qualified staff in adequate numbers and individual treatment plans. Some mental hospitals opted to release patients rather than provide quality treatment.

Occurring simultaneously was the amendment to the Social Security Act that provided a monthly allotment for disabled persons under the auspices of the Social Security supplemental income.[3] This allowed mentally disabled persons, who had been dependent upon the state because of lack of financial resources, to be discharged from state facilities and returned to the community with some sense of financial support. This event, coupled with the Supreme Court decisions, established mental health and social policy and shaped the delivery of deinstitutionalized mental health care services.[13,22]

RESPONSES TO THE SUPREME COURT DECISIONS

State and local governments responded favorably to the Supreme Court decisions of deinstitutionalization as evidenced by changes in commitment and discharge processes and the strong ethical and social policy for adopting the principle of the least restrictive alternative. Because the financial and administrative resources and supports have not been available, state and local governments have been unable to implement the Supreme Court ruling.[23,24]

Most of the legislation developed or enacted since the formation of the National Institute of Mental Health has focused on an environmental approach, ie, promote patient discharge from the institutions to the community.[25,26] The problem with the effective and humane deinstitutionalization of the individual has been the lack of financial support to either the communities who receive the patients or the patients themselves.

By the end of the 1970s the economic condition of the United States was threatening the Community Mental Health Center. In response to the demise of community mental health services and the Supreme Court ruling, President Carter proposed to Congress the **Mental Health Systems Act.** The purpose of this act was to provide direction for states to review and revise mental health laws to ensure that clients' civil rights were protected, and that they received needed services. Funding of community mental health centers would be authorized to provide services for high risk populations, ambulatory mental health centers, prevention units, etc. The Mental Health Systems Act was designed to coordinate a two-tiered system of mental health care that had evolved since Kennedy's 1963 Community Mental Health Center Act. Before the Mental Health Systems Act could be implemented, the political climate changed, significantly altering the role of the federal government in the nation's mental health.[3,5]

Impacts on the Nurse, the Consumer, and Society

THE NURSE

The development of psychiatric nursing practice and education during the past 40 years has been related to sociopolitical and economic forces and concomitant mental health legislation. The deinstitutionalization movement impacted nursing in that, as specific mental health needs were identified, training needs of mental health workers were developed. Mental health legislation enacted during the 1950s and 1960s has been viewed as the most significant piece of legislation affecting the development of graduate training programs in psychiatric nursing and in the development of psychiatric content in baccalaureate nursing programs.[27-29]

The quality of nursing care given to patients and the research of patient care were influenced by this legislation. Since the passage of the **Community Mental Health Centers Act of 1963,** psychiatric nursing has been characterized by innovation with new roles for psychiatric nursing emerging. For example, the scope of psychiatric nursing has broadened to include not only administration, teaching, and management, but intervention and treatment of various levels of mental health and illness in community and institutional settings. Psychiatric nursing has developed in response to the growth of the professional organization and the recognition by society of the need for qualified, well-educated nurses to provide psychiatric mental health care. Furthermore, the Community Mental Health Center Act legitimized the advanced practice role of the psychiatric-mental health nurse and released it from medical/institutional domination. The Community Mental Health Centers Act of 1963 not only moved the patient into the community, but it moved the nurse into the community as well. As can be seen, the roles of the psychiatric mental health nurse and public health (community) nurse developed and advanced more as a result of this legislation than any other legislation to date.

The passage of the mental health legislation described thus far has not been without struggle for autonomy and independence in the acceptance of nursing. Psychiatric nurses, concerned about health care planning, policy development, and the humanistic care and treatment of individuals, found themselves in adversarial positions and "ethical" dilemmas with patients or with the judicial-legal-psychiatric system. For example, the professional nurse is an advocate for the patient and in that role should protect the patient's civil liberties and dignity while at the same time promoting patient rehabilitation and facilitating effective delivery of coordinated services. Oftentimes, these roles are in opposition to each other, resulting in ethical dilemmas for the nurse.

Nurses have responded to these conflicts by involving themselves in health care policy development. Nursing has assumed an aggressive political position as evidenced by election to congressional seats, involvement in local, state, and national mental health associations, development of support groups for the chronically mentally ill, and identification and utilization of resources for the mentally ill.[30]

THE CONSUMER AND SOCIETY

The consumer and society have been impacted by the deinstitutionalization programs that were launched in an incremental fashion with little analysis of the practical limitations of the programs or the long-term consequences of the program. To illustrate, the patient has become lost in the system, or worse yet, become a victim of the system. Instead of being deinstitutionalized and treated in a humane manner, the mentally disabled have been deinstitutionalized in other facilities, not always the least restrictive alternative.[31]

Newspaper articles have described former mental patients who are homeless or without support systems who become victims of crimes or lost in the system. In order for the chronically mentally ill to be humanely deinstitutionalized, community support systems that strengthen the individual's chances of successful adaptation to the community are mandatory. These include group homes, lodge programs, or other sheltered living environments. Employment opportunities that are not competitive and that enhance the individual's sense of self-worth are essential to the patient's successful adaptation to community living.

The case of David (a pseudonym), a 27-year-old, single Caucasian male with chronic mental illness, illustrates this point. Due to the nature and chronicity of David's illness, and numerous involuntary commitments to state institutions, all family supports and community resources had been exhausted. He had limited social supports and little hope of remaining outside the state mental hospital for any prolonged period of time following discharge. He had been hospitalized 12 times since age 20. During one of his hospitalizations at a state facility, an attempt was made to find a structured living and work environment for him, knowing that his success in the community depended upon such a placement. David had no financial resources. Aware of the Supreme Court decisions and his civil liberties, David, along with his court-appointed attorney, demanded release from the hospital rather than wait for financial aid to be approved or for a group home vacancy to materialize. Within 30 days post discharge, David came to the attention of law enforcement officers and subsequently, mental health personnel, when he was found wandering the city streets inadequately clothed in the subzero temperature and in a confused and delusional state.

During his rehospitalization, application was made and granted for **Social Security Disability Income (SSI)**. (This entitlement allows individuals with chronic illnesses who have no financial resources to receive a monthly allotment.) David was eligible for discharge seven months before his actual discharge date. Critics might say that David's civil liberties had been violated when he was not discharged after he recompensated (he no longer evidenced psychotic behavior) 45 days after admission. Other critics would offer a similar comment when mental health professionals discharged him into the community without available resources or supports.

David remained out of the institution in a structured group home for three years. In 1981 the federal government withdrew all monies from SSI participants 55 years of age and younger who were receiving SSI monies, until a formal review of the individuals' chronic illness and disability could be verified. When David's money was gone and there were no other resources available to him in the community, David returned to the hospital. Although deinstitutionalization was intended to humanize the delivery of psychiatric services and to improve the lot for the psychiatric patient, David's situation is clearly an example of deinstitutionalization working in theory, but not in practice.

Programs aimed at deinstitutionalization and protecting the individual's civil liberties failed in the face of changes and unanticipated circumstances. This has been due, in part, to the decline in tax revenues during the last eight to ten years and to the increase in health care costs. In addition, people are living longer and are subject to chronic or long-term illnesses that require multiple resources.

Advances in medical technology have improved early diagnoses and treatment of physiological disorders and prolonged life for both the physically and mentally ill. Likewise, mental health advances have resulted in earlier diagnoses and treatment of mental disorders and subsequently resulted in prolongation of the lives of the mentally ill. Consequently, the population of chronically mentally disabled adults is rapidly increasing. Chronically mentally disabled individuals are often between the ages of 18 and 35 when they experience their first psychotic episode that requires hospitalization. They suffer persistent disability in their psychological and social functioning, so much so that they need the help of mental health and other social agencies in a variety of ways over a period of years. Because of the nature and chronicity of their diseases they require individual, creative, and flexible treatment approaches. For example, many chronically mentally disabled adults resist community mental health treatment programs because of the bureaucracy. These same patients have responded favorably to treatment programs developed in (nonbureaucratic) coffee houses.[1,32-33]

State hospitals, because of their bureaucratic organization structure and due to Medicare and Medicaid changes, found themselves in direct competition with the community for the dollar. Consequently, there were no collaborative efforts towards successful integration of the patient into the community in the least restrictive alternative. In the absence of funding, the message was clear that mental health care and treatment were not a priority. State institutions were inadequately funded, as were community mental health centers.

Not all mental health policies have failed. Those that succeeded for a short time did so during periods of economic stability or during periods when the ethic was one of moral humanitarianism. Current programs and policies have failed because the policy makers have not taken into consideration the reluctance of the public to allocate sufficient resources for the ever-expanding population of the chronically mentally ill.[13]

Litigation, or a law suit, is a crude tool to change the mental health system. Usually judicial decisions are based on constitutional question or on statutory intent, which require executive and legal actions. While litigation has changed the mental system and patients have been released (deinstitutionalized) in significant numbers from state hospitals, these decisions have not always resulted in appropriate alternatives to institutional care. Similarly, individual's rights have not always been safeguarded as was intended.

There is an agreement, among mental health professionals and the judicial system, that it is inhumane to keep people with chronic, severe mental illnesses in hospitals when they are not getting better or when all that can be done has been done. Nevertheless, it is also inhumane to discharge the chronically mentally disabled individual, who even in remission exhibits extreme dependency on the mental health system, without adequate community support or resources. These individuals are often socially isolated, with limited social supports, and with little hope of lasting success, despite their aspirations and motivations.[33,34] Discharging the mentally disabled patient from the hospital as soon as he/she has received "maximum hospital benefit" protects his/her civil liberties, but to do so without legislative and social or community support is inhumane and contributes to the decline in the quality of life.

Future Considerations

Administrative "buck-passing," as well as the absence of funding, obstruct the mandate of change, and hinder the determination of priorities and the direction of policy formulation. In order for policies to be implemented, communities need "start-up" dollars and flexible funding to support the treatment of the mentally disabled. Currently, the financial structure for each state's mental health program is based on **block grants.** The concept of block grants was developed in the 1970s under the guise of "new federalism."

Block grants decentralized federal social programs to state and local governments. The rationale: to limit federal involvement in these programs and to boost the fiscal and political responsibility of state and local programs.[35] Block grants were designed to increase the decision-making activities of the local and state governments. However, because of the flexibility that block grants afforded states, great inequities in the same program occurred across the states. As a result, uniform benefits for the deinstitutionalized, chronically mentally ill have been lacking. Furthermore, because the deinstitutionalized chronically mentally ill are heavily dependent on state determined benefits, they are vulnerable in periods of economic flux. The overall result of block grants has been reduction in programs and services for the mentally ill.[35]

For mental health policies to work successfully, both fiscal and programmatic interventions must be effected by the experts in these areas. Therefore, what is needed are small, centrally located, therapeutically oriented programs available to the individual in the community residence. Community residences should be available with multimodal treatment, supervised living arrangements, and sheltered employment. The state of Wisconsin has developed a community-based service for the deinstitutionalized adult. Over time, Wisconsin evolved a mechanism for funding and methods of fixing of responsibilities that have made it fiscally and organizationally possible for counties in the state to develop comprehensive community programs for chronically mentally ill persons.[36,37] Involuntary commitment to outpatient treatment may be another approach to treating the deinstitutionalized chronically mentally ill.

As chronic illnesses, the financing of indigent health care, and the provision of health care needs are examined, mechanisms for rendering mental health care services must also be evaluated. Currently, there is no congressional proposal of national health insurance that contains significant mental health benefits.[5] Furthermore, the opposition to national health insurance precludes one from assuming this to be a viable solution to the health care of the mentally disabled. Yet the current Supreme Court rulings must be maintained and monitored, placing the mental health professional, civil liberty attorneys, and state legislators in a "Catch-22" situation. Monitoring professional standards in care and practice of health care providers (nurses, psychiatrists, psychologists, social workers) through the professional organization (ANA, APA, JCAH, AHA, ACSW) is one way to maintain the Supreme Court rulings in a humane manner. Health care professionals are in key positions to prepare for policy changes by conducting research relative to treatment in the least restrictive alternative.

Limited research has been done to provide a precise picture of the chronically mentally ill patient and his/her interaction with or response to a variety of mental health services and the consequences of these services. Instead, the literature is replete with studies and reports on medication compliance/noncompliance and recidivism rate.[38-40] Such research would provide the empirical data on the efficacy of treatment interventions and therapeutic environments.[22,40]

Identification of the needs of the community and involvement at the grass roots level to carry out the least restrictive alternative policy are clearly roles for the professional nurse.[30] Conveying these needs to city councilmen, state legislators, and the relevant publics will enhance the development of policy changes. Coupled with empirical evidence, policy changes then will not only be supported, but more importantly, the short-term and long-term consequences of the policy can be evaluated.

Finally, the health care professional must remain an advocate for the mentally disabled to ensure that community and institutional resources are in place. The role of the advocate should be to protect the patients' civil liberties and dignity, while promoting patient rehabilitation and facilitating effective delivery of coordinated services. In this specific issue the posture of professionals as advocates is supported by the Supreme Court.

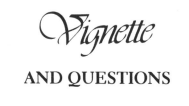

Vignette

AND QUESTIONS

Polly, an 18-year-old single female, had been in and out of state institutions since the age of 11. She is the oldest of four children. Her siblings, who were "normal," lived with their natural parents in a nearby community. Polly sometimes lived with a maternal grandmother when she was not in institutions. Her grandmother died when Polly was 16.

Polly's diagnoses included attention deficit disorder with hyperactivity, psychotic-like behavior, and oppositional behavior. Academic and intellectual assessments indicated that Polly's IQ was 99 and that her academic performance was at fifth-grade level. Polly was assessed as socially deprived.

Coincidentally, when Polly turned 18, the Supreme Court handed down decisions relative to the rights of mental patients, such as the right to the least restrictive environment. In light of these rulings, civil liberties attorneys reviewed all patient records within the institution where Polly was hospitalized and initiated legal action to discharge patients from the hospital. One such patient was Polly.

The state in which Polly resided had narrowly defined laws that made involuntary commitment possible only when mental illness existed along with dangerousness to self or others (suicidal/homicidal). Hospital professionals argued that Polly was a danger to herself because she lacked the necessary skills to survive independently; she had no employment skills, limited financial resources, and no problem-solving or critical thinking skills. Polly's attorneys cited two incidents in which Polly left the hospital and was gone for three days on one occasion and one week on another occasion without harm coming to her. In addition, they substantiated that Polly received $170.00 SSI per month. Therefore, she not only had the financial resources to support herself, but the capacity to survive on her own independently.

Hospital personnel testified of Polly's learning disability and social deprivation, which necessitated her living in a structured group home. They pointed out that to discharge Polly into the community without any resources for her would result in her falling victim to society, being abused by society, or perhaps worse. The hospital contended that the meager SSI income was not enough for Polly to survive on in the community. No other resources were available. The hospital's alternative was to continue to work on a placement in a group community home where former patients live together and work at their own janitorial business. Placement in this facility would take three to six months, as a site for the group home had not been found and community members were opposed to a group home.

According to the Supreme Court decisions, all mental patients have the right to maintain the greatest degree of freedom, self-determination, autonomy, and integrity of body, mind, and spirit. The mentally ill are entitled to a full compliment of personal and civil liberties while being protected from the public. Patients' civil liberties should be upheld to the extent that to do so does no harm to the patient or society.

Society wants a mentally ill individual where he/she will cause the least harm. Society wants protection from the mentally ill or mentally retarded.

Mental health professionals support the right of mental patients and in particular support their discharge to less restricted environments. They oppose discharge without adequate resources.

1. Should Polly be discharged from the hospital? Support your answer.

2. Support the premise that a chronically ill patient should be treated in an institution.

3. Discuss the professional nurse's role in resolving the complex problem of the deinstitutionalization of the mentally ill.

INFORMATION SOURCES

Nurses and other mental health professionals can and do participate in any number of national associations and advocate for the mentally ill. Local and state chapters are in existence in many areas. Interested persons should contact their local mental health association for more information. Listed below are national organizations/groups that can be employed when advocating for the mentally ill.

National Alliance for the Mentally Ill (NAMI): NAMI is a national organization for family members of psychotic persons. There are local and state groups of NAMI.

National Center on Child Abuse and Neglect: This is a national organization with local and state chapters.

National Mental Health Association: This national organization is a political force in effecting national mental health legislation. Local and state chapters are also instrumental in effecting changes in state mental health laws.

National Commission for the Protection of Human Subjects of Biomedical and Behavioral Research: This commission has developed ethical principles for the conduct of research involving human subjects and developed guidelines to ensure that such principles are followed. This information can be used by the mental health professional to ensure the patient's constitutional rights.

American Nurses' Association, Division of Psychiatric and Mental Health Nursing Practice.

Local legislators and elected senators and congressmen. Get to know your representatives and acquaint them with mental health issues and the development of mental health policies.

REFERENCES

1. Bachrach LL: Is the least restrictive environment always the best? Sociological and semantic implications. Hosp & Comm Psych 31: 2, 1982

2. Donahue W: What about our responsibility toward the abandoned elderly? Gerontologist 18: 2, 1978

3. Harding TN, Curran WJ: Mental health legislation and its relationship to program development: An international review. Harvard Legislation 16: 1, 1979

4. Chamberlin J: The role of the federal government in development of psychiatric nursing. Psychosocial Nurs Ment Health Serv 21: 4, 1984

5. Morrissey JP, Goldman HH: Cycles of reform in the care of the chronically mentally ill. Hosp & Comm Psych 35: 89, 1984

6. Stone A: Recent mental health legislation: A critical perspective. Am J Psych 134:273, 1977

7. Yardy K: New directions in federal policies for health care: A critique. Bull Acad Med 59: 4, 1983

8. Ewalt J: The mental health movement. Mill Mem Fund Quart 57: 4, 1979

9. Mechanic D: *Future Issues in Health Care*. New York, The Free Press, 1979

10. Fagin C: Psychiatric nursing at the crossroads: Quo vadis? Perspec Psych Care 19: 3, 1981

11. Hedlund N, Jeffery F: Historical development in mental health psychiatric nursing. In Beck C, Rawlins R, Williams S (eds): *Mental Health Psychiatric Nursing*. Toronto, CV Mosby, 1984, p3

12. Dumas R: Social, economic, and political factors and mental illness. Psych Nurs Ment Health Serv 21:3, 1983

13. Morrissey JP, Goldman HH: Cycles of reform in the care of the chronically mentally ill. Hosp & Comm Psych 35: 89, 1984

14. Robbins H: Influencing mental health policy: The mental health approach. Hosp & Comm Psych 31: 9, 1980

15. Annas GJ: Refusing medication in mental hospitals. The Hastings Center Reports, 1980

16. Speece, RG: Preserving the right to treatment: A critical assessment of constructive development of right to treatment theories. Arizona Law Review, 1979

17. Developmentally disabled assistance and bill of rights, PL 94, 1975

18. Bradley V, Clark G: *Paper Victories and Hard Realities: The Implementation of the Legal and Constitutional Rights of the Mentally Disabled*. Washington, Georgetown University Health Policy Center, 1976

19. Hoffman R: Treatment of the mentally ill. San Diego Law Rev 14: 28, 1977

20. Zlolnic D: First do no harm: Least restrictive alternative. W VA Law Review 83: 3, 1981

21. Hiday V, Goodman RR: Least restrictive alternative. Int J Law Psychiatry 10: 159, 1982

22. Yohalem JB, Manes J: The rights of the mentally disabled and progress in the face of new realities. Trial 80: 12, 1983

23. Binkley TC: The mentally ill: A discussion of rights. Trial 79: 7, 1982

24. Eth S, Levine ML, Lyon-Levin M: Ethical conflicts at the interface of advocacy and psychiatry. Hosp & Comm Psych 35: 7, 1984

25. Flagg J: Public policy and mental health: Past, present, and future. Nurs & Health Care 4: 5, 1985

26. Navarro V: Selected myths guiding the Reagan administration's health policies. J Public Health Policy 5: 1, 1984

27. Peplau H: Principles of psychiatric nursing. In Arieti S (ed): *American Handbook* vol 2. New York, Basic Books, 1959, p1856

28. Sills G: Psychiatric mental health nursing: Historical developments and issues. In Leininger M (ed): *Contemporary Issues in Mental Health Nursing*. Boston, Little, Brown, 1975, p74

29. Brophy E, Hedler DK: Quality assurance. In Beck K, Rawlins WS (eds): *Mental Health Psychiatric Nursing*. Toronto, CV Mosby, 1984, p1350

30. Moccia P: The Nurse as a policymaker: Toward a free and equal health care system. Nurs Health Care 5: 480, 1984

31. Pepper B, Ryglewicz H: An uninstitutionalized generation: Psychiatrically disabled young people in the community. An unpublished paper presented at the Conference on the Young Adult Chronic Patient, Capital District Psychiatric Center, Albany, NY, June 3, 1981

32. Miller RD, Fiddleman PB: Outpatient commitment: Treatment in the least restrictive environment. Hosp & Comm Psych 35:2, 1984

33. Bachrach L: Young adult chronic patients. Hosp & Comm Psych 32:3, 1982

34. Reich R, Siegel L: The chronically mentally ill shuffle to oblivion. In Bonnie R (ed): *Psychiatrists and the Legal Process: Diagnoses and Debate*. Dearborn, Michigan, Insight Communications, 1977, p276

35. Lee PR, Estes CL, Ramsey NB: *The Nations Health*. San Francisco, Boyd & Frasier, 1985, p373

36. Stein LI, Gasser LJ: The dollar follows the patient: Wisconsin system for funding mental health services. *New Directions for Mental Health Services* 18: San Francisco, Jossey-Bass, 1983

37. Stein LI: Test mental health community treatment of the young adult patient. In Pepper B, Ryglewicz H (eds): *New Dimensions for Mental Health Services*. No. 14. San Francisco, Jossey-Bass, 1982

38. Fine SB: Psychiatric treatment and rehabilitation: What's in a name? J Nat Assoc Prev Psych Hosp 11:5, 1980

39. Miller RD: Beyond the old state hospital: New opportunities ahead. Hosp & Comm Psych 32:1, 1985

40. Caton CLM: The new chronic patient and the system of community care. Hosp & Comm Psych 32:7, 1981

HAZEL W. JOHNSON-BROWN, RN, PhD, FAAN

With Vignette by Donna Rae Richardson, RN, JD

CHAPTER 24   *To Understand and Participate in Public Policy Formation: A Challenge to Nursing*

Background and Overview

HISTORY OF THE DEVELOPMENT OF FEDERAL HEALTH CARE POLICY IN THE US

Significant forces are shaping US federal health care policy during the 1980s and will continue to affect it through this century. The most influential forces are national socioeconomic and political trends, as well as trends specific to health care.

Writers identify numerous trends. Milton Roemer (1985) cites 12 major trends in society, economics, and politics, and lists 15 major health trends on which the nation is basing current health care strategies. Although each trend affects health policy, the most important for the purposes of this chapter are:

- Advancing technology, the allocation of resources, quality of life
- Economics and control of the rising cost of health care
- Population—growth, movement, and aging
- Health promotion for cost containment[1]

433

But merely to identify trends or debate their significance is to miss the target. Trends and significance do not lead to policy. The focus of US health policy remains fragmented and diffuse. Through their involvement in effective policy formation, nurses can help the nation anticipate and respond to the most significant trends.

As described by Hawkins and Higgins, early US efforts in health care were also fragmented. Early American history recounts that individual communities took responsibility for their own health care. Communities cared for diseased patients and responded to particular epidemics and injuries. As the communities grew and became more diverse, diseases and injuries increased. Hospitals and "pest houses" emerged, centralizing control and determining the care to be delivered. Over time, government— local and city—began to decide health issues.

The federal presence in health care dates back to 1798, when Congress established the Marine Hospital Service for the Relief of Sick and Disabled Seamen.[2] As part of a national policy, the earliest federal movement toward prevention occurred after the cholera epidemics of the 1800s.[2]

As policies evolved from 1905 to 1965, the federal government increasingly subsidized varied aspects of health care. In fact, this period witnessed major progress in setting national health policy. Weeks and Berman provide a time stream of events that underlie the programs of the 1980s, the effects of which will continue into the 1990s. The events read like a history of public health policy development, but without a focus:

- 1910. Abraham Flexner presents his study of American medicine, marking a major turning point in medical education and health care delivery.
- 1912. Theodore Roosevelt, the first presidential candidate supporting a national health insurance proposal, advocates social reforms and health insurance for industry.
- 1900–1929. The discovery of insulin and penicillin opens new avenues for treatment and prevention. Also, the cost of certain treatments or procedures is initiated; World War I affects health policy.
- 1930–1965. The most significant period for American health policy. Prepaid hospital plans develop; funds are provided indirectly for medical care for the needy; the Social Security Act passes in 1935; the Hospital Service and Construction Act passes in 1944; the Hill-Burton Act of 1946 lays the foundation for the development of an integrated and balanced system of hospitals throughout the country; a national conference on aging takes place; in 1950 an amended Social Security Act provides direct state payments to physicians and other providers; the Salk vaccine is developed; military health services begin for dependents; the Kerr Mills bill

provides monies for health services to the medically indigent; and, in 1965, Medicare and Medicaid become part of the Social Security bill.[3]

In the 1980s, what new conditions in the United States clamor for the development of public health care policies? What situations will arise in the 1990s? How can nursing professionals help develop a national health care policy that will provide guidance for dealing with these emerging trends?

Although the United States is a highly populated country, immigrants, legal and illegal, continue to enter the country at a rapid pace. The health of these individuals will profoundly affect the nation's resources. Furthermore, the US population is aging. A substantial number of Americans are over 100 years of age now. By the year 2010, this centennial population is estimated to reach approximately 30,000. Another significant change that strains US health policy is the transformation of the lower social classes by largely nonwhite peoples and those whose primary language is not English. This trend is exacerbated by unemployment, malnutrition in children, and a large and growing number of medically indigent people.[4]

But in health care, the most vexing issue today is the soaring cost of care. In 15 years, this cost has nearly quadrupled. The percentage of the gross national product represented by health care has risen from approximately three percent in 1965 to approximately 12 percent in 1987.

The nation will need to make effective policy decisions around such major issues as a swelling immigrant and aging population, changing class structures, limited resources, advancing technology, quality of life and care, and spiraling cost.[5]

Yet all the evidence suggests that merely solving specific health care problems—putting out brushfires—fails to produce a clear national health care policy. In an atmosphere of limited resources, cost containment, shortages of health care personnel, and expanding technology, the need to articulate a clear, effective direction is critical. In the last two decades of the twentieth century, what role can nursing professionals play in defining and shaping national public policy?

To understand their potential and bring their influence to bear effectively, nursing professionals must firmly grasp what national health care policy is and how it is defined. Further, nurses must identify and make the unique contributions they can offer in federal policy formulation. ? → such as?

In particular, both because of their education and professional aura, nurses bring a holistic view to public policy development. On the patient level, they view health care in terms of the whole person, not in terms of specific diseases, in terms of the family and the community, not in terms of specific treatments. This unique approach civilizes the health care system and brings rationality and humanity to patient care. Through a nursing approach, nursing professionals should begin to do the same for the development of public policy.

If nurses fail to involve themselves, policies will nonetheless affect them. As professionals, nurses see how policies affect their patients, and how policies modify the systems of delivery in which they work. Unless nurses elect to follow, they must take the lead in public policy formulation. This chapter focuses on their participation in policy development at the national level.

FORMULATION OF FEDERAL HEALTH CARE POLICY

Ultimately, policy-making means making a choice: choosing a direction and presenting a framework for action. Although public policy has been defined in a number of ways, the definition that **public policy** is "whatever governments choose to do or choose not to do" remains clear and simply stated.[5] Health care policy represents both choices for the public good and how the society formulating the policy expresses the value of health.[5]

One of the most important aspects of policy development is how the decision is made. The method of identifying the problem is as important as the problem. Equally important is who offers advice and/or applies pressure for decisions.

Within the federal system, a set of processes determines **policy formation.** Kingdon indicates that policy is formulated through such processes as "setting of the agenda, the specification of alternatives from which a choice is made; an authoritative choice among specified alternatives, such as a legislative vote or a presidential decision; and implementation of the decision."[6]

Agenda setting is the process that narrows and focuses the list of problems or issues. A number of influences can shape agenda setting:

- A crisis draws national attention.
- Knowledge accumulates in a particular area.
- Political influences precipitate policy formation.

Alternative selection can be made preemptively either by a presidential choice or a vote of the Congress. Usually this occurs after serious review, data gathering, and analysis. Alternatives are usually narrowed to those that should be considered seriously.[6]

To steer through the system of formulating policy is to review how a problem becomes a proposal, to examine the influence of interest groups, and to look at decision-making and the development of financing for the new program. Although these activities take place concurrently, for the sake of clarity each appears here separately.

How the Problem Becomes a Proposal.   A problem or issue can be identified in different ways. A group or commission may identify issues and make recommendations. Any one of the recommendations can become the issue from which a proposal develops. Problems result from an event; a problem can be a long-standing issue that sooner or later finds its time. Proposal formation requires as much attention and support in its initial phase as it does when it has evolved into a bill before Congress.[5]

Influence of Special Interest Groups.   The role of interest or influence groups is to inform and educate legislators. **Interest groups** range from those who represent organized labor to those representing business, from professional associations to specialty groups, from individual citizens to civic groups. These clusters present an array of interests and abilities to influence legislators. Each group has its own grass roots power, because grass roots individuals represent voters and potential supporters in their home states or towns.[7] Interested professionals rely on their status for influence and effect.

Florence Nightingale was the first nurse to lobby or exert public policy influence. During the Crimean War, Nightingale knew that if she could demand sanitary conditions, she could save lives. With zeal and determination, she pursued her mission. But her policy contributions extended well beyond her work in the hospitals during the war. For example, Nightingale played a role in the establishment of the British Sanitary System as well as making other contributions to public health.[7]

Another pioneer nurse exerting influence was Lillian Wald. Wald used the power of the social and political system to cause major changes in the health and welfare of children and women. Although well known for her work in the establishment of the Henry Street Settlement, Lillian Wald's greatest contribution to the health policy of the nation came in her work with the Congress in the passage and establishment of the **Children's Bureau;** the Bureau had a mission to fight the exploitation of child labor and ensure the health and welfare of children.[8]

During the past ten years, the nursing profession has begun to forge a visible and powerful role in health policy development. This developmental function has stimulated activism and education of legislators at the local, state, and federal levels on such issues as protection of human rights, distributive justice in allocating health resources, and direct reimbursement for nursing services.[9]

To further establish itself as an interest group with clout, the professional nursing organization—the American Nurses' Association (ANA)—established eight long-range goals. The ANA also developed a new organizational mission statement: "To improve nursing services and access to those services and to promote, advance, and protect the interest of nursing, thereby increasing the overall quality of health care by providing:

- leadership and representation for the profession in both national and international affairs,
- information, research, and resources relevant to the development and advancement of nursing practice, nursing education, nursing services, nursing research, and economic and general welfare of nurses;
- for a coordinated system of credentialing for the nursing profession."[9]

This mission statement sets the tone for ANA action in public policy and can guide individual nurses in their public policy involvement.

Decision-making.   Decision-making in federal policy development is complex. Looking to history, when the US system for decision-making was being formulated, its developers deliberately made it complex. In his review of the system of decision-making, Charles Jones suggests that the framers of the Constitution and of democratic government "were more concerned with preventing tyranny than they were about facilitating policy development."[11]

Jones's statement illuminates the reasons why the decision-making process in the United States is ambiguous. Jones explains that proposals are typically filtered through decision-making processes characterized by:

- An incremental style (build on the base, rely on marginal decisions)
- A search for analogies and precedents (new problem? how did we handle a similar case? any precedent for the proposal?)
- A highly segmented organization (highly balkanized, bureaucratic structure in the executive, committee/subcommittee system in the legislative and in triplicate in the federal system)
- Differential group access to Congress and the executive, eg, policy-centered networks (communication and contact overtime among those interested and involved in a subject)
- Bargaining expectations leading to compromise (thus encouraging incrementalism)
- Short-run orientation (dictated in part by the two-year election cycle of the House of Representatives)

The result is policy-making that is obtuse, indirect, circuitous, and fragmented. Program implementation is characterized by unsystematic experimentation (administrators gain experience in implementing a program, then propose further increment; both good and bad programs often survive). Program evaluation often reads "program justification." Even bad programs develop a supporting clientele.[11]

Jones suggests that if this description is accurate, a comprehensive proposal is moderated, compromised, and de-escalated by special interest groups. Social, economic, and political conditions will and do influence the process.[11]

Another observation can be made about incremental decision-making: the model is conservative. It retains the status quo while minute changes occur. Thus, as a nation, Americans accept the legitimacy of established programs and existing structure. D. G. Gil proposes that the incremental decision-making process fits the American social model and its dominant values. The social, political, and economic systems stand structurally correct and do not allow problems, issues, and proposal decision-making to change or disrupt the basic model.[12]

Financing the Development of the New Program.   In his 1986 State of the Union address, President Reagan spoke of two major proposals he would place before the Congress and the American people during his final two years in the White House. The next day, while applauding the merits of the President's ideas, his cabinet and advisory committee immediately began raising the issue of financing the programs and subsequent proposals that would emerge.

Public policy development never ends. It is important not only to develop the idea for treating a problem or responding to an issue, but also to develop the necessary funding plan—the budget. Once identified, the budget demands a financing plan: from where will the money come?

"Budget is at the heart of the political process" writes Aaron Wildavsky in *The Politics of the Budgetary Process*.[13] This statement is certainly borne out in any review of proposals and programs facing Congress. Confronting the largest deficit in history, the people and the Congress must determine how much money to authorize and appropriate for each program. In other words, representing the people, the Congress and the President must decide what to do (**authorization**), that is, which programs to approve.

The second question is how much money will be spent implementing these programs (**appropriation**). A third question also demands an answer. Where will the money be obtained: the private sector, the government (state or federal), taxes, bonds?

In the federal system, funds for program financing move through a number of steps before they become available. The first budget step is simultaneous formulation within the executive branch, the Office of Management and Budget (OMB), and in the Congressional Budget Office (CBO). These two offices decide what programs will be funded and what programs will not.

The OMB and CBO funding work begins from nine and a half to at least 19 months prior to the fiscal year. So a new program, identified and passed by Congress and signed by the President, may not be implemented immediately.[11] Another method of funding, however, may be used to start the program: tapping monies from prior years that were appropriated for a similar activity, but not used. Usually this money must be spent within a prescribed time or it reverts to other programs or to general revenues.

Wildavsky's statement that budget is a highly political process is clearly demonstrated as the Congress and Executive Branch work out their differences (**reconciliation**) and come to agreement about what will get funding and when and how much. This is the authorization process.

Following authorization, the House and Senate engage in the appropriation process, which involves similar political overtones. In this ambiguous situation and with difficulty, the committees of both the House and Senate decide to appropriate funds to programs that build on the larger plan, while holding costs within budget where possible.

During the Reagan years, another source of funding has developed—the private sector. Programs and proposals in the best interest of business and industry have stimulated active participation in public policy. Employers and unions alike are interested in holding health care costs down. Programs that offer the opportunity for cost effective quality health care gain support from the private sector.

A case in point is catastrophic health care. As the task force recommendations and the secretary of health and human services plan were being introduced, the President reminded the task force to look to the private sector first for financing of the recommendations and to the government only as a last resort.[14]

In a review of the process of financing programs, the observer is struck by the fact that getting an agreement or decision to accept a program or proposal constitutes only the first five innings of the ball game. The next four innings take place in the complex arena of the budgetary process. This process may cause the game to go into extra innings, delaying implementation of a hard-won program. Regardless of the worthiness or unworthiness of a program, this remains the game.

Program Implementation and Evaluation.   The dictionary defines implementation and evaluation in the following words: **implementation** provides a definite plan or procedure to ensure fulfillment of something or some process; **evaluation** is the examination, judgment, or calculations in numerical value of some thing or process. In the policy arena, however, Jeffery Pressman and Aaron Wildavsky define "implementation as a set of interactions between setting goals and the actions geared to achieve them."[13] In that same policy context, evaluation is a judgment of the merits of a program or decision.

Implementation.   In the policy arena, implementation demands a complex strategy. Because of the seamless web of connections, actions, and goals, clarity dims as the process moves from decision to the operation or initiation of a program. To arrive at a reasonable resemblance of what was intended by the decision is the thrust of the implementation plan.[11]

To consider a program's implementation, examine the "Non-Smoking Society by the Year 2000," a program proposed by Dr. C. Everett Koop, the Surgeon General, in a speech to the American Lung Association in 1984. Although the program's implementors at first faced significant obstacles, they started the program on a variety of fronts. By 1987 the success of the implementation could be measured in the reduction of adult smokers, private sector initiatives to ban smoking in meetings and other public and private places, and in government actions to reduce smoking in government-owned buildings. Even though far-reaching, the effects of this program remain limited. Implementation usually only means arriving at a reasonable expectation intended by the decision.

The nonsmoking program failed to ban the manufacture of smoking materials or reduce the export of the commodity. So, on the international scene, the World Health Organization program for a smoke-free society has met with less success in implementation.[5] Why? Jones suggests that the constant and numerous challenges facing implementation must be recognized: "Problems and demands are constantly defined and redefined by the policy process. Programs requiring intergovernmental and public participation invite variable interpretations of purpose. Programs may be implemented without provisions for learning about failure. Programs may reflect an attainable consensus rather than a substantive connection."[11]

Add to these challenges the difficulty of determining who has responsibility and authority for a program or decision implementation. Delegation of authority sometimes leads to absence of leadership and lost purpose. Some programs become subject to a variety of interpretations, they lose in competition with other programs, or they flounder in ambiguity. The result? The programs miss their original goal.

Evaluation. Effective policy development hinges on evaluation. In an era of budget deficit and demands for cost effective programs, evaluation is gaining greater force in program implementation and continuance.

In most programs, some form of evaluation occurs from policy development through implementation. However, formal evaluation is often avoided until the project ends or needs refunding.

Program evaluation occurs in three stages: needs assessment, formative evaluation, and summative evaluation. The needs assessment is usually evident during policy development. **Needs assessment** responds to questions of intended goals, outcomes, and population identity and distribution, and it identifies opportunities for successful implementation.

Formative evaluation involves monitoring the program for adequate resources to accomplish objectives; it questions whether the services needed are the services identified; it looks at other populations affected, and at other variables that surface during the program. An important question that formative evaluation may identify is what is actual cost and how does this cost reflect projected cost? Formative evaluation permits changes in course and reallocation of resources to meet unexpected needs. Formative evaluation may also help identify compliance and noncompliance activities.[15]

Summative evaluation is a more familiar process. It usually occurs at specified end periods—the requirement for continuation and/or additional budgetary needs is identified.[16] Summative evaluation can be rigorous research because it is retrospective and seeks to determine where the actual outcomes reflect the outcomes as projected; and if not, why not? If outcomes are as projected, should the program be continued? If so, why?

Although most people consider evaluation an objective, straightforward process, it involves values and can be strongly political. The outcomes of an evaluation are influenced by who is doing it, who is paying, what purposes are identified, and by whom. Although program evaluation should provide guideposts to appropriate decision-making in public policy, it entails judgment, power, and influence.

As the public continues to demand cost effective and quality service, productive evaluation should assist in the development and continuation of effective health policies. It should establish clear outcomes and define expected organizational and program performance; assess continually, identifying deviations; suggest changes when appropriate; and clarify and strengthen communication to establish support program continuation or discontinuance.[15]

Nursing recognizes that continued support and funding of health care programs must be based on relevant outcomes. Nurses must identify which outcomes are important and significant to the health of the nation. These outcomes include legislation that focuses on major health problems, safety and improved working conditions, military improvement, and the like.

In an era of information and technical development, policy development, maintenance, and continuation cannot rely on common sense, conventional wisdom, or intuition. To assist in better decision-making in the policy arena, it is increasingly reasonable to expect formal program evaluation that ensures more objectivity.

Impacts on the Nurse, the Consumer, and Society

THE NURSE

In health care as well as in industry, business, and science, public policy is a never-ending process. Interacting with federal, state, and local government is a way of life. Recognizing the need to be concerned and involved in public policy, nurses are preparing themselves formally and through on-the-job opportunities to participate in the total process.[17]

In an interview in the March 1987 *American Nurse*, Virginia Henderson observed the following about the need for nurses' involvement: "The World Health Organization's goal, 'Health for all by 2000,' reflects a universal belief that health care is a human right. Nurses, with other health care providers, will work with citizens in every nation to produce resources making it possible to offer health services for all at the lowest cost and emphasize disease prevention, health education, and self-care."[18]

Involvement.   Nurses have learned that to realize their goals, they must understand and become involved in public policy formation, in implementation, and in evaluation. For instance, they have learned the importance of public policies that determine *where* health care is delivered. As an industry, health care is experiencing profound change: "There is a shift from the insular self-contained industry to a highly competitive mega entity, multi-hospital, multi-provider industry; a shift from treating and maintaining to preventing and promoting health."[19] Those policy shifts dramatically affect nurses and their practice.

In writing about the evolution of health care, Ehrenreich and English salute the early attempts of nurses to influence health care and shape their role in the health industry. They admonish today's nurses to realize that they too must be active—not bystanders—in the shaping of health policy. Risk-taking by involvement in public policy formulation is the wave of the future. Nurse participation in policy formation is the key in progress toward future roles in the health industry.[20]

Although nurses are the largest group within the health professions, their influence on public policy development fails to measure up to their numbers and potential. Branded a "sleeping giant" by the media, nurses have begun to awaken from a long nap. Nearly two million strong and still growing, their potential is awesome. Yet in today's competitive environment, they are only just beginning to realize their power and influence.

Nurses clearly understand that health policy for all Americans is determined by those who include themselves in the decision-making processes. Changes in the perception of women's roles in society have energized nursing. The working woman is a reality. In addition, more than ever before, women are remaining in the work force, marrying, raising a family, seeking further education, and accepting and performing work at higher levels in industry and business.

However, Aydellote suggests that more of the two million nurses must develop new attitudes to have major influence in the public policy arena. These attitudes include developing respect, trust, and openness when working with each other and other professionals; recognizing the reality of conflict and confrontation when negotiating competing ideas and positions; a willingness to learn new languages, symbols, and values in a rapidly changing world; the ability to shift leadership styles in response to different situations; and an active awareness that all human beings need support and approval.[9]

To assimilate these new attitudes into the nursing profession, Aydellote advises that nurse leaders in education and service overcome their differences, collaborate, and clarify the definition of nursing; and in addition create new markets for nursing services; institute educational policies in nursing that recognize and support social mobility; develop work policies that take into account issues that affect men and women: salary equity, maternity leave, child-care services, and working conditions during the childbearing or procreation ages of men and women; and finally work toward a unified public image by supporting nursing organizations that can speak on the various major issues that confront nursing.[9]

Nurses are beginning to tackle Aydelotte's challenges. The **Tri-Council for Nursing** demonstrates a coming together of nursing leadership. The council consists of four major organizations: the American Nurses' Association (the professional registered nurse); the American Association of Colleges of Nursing and the National League for Nursing (education); and the American Organization of Nurse Executives (administration). The Tri-Council serves as an arena for discussion of major health issues and a body for developing strategies for collective action on legislative and regulatory issues, such as the nursing education bill, the establishment of the National Center for Nursing Research, and catastrophic health care.

The National Federation of Specialty Organizations also participates in policy formulation by lobbying legislative representatives on issues of importance to their special interests and to the entire profession.

These endeavors symbolize nursing's growing and developing political savvy. As the grass roots of the nursing profession become more aware of their political potential, leadership is capitalizing on this readiness to provide opportunities for building the necessary confidence and skill in the political arena.[8]

Legislative Action.   In this decade and the next, the challenge for nurses and the profession is to develop individuals who will engage fully in the political and legislative process. However, before nurses can become involved in legislative actions, they must understand the steps of the **national legislative process.**

For a national bill this process includes:

- Formal introduction in House or Senate
- Referral to a standing committee or subcommittee; most bills go only this far
- Hearings by a subcommittee
- Marking up—changing the bill's language
- Reporting the bill to the floor

- Debate on the bill, including consideration and acceptance or rejection of amendments
- Final passage of the bill and referral to the other house, for a similar process
- After passage by both houses, referral to the Conference Committee if the language of the bills differs
- Final vote of acceptance in the Conference Committee Report, reconciling differences
- Signing or veto by the President
- If a veto when Congress is in session, referral back to Congress; if both houses vote to override, the bill becomes law.[17]

THE CONSUMER AND SOCIETY

The rising costs of health care are heightening consumer interest and concern and are forcing consumers to become more educated about health care. Overall, this decade is producing consumers concerned and articulate about health care and ready to demand quality in its delivery.

Realizing strength in numbers, consumers are seizing upon participation and membership in consumer groups such as the American Association of Retired Persons, the Gray Panthers, and others, to make major contributions to policy development and implementation. These consumer contributions have included development of catastrophic care programs.

Access to care for all segments of the population is another growing consumer concern. The groups most affected by access issues are the aged, the underemployed, the unemployed, the indigent, the minority populations, people with catastrophic illnesses, and a large segment of people who are not citizens and are usually referred to as "illegal." Although a health policy must address both quality and quantity of services for these populations, this consumer issue is being addressed in a fragmented way. Who can speak for these less advantaged consumers?

The availability of health care to all segments of the population is another compelling social issue. Society as a whole must be involved in the policy decisions. Why? Because the society of tomorrow is influenced by the decisions of today. Perfectly reasonable decisions can have negative effects on the future. These negatives can arise from unanticipated developments or from subtle trends that fail to be recognized. Therefore, today's health-care-policy decision-makers must also have a clearer and holistic vision of the future that will be preferred in health care delivery.[8]

Of leading importance to consumer health care decision-making is the economics of delivery. The economics of health care delivery includes personnel resource management, control of scarce commodities, facility maintenance, education of personnel, and cost of care. These issues and more must be part of the decisions that society will make about health care.

Recent surveys indicate that most Americans believe that their health care is good and that they have access. Even those who identify themselves as without access estimate that if they needed health care, it would probably be of good quality.

Most individuals receiving health care under varied health plans express concern about rising costs. They too want to confront not only the question of cost but also the question of universal access to the system. Access is obviously an issue of major concern.

Another major issue, related to cost and impacting on consumers and society, is the ethical dilemma emerging from an era of scarce resources. How do you spread limited resources to respond to all individuals with health care needs? This question still awaits direction and a plan for the future.

Groups and **coalitions** (a body of alliances) that address and plan for the future of health care delivery represent society's approach to the consumer health care problems of access and cost. This approach provides opportunities for monitoring health policy development from the initial idea to its implementation. Health care is big business; its impact across the entire spectrum of society is great. Therefore, decisions cannot be left to a few individuals. Participation, cooperation, compromise, and a collaboration among and between all segments of society will lead the nation to a rational policy that contains costs and maintains quality and access. Nurses must play a role with the consumer in the policy arena.

Future Considerations

Today's realities are the foundation for the future. The trends are clear: a recession in the hospital industry, admissions declining, increased competition for "good" patients, and a decrease in the safety net previously enjoyed by hospitals. Care is being delivered through a network of systems rather than by free-standing hospitals.

Physicians are moving into group practice and choosing to work in those facilities that let them share in the risk and the profit. A strong movement argues for greater control of health care practice. A new approach to the consumer is emerging. Management is more image conscious and is spending funds to promote strong public relations programs. These trends will continue into the immediate future.[21]

The health needs of the consumer are changing. The client is older, sicker, and less able to pay for costly care. The hospital itself is promoting the development of new and different community care facilities. Home health care is growing and developing its own constituency while regulation and control of this delivery system are materializing.

In 1984, to determine the direction of health care, Arthur Anderson and Company completed a study for the American College of Hospital Administrators. Experts representing nursing, medicine, health administration, legislation, regulation, insurance, and health goods supply participated. The results of this survey included the following predictions:

- More outpatient and urgent care centers emerge, reflecting the desire of patients to remain out of hospitals and the desire of the health industry to increase competition and drive down costs.
- Older Americans absorb much of the federal/state dollars for chronic and acute care.
- Advances in technology improve quality of care, while the ethical issues and social concerns around the issues of limited resources increase.[22]

To deal with the Anderson predictions, alternative health care delivery systems such as home health care, health maintenance organizations, and preferred provider systems are growing and expanding, and will continue to develop.

In this responsive environment, professional nursing is looking for the opportunity for significant participation. Kathleen MacPherson, Professor, University of Southern Maine, writes that the "emerging preferred provider organizations provide nurses with the opportunity to promote a health policy that will allow them to market their services as autonomous health care providers."[23] She observes that nurse-controlled PPOs can provide society with a life-enhancing alternative form of health care.

Dr. MacPherson proposes that nurses view involvement in health care public policy as the challenge of the decade. This challenge includes promoting nurses as providers of value and worth. This stance demands involvement in politics to develop policy. MacPherson advises against separating policy from politics. Health policy, like other policy decisions, she warns, is inextricably linked to the political-economics domain.[23]

Political and policy decisions derive from values, perceptions, and complex interrelationships. During the past five years, the nursing profession participated in the **Health Policy Agenda for the American People** (1982), a program initiated and led by the American Medical Association. Approximately 172 different health, health-related, business, government, and consumer groups participated in the Health Policy Agenda. The mission of this group was to examine present health concerns and anticipate issues of the next decade and the next century.[24]

The policy areas addressed by the Health Policy Agenda are important to understanding which issues can affect policy formulation: supplying professionals, providing technology and facilities, organizing resources, communicating health information, ensuring quality, paying the bill, and preparing for the future through research."[24]

During this same time period, the American Nurses' Association (ANA) was engaged in developing its own long-range plans and agenda for health care delivery and the profession's role in that delivery. In 1986 the House of Delegates of the ANA adopted the following goals for the future: expand the scientific and research base for nursing practice; clarify and strengthen the educational system for nursing; develop a coordinated system of credentialing for nursing; restructure organizational arrangements for delivery of nursing services; develop comprehensive payment system for nursing services; achieve effective control of the environment in which nurses practice and offer services; enhance the organizational strength of the ANA; maintain and strengthen nursing's role in client advocacy.[10]

Finally, anticipating the distant future and determining how nurses can participate in health care public policy, it is helpful to see what forecasts emerged from the Center for Nursing Excellence Work Group—Nursing 2020. Myrna Warnich, chairperson of Project 2020, suggests, "Without plans and vision for our future, others could and will shape the future for nursing."[25] The Center group gave these forecasts a high probability of occurring by 2020:

- Because occupational health will become a major focus, nurses will be involved in keeping workers well and productive.
- Greater numbers of nurses will see themselves as health consumer advocates and will play a larger role in consumer legislative and regulatory activities.
- Nurses are knowledge workers rather than technical workers and will use technology to enhance patient care as well as substitute technology for non-patient care functions.[25]

Health care planning is the basis for public policy development. Nurses have an inherent role and responsibility in planning, policy initiation, development, implementation, and evaluation. Their role is rooted in history and practice. Yet it is a function that in the past has been accepted by only a few. The future dictates that it is every nurse's responsibility and right to be involved. Public policy is inextricably interwoven with politics. As nurses become more politically active and astute, they will influence policy more effectively.

The "sleeping giant" is awakening!

Susan Beckwith, a senior nursing student at a major southern university, is enrolled in Nursing 420, Nursing and Infectious Diseases. Charles DiPerrillo, a policy analyst from the Department of Health and Human Services, is giving a guest lecture to the class on the topic of social conditions that force changes in public policy. Concluding his lecture, he says the following:

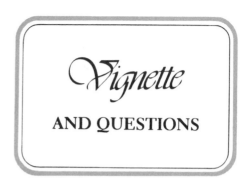

During the public health crisis regarding Acquired Immunodeficiency Disease Syndrome (AIDS), we have recognized that a cure or vaccine is at least a decade away. Almost universally, health professionals acknowledge that the only way to prevent the disease from spreading further is to educate the public about it, about its transmission, and about protective measures to prevent personal contact with the Human Immunodeficiency Virus HIV-II.

The public health implications of the fatal disease are compounded by its modes of transmission. Although AIDS is a blood-borne disease (like hepatitis), and is contracted through contact with blood and body fluids, the public has associated the disease with homosexuality and illegal drug use. Why? Because it was initially identified in the US by the Center for Disease Control (CDC) after a pattern of deaths in the homosexual community.

To accomplish its mission of public education, public health officials are advocating sexual abstinence, monogamy, and, failing that, "safe sex." Safe sex involves the use of condoms during intimate sexual contact between partners who do not know their HIV status. Intravenous drug use, which is an illegal practice, is admonished, but we have realistically noted that drug addicts won't stop drug abuse. So we are reluctantly recommending nonsharing of needles, or needle sterilization.

Additionally, some public health officials, politicians, and religious leaders recommended testing individuals to determine who has been exposed to the HIV virus. Public health estimates indicated that in 1987, 1.5 million people were exposed, but less than half were aware of their seropositivity. Proponents of testing stressed that since AIDS is an infectious disease, it should be treated like other communicable diseases (like tuberculosis, or other sexually transmitted diseases, such as syphilis or gonorrhea) and that once reported require contact tracing of intimates.

1. What is nursing's role in addressing a public health epidemic?

2. Are education and prevention the most effective ways to fight an incurable infectious disease? Are other measures necessary?

3. If the disease is not spread through casual contact, is quarantine needed?

4. Should public health officials consider nonmedical/health concerns, eg, costs, human rights, or morals in determining health care policies regarding AIDS?

5. If testing can determine exposure but not provide other results, should it be considered an effective disease prevention tool?

6. Is a testing policy appropriate? How extensive should it be? everyone? high-risk individuals? certain age groups? hospital patients? health care workers?

7. What follow-up should occur after testing?

8. Should testing results be reported? to whom? patient? spouse? contacts? employers? public health officials?

9. How should these decisions be made? by public health officials alone?

10. If AIDS is a national crisis, should states be allowed to address it singularly? Is one national policy appropriate?

11. Should legislators determine specific health care policy, eg, treatment modes, health education content, and public health procedures?

12. If state compliance with federal policies is required for financing medical programs, does voluntary noncompliance effectively disenfranchise certain citizens from health care systems?

13. Are official policy-making bodies needed? If so, what groups should be represented? providers? consumers? legal experts? ethicists? institutional representatives?

14. What could nursing bring of special value to these discussions?

15. The assumption is made that physician participation represents health care. How would nursing assure separate representation? why?

INFORMATION SOURCES

The list of information sources includes the articles and books in the reference section below and the following:

Fifty Years of US Health Care Policy. Hospital, May 5, 1986, p95

Health Care Policy—Advances in Nursing Science. 9 (3), April 1987. Aspen Publications, 7201 McKenney Circle, Frederick, MD 21701

Healthy People: The Surgeon General's Report on Health Promotion and Disease Prevention. Washington, DC, National Health Information Center, ODPHP, P. O. Box 1133, Washington, DC 20013-1133

Joint Center for Political Studies, 301 Pennsylvania Avenue, Suite 400, Washington, DC 20024

Solomon SB, Roe SC: *Integrating Public Policy into the Curriculum.* New York, National League for Nursing, 1986. (An excellent listing of information sources appears on pp92–101.)

REFERENCES

1. Roemer MI: *National Strategies for Health Care Organization: A World Overview.* Ann Arbor, Health Administration Press, 1985

2. Hawkins JBW, Higgins LP: *Nursing and the American Health Care Delivery System,* 2d ed. New York, Tiresias Press, 1985

3. Weeks LE, Berman HJ: *Shapers of American Health Care Policy: An Oral History.* Ann Arbor, MI, Health Administration Press, 1985

4. Jonas S: Introduction. In Jonas S. (ed): *Health Care Delivery in the United States,* 3d ed. New York, Springer, 1986, p1

5. Dye TR: *Understanding Public Policy.* Englewood Cliffs, NJ, Prentice-Hall, 1984

6. Kingdon JW: *Agendas, Alternatives and Public Policies*. Boston, Little, Brown, 1984

7. Kalisch PA, Kalisch BJ: *The Advance of American Nursing*, 2d ed. Boston, Little, Brown, 1986

8. DeBella S, Martin L, Siddall S: *Nurses' Role in Health Care Planning*. Norwalk, CT, Appleton-Century-Crofts, 1986

9. Benoliel JO, Pacjard NJ: Nurses and health policy. Nurs Admin Q 19:1, 1986

10. American Nurses' Association: Report of House of Delegates: Summary of Action Reference, Hearing B. p36, 1986

11. Jones CO: *Introduction to the Study of Public Policy*, ed 3. Monterey, CA, Brooks/Cole, 1984

12. Gil DG: *Unravelling Social Policy*, 3d ed. Cambridge, MA, S. Cheatman Books, 1981

13. Wildavsky A: *The Politics of the Budgetary Process*, 3d ed. Boston, Little, Brown, 1979

14. Fox PD, Goldbeck WB, Spies JL: *Health Care Cost Management*. Ann Arbor, MI, Health Administration Press, 1984

15. Rossi PH, Freeman HE, Wright SR: *Evaluation: A Systematic Approach*. Beverly Hills, Sage Publications, 1979

16. Wholey JS, Abramson MA, Bellairta C: Performance and Credibility: *Developing Excellence in Public and Nonprofit Organizations*. Lexington, MA, Heath, 1986

17. Kalisch BJ, Kalisch PA: *Politics of Nursing*. Philadelphia, Lippincott, 1982

18. McCarty P: How can nurses prepare for year 2000? Interview of Virginia Henderson in Amer Nurse, March 1987

19. MacNerney W: As I see it. Amer Nurse, March 1987

20. Ehrenreich B, English D: *Witches, Midwives, and Nurses*. Old Westbury, Feminist Press, 1973

21. Fagin CM: Nursing's Pivotal Role in American Health Care. In Aiken LH (ed): *Nursing in the 1980's—Crises, Opportunities, Challenge*. Philadelphia, Lippincott, 1982, p459

22. Health Care in the 1990's: Trends and Strategies. Study done by Arthur Anderson & Co. for the American College of Hospital Administrators, 1984

23. MacPherson KL: Health care policy, values and nursing. Advances Nurs Sci 9:1, 1987

24. *Health Policy Agenda for the American People*. Chicago, American Medical Association, 1987

25. Executive Summary of the Nursing 2020 Project: A Study of the Future of Nursing. New York, National League for Nursing, 1988

BEVERLY C. FLYNN, RN, PhD, FAAN

JOANNE MARTIN, RN, DrPH

CHAPTER 25 *Demystifying Political Involvement*

[Political activity] is a mixture of science, craftlore and art. The science is the body of theory, concepts, and methodological principles: The craftlore the set of workable techniques, rules of thumb, and standard operating procedures: The art, the pace, style and manner in which one works.[1]

More and more nurses are urged to become politically involved. This chapter examines why nurses should be politically involved as individuals; as members of a professional group; and as providers of care to people, many of whom are underserved and underrepresented. We also will discuss the different arenas of political activity; the various important roles actors play; and how nurses can more effectively participate in the political scene.

Background and Overview

Before addressing how nurses might go about becoming politically involved, we need to entertain the question of whether or not we believe it is possible for nurses to influence the policy-making process. After all, the reason nurses want to become involved in politics is that they want to influence the policy decisions that are made by others, especially the decisions that impact the way nurses practice or affect the people nurses want to help. Not only do nurses need to react to policies in a timely manner by using their influence as policy advocates, but also nurses want to be proactive and

453

involved in initiating policies. In order to participate effectively, nurses need to be involved in the various phases of the policy process, including policy analysis, policy formation, policy advocacy, and policy action.

ELITISM VS. PLURALISM

There are two competing schools of thought, neither of which has compiled compelling evidence that its view is entirely accurate. **Elitism** contends that the policy-making process is controlled by a few powerful individuals who set the agendas, decide which issues will receive attention and action, and select the approaches or potential solutions to the problems as they have identified them. The elites control the policy-making process by controlling the resources, determining what research is needed and what will be funded through government or foundations, creating public opinion, and making the decisions and laws that impact our lives. The elite decision-makers at the federal level include: the President, Vice-President, presidential appointees, staff of the executive branch, congressional leaders, other members of Congress, congressional staff, the Supreme Court, powerful private interests, influential leaders, foundation executives, policy planners, persons representing the media, and people involved in large coalitions. An analogous list could be compiled at the state and local level, and a similar cadre of "in group" individuals or positions could be identified in the workplace. A key provision of the elite school is that the same group of powerful decision makers exert influence over virtually all decisions.[2] For example, the same set of actors influence decisions regarding land use and education, transportation, and health care. Moreover, although the elites may differ in their priorities, they share a common worldview that is shaped by their common backgrounds and their similar sets of experiences. Given their worldview, some problems and potential solutions are excluded from among the options the elites are willing and capable of considering.

The contrasting school of thought is called **pluralism,** and a leading proponent is Robert Dahl. Pluralism fits more closely with how American democracy is designed to function and, according to Dahl, it does work in that fashion.[3] Pluralism recognizes that some individuals or groups are more influential than others, but, in contrast to elitism, pluralism asserts that the people who have influence in one area are not the same people who have influence in other areas. Those who are influential in health are not necessarily influential in transportation, land use, or education. Some overlap may occur and some individuals may be active in most areas, but this tends to be the exception, not the rule, as the elitist school believes. From the pluralist point of view the system is much more permeable to influence from a broader group of individuals and groups.

Both elitists and pluralists agree that influence over political decision-making is unevenly distributed. There is great variability in the level of individual and group resources, skills, and incentive. The difference lies in whether or not a non-elite individual or group can ever expect to have any significant influence over policy-making. Elitists claim that they are influenced only by other elites; pluralists claim that non-elites can influence policy through the skillful use of their resources. Depending upon the viewpoint that is adopted, it appears that nurses either need to become part of the elite or they need to increase their resources and skills in order to be influential.

Clearly nurses can influence the policy process if they work as a group in coalition with other groups that share common interests. For those who believe that it is necessary to become part of the elite in order to wield influence, nurses can do so by being leaders within a large coalition. This is not to suggest that nurses cannot or should not strive to become part of the elite decision-making group through being elected to Congress or serving as a presidential appointee or staff to Congress. However, those positions are limited, whereas coalition activity is by definition more broadly based, more inclusive, and more likely to allow participation by greater numbers of nurses. From the pluralist perspective, coalitions afford the opportunity to do just what is needed to be influential. By joining together as nurses and by working with other organized interest groups, nurses can enhance their influence by increasing their resources and developing greater skill in the effective deployment of the resources they have.

INTERESTS AND INTEREST GROUPS

The responsibility for nurses to be involved in the political process stems from the fact that it is the "American way"; it is the way our democracy was designed to work. A cornerstone of American political tradition is an understanding of the role of self-interest in human activity. Because the founding fathers of our democracy recognized that human behavior is guided by self-interest, they believed that government should be responsible for providing an orderly process for individuals to pursue their own ends.[4] Looking after our own professional interests or speaking in behalf of those we serve is not viewed as overly self-serving. On the contrary, nurses are expected to try to influence elected officials about issues that affect them and the people they try to help. In this regard nurses are no different from any other special interest group.

If it is legitimate and desirable to promote particular interests, it is important to understand how interests are defined and by whom. Two competing approaches can be complementary. One approach asserts that interests are best defined subjectively by those who are affected. Most situations require complicated trade-offs and not everyone shares the same set of priorities. Outsiders who do not share the preferences of those who are involved may define interests differently simply because "beauty is in the eye of the beholder." The other approach claims that an informed, unbiased outsider can objectively identify the interests of another person or group by assessing what will benefit that person or group. Although this approach risks patronizing overtones, it is necessary because those who are most affected can be unaware or misinformed. For example, a 1984 survey conducted by the American Association of Retired Persons found that 79 percent of the members who responded believed that Medicare provided coverage for long-term nursing home care, when in fact this was not the case.[5]

As helping professionals, nurses may wonder why people often don't appear to want what they need or why people don't always prefer what seems to be in their best interest. Outsiders may pose the same questions about the nursing profession. We are faced with a dilemma when we try to explain why individuals or groups fail to pursue a particular interest. On the one hand, it may be a failure to accurately assess their interest due to lack of knowledge, complexity of choice, or societal limits placed upon behavior. On the other hand, they simply may have different preferences.

Depending upon the issue, interest is defined at different points along the subjective-objective continuum. When nurses examine issues that relate directly to the nursing profession, interests are defined subjectively as preferences. If policy-makers want to know what is good for nursing, just ask nurses. This approach reinforces the need for nursing to speak for nursing. But what happens when nursing advocates for other groups such as the elderly, the handicapped, or the poor? We move more toward the objective end of the continuum and argue that nurses can determine another group's interests by assessing what will benefit their group.

Working in partnership is one way to avoid the potential pitfalls of either the subjective or objective approach. In defining the interests of the nursing profession, partnerships with other groups, including consumer, political, and other professional groups, can provide nursing with additional knowledge from different perspectives and help nurses to more accurately assess their own interests. Likewise, working in partnership with the groups nurses try to help facilitates sharing the special knowledge nurses have, yet avoids a paternalistic attitude regarding the groups best interests.

INFLUENCE THROUGH RESOURCES, SKILL, AND INCENTIVE

Effective political involvement depends upon the amount of influence individuals and groups have, which in turn depends upon their differing levels of resources, skill, and incentive.[6] It is clear that all groups do not have the same level of resources such as money or manpower, but even when they do, some groups exhibit more skill in using the resources they have. In fact, groups with limited resources can use their resources so skillfully they overcome the initial disparity. To go one step further, the skillful use of resources does not occur unless there is some incentive. The most powerful special interest groups or individuals do not become politically involved unless they have some reason to do so. Incentive, resources, and skill are linked. When the incentive is great, people find the resources and develop the needed skills. And having the resources and skills readily available increases the incentive because the efforts are more likely to be effective.

At all levels the incentive to become politically involved is greatest when individuals or groups believe that they stand to gain or lose a great deal by a particular policy decision. Assessing who will benefit from the decision and who will bear the costs of the decision helps to predict which individuals or groups will become politically involved. Both the benefits and the costs of a policy can be described along a continuum from concentrated to distributed. The placement of costs or benefits depends upon the degree to which it is narrowly concentrated on members of a segment of society or widely distributed among most or all members of society.

For discussion purposes examples will be given for the four categories of costs and benefits: interest group politics (concentrated benefits, concentrated costs); client politics (concentrated benefits, distributed costs); entrepreneurial politics (distributed benefits, concentrated costs); and majoritarian politics (distributed benefits, distributed costs).[4]

Table 25-1 shows the four combinations of costs and benefits.

The first situation illustrates why special interest groups such as the American Nurses' Association have great incentive to become involved when the costs or the benefits are concentrated on the people they represent. Consider the case of a bill that was introduced in Florida and became law in 1986. The legislation allowed nurses to prescribe and dispense medication under standing orders. The benefits are concentrated on one group, nurses, and the costs are concentrated on a different group, pharmacists. In this situation it should not be surprising that the highest level of political involvement was with the respective professional associations, since it was their members who stood to gain or lose the most. Although consumers also may benefit from legislation that results in easier access to needed medication, the general public tends to be indifferent to this type of debate because potential benefits are minimal for most individuals.

In another situation the benefits may be concentrated on a few, but the costs are distributed among many. Typically, the benefits are given to a small but vulnerable group such as high risk infants, families who have experienced sudden infant death syndrome (SIDS), the handicapped, or the

TABLE 25-1

*Distribution of Costs and Benefits**

		BENEFITS	
		CONCENTRATED	DISTRIBUTED
C O S T S	Concentrated	Concentrated Benefits Concentrated Costs	Distributed Benefits Concentrated Costs
	Distributed	Concentrated Benefits Distributed Costs	Distributed Benefits Distributed Costs

* Table based upon James Q. Wilson's conceptual framework as discussed in Schlotzman and Tierney (1986), pp 83–85

frail elderly. The costs are distributed to society as a whole: taxes that are collected from most people are designated for a particular category of needy persons. Although the groups that would receive the benefit sometimes are active and organized, often they are unorganized and unfocused. Their interests may need to be articulated by the helping professionals. Professionals such as nurses become their advocates through professional associations, public interest groups, and organizations such as hospitals and universities. Opposition is lessened when the costs are distributed because no single group feels the burden.

A third situation occurs when the benefits are distributed to much of society, but the costs are concentrated on a few. Organized interest groups have great incentive to protect their members or organization, but the general public has little reason to become involved because benefits are relatively small for each individual and the cumulative benefits may not be appreciated. Classic examples are found in environmental legislation and seat belt laws. In both cases industry perceived that they were going to pay the costs for society's benefits. Reducing the costs of medical care is similar; the benefits are disbursed to most of society, but the costs are concentrated on physicians and hospitals. The American Medical Association and the

American Hospital Association should be expected to oppose decisions that could adversely affect their members, even if the public will benefit. The general public is difficult to arouse because those who stand to benefit may not be aware or informed and the element of uncertainty regarding future needs for medical care leads some to doubt that they would ever benefit at all. In this example the use of the term *medical* care rather than *health* care is purposeful. Health care comprises relatively little of what physicians and hospitals actually do or receive reimbursement for, and the efforts for cost containment are directed toward the reduction of high costs medical care.

The last situation concerns benefits that are distributed to most of society, with the costs also distributed to most of society. Since the benefits and costs to each individual are minimized, the debate is formed along ideologic grounds. The argument is not between or among organized interest groups, but between the major political parties. Issues related to national defense, social security, the national debt, and the role of government can be expected to be resolved through partisan politics. If nurses want to be politically active on these issues, they should do so by supporting the candidates who express views they agree with and share.

TARGETS AND TIMING

Supposing a group of people have incentive and resources to promote or oppose a policy effort, how can they skillfully use their resources to be effective and efficient? Many excellent references discuss various tactics that have been employed successfully in the past, including coalition formation, letter writing campaigns, and demonstrations. Tactics work well when they are directed at the right target, at the right time, and for the right purpose. Skill involves knowing who to approach and when. Directing pleas to the wrong person or group at the wrong time is not an efficient use of limited resources and even may be detrimental to the overall cause. It helps to understand that each person or policy actor has a particular role to play within a defined period of time during the course of the policy effort. Hayes[7] reported that policy actors are usually ineffective when they attempt to play a role that is not assigned to them.

Let us examine three scenarios. First, consider the issue of health care as a right and argue that access to the health care system should be assured through some form of national health insurance. This is what Hayes[7] refers to as a **high level issue;** one that focuses on social values. The policy effort is to make health care a **political issue;** that is, a legitimate object of government action. The debate will focus on the principles of social justice; the responsibilities of institutions; and the philosophy of government. The main actors will be powerful national figures, such as the President, congressional leaders, powerful private interests, large coalitions, and the media. Until this debate is settled and health care as a right is on the national agenda, lobbying freshman congressmen and writing to the United States Department of Health and Human Services are not likely to have much impact.

Second, suppose an existing program, such as the National Health Service Corps or Migrant and Community Health Centers, is up for reauthorization. This would be considered a **middle level issue** in which the debate revolves around the allocation of resources and assignment of authority. Statements based upon statistics will be used to try to answer questions of efficacy, efficiency, fairness, and administrative competence; for example, "every dollar spent on community health centers saves three dollars in the Medicaid budget." The major actors will be presidential appointees, members of Congress, and smaller coalitions. In this example, one would expect to interact with actors from the Bureau of Health Care Delivery and Assistance, which is part of the Health Resources and Services Administration in the Department of Health and Human Services; congressmen who sit on committees such as the Senate Labor and Human Resources Committee and the House Subcommittee of Health and the Environment, which authorize the legislation; or committees such as the House Subcommittee on Labor, Health, and Human Services, and Education, which appropriates monies for implementing the legislation; and lobbyists representing groups such as the National Association of Community Health Centers.

Third are the **low-level issues,** most of which receive little or no attention from elected officials because they focus on the implementation phase. Alternative approaches are evaluated by legal, financial, and technical experts and constituents who have a narrower focus and a strong interest in the decisions that will be made. Regulations that specify the qualifications health personnel must have in order to provide services and regulations that determine which services will be reimbursed and required are typical of low level issues that can greatly impact the kind and amount of health care that is available.

Each level is important in its own way. At each level there is an opportunity for policy to affect nursing practice, consumer care, and societal needs. Each level also affords opportunities for providers and consumers to influence policy, if they wish and if they skillfully use their resources.

Impacts on the Nurse, the Consumer, and Society

The increased political involvement of nurses has the potential to shift power relationships that currently exist, and move nursing into a much stronger position in the health field. Nurses' political involvement will be discussed in terms of the impacts on the nurse, on the consumer, and on society.

THE NURSE

Political involvement by nurses enhances the professionalism of nursing. A brief analysis of nursing as a profession will clarify this statement. The characteristics of a profession have been presented in the literature. For example, Barber[8] indicates that there are four attributes that characterize a profession: a high degree of knowledge, primary orientation to community interest rather than self-interest, high degree of self-controlled behavior that is based upon an ideology and a code of ethics, and monetary and honorary rewards.

These characteristics are congruent with those of nursing as a profession. Diers[9] asserts that "nursing is an independent profession that has a set of activities, theories, and practices requiring intellectual and clinical autonomy." Nursing's code of ethics points to responsibilities for the nurse's political activities: "The nurse collaborates with members of the health professions and other citizens in promoting community and national efforts to meet the health care needs of the public."[10] These responsibilities for nurses are also consistent with those stated in the purposes for the American Nurses' Association's (1985) *Report of N-Cap to the House of Delegates*[11] and the American Nurses' Association's *A Social Policy Statement.*[12] In essence, there is a general professional mandate for nurses to be involved in the political process in collaboration with other health professionals.

As nurses become involved in political activities with other disciplines, they are forced to clarify their values. As nurses realize the need for greater unity and cohesion, they need to decide what they believe in and state these beliefs. In particular, nurses need to examine how their professional values match the existing social agenda. For example, one of the most important policy agendas in health care today is controlling costs. Nurses have the ability to offer health care alternatives at a lower cost while providing a continuum of quality services within a fragmented health care system. Professionals are concerned with community interests; therefore as professionals, nurses need to understand the sociopolitical and economic factors related to health problems. If concern is with community interest rather than self-interest, then nurses need to support and promote policy initiatives that are aligned with the profession's ideology and ethics. For example, nurses have been acutely aware of how much health policy affects nursing education since the 1970s, when federal allocations to the budget for nursing education were severely cut. Concern with community interest surfaces as budget allocations direct not just the types of nursing education programs that are offered, but ultimately the nursing services offered within our health care system. Nurses must be alert to these budgetary issues and use their political skill to influence policy-makers to support nursing education and service programs that promote the health of populations at greatest risk to health problems. Nurses need to be concerned with the total health care system, of which nursing is a part.

The opportunities for expanding monetary and honorary rewards are more likely to result for the profession as nurses become more involved in political activity. Fagin[13] reviewed studies on nursing over the last 20 years and concluded that nurses have contributed to reducing morbidity and mortality, improving the quality of life as well as reducing costs, yet these findings are rarely presented during policy making. With the change in Medicare reimbursement from retrospective to prospective payment, nurses are presented with an opportunity to articulate how they provide quality health care at less cost than medical services. When Walker[14] separated nursing costs from the hospital bill, it was found that nursing costs were smaller than expected. Nurses need to use the research findings they have to enhance professionalism. Not only will nurses increase control over their own work, but nurses will have the opportunity to receive appropriate monetary rewards for that work. This is congruent with society's great need and limited ability to pay because a large part of the revenue produced by nursing services is not received by nurses. These dynamic factors in the health policy arena will impact greatly on the future practice of nursing. Therefore, nurses need to be involved in the political process so that they have some control over their own destiny.

At the same time the political process provides society the mechanism to retain some control over the profession by holding nurses accountable for their own actions. It is when responsibility, accountability, and economic rewards merge that professionalism can be enhanced. Nurses can make this happen through their political involvements, which are not only sanctioned by the profession but necessary for enhancing professional status.

Frequently, when becoming involved in the political process, the action involves proposed legislation either at the federal or state level. Since such legislation may take the form of a bill, nurses need to understand the process of how a bill becomes a law. The processes in almost all states mirror the federal level and are outlined clearly in many resources, for example Bagwell and Clements.[15]

Professional organizations such as the American Nurses' Association take pride in preparing their members for political action through formal conferences and through their mailings about legislative issues. The American Nurses' Association's network of congressional district coordinators identifies and organizes nurses to work on campaigns of federal candidates who are friends of nursing.

At the state level members of the state nurses' association and the state public health associations also provide testimony and lobbying on legislative issues. There are many opportunities to participate in these efforts first hand either as an observer or as one who is involved in the political action. Additional members on legislative committees of these state organizations are usually welcomed, as there are many issues to follow and much work to be done. These committees can provide information, such as the names and addresses of elected officials and how to attend sessions of the legislature. Practical tips in communicating with legislators and participating in networks, coalitions, and political action committees can be found in resources such as Bagwell and Clements[15] or Mason and Talbott.[16] Some national and state political resources also are listed in those resource books.

Success breeds success. As nurses increase their political involvements through networks, coalitions, political action committees (PACS), and meetings with legislators, they gain political clout. Nurses gain power in the decision making process by looking beyond nursing and nurses for political support. Political action committees, eg, ANA-PAC, have given access to elected officials who support nurses' concerns and positions on issues. For example, 88 percent of the candidates endorsed by ANA-PAC in 1984 won their elections. This is an outstanding record; by comparison the AFL-CIO was pleased when 60 percent of the candidates they endorsed won.[11]

Nurses are skilled in the nursing process, which is no different from the decision making process. This can give power. Other skills needed for building power include communication, persuasion, negotiation, leadership, parliamentary procedure, group dynamics, and networking.[17] In essence, the skills needed in political activity are the same as those needed for good interpersonal relations.

Nurses who have learned to work within the system need to learn to work toward changing the system when change is appropriate. For example, although nurses may view the development of a national health insurance program as beneficial to all persons in society, particularly the poor, they realize such a development will require vast changes within the health and medical care complex. Yet nurses can learn to use their expertise to support such changes of the system. For example, nurses know how to communicate with multiple audiences. They can use that skill to communicate through the media. But first they need to learn how to use the media to their advantage. When nurses speak to the general public about what has been done within nursing practice and nursing research, they need to speak in common English and to convey the message in 30 seconds or less. By becoming involved in political activity, which is a mixture of science, craft, and art, nurses will gain political savvy.

THE CONSUMER

In considering the impact of health policy on the consumer, we can refer back to Figure 25-1, which indicates four combinations of costs and benefits. Much of the desired effect of health policies relies on impacting the consumers, as individuals, to change their own behavior. In some cases there are policies that benefit a few and costs that are distributed to a few. Policies that emphasize lifestyle changes or the third-party reimbursement for the delivery of personal health services do not affect all persons. For example, policies that support parental leave from work really only benefit working people of childbearing age and the costs are borne by businesses who have such workers. The unemployed or part-time employees will not benefit from these policies, as they do not qualify for them. This same scenario can be seen in employer contributed health insurance benefits, which definitely are advantageous for the employed. Not only do the employed worker and family members have hospital and other medical insurance, but the workers also may be covered for occupational health programs that aim at health promotion and disease prevention. Although the intent of many of these policies is laudable, the effect is a widening of the health status gap between the "haves" and the "have nots" and a false impression that what is available for some is available for all.

Other laws emphasize individual consumer behavior change; for example, laws that require the individual to wear a seat belt; to wear a motorcycle helmet; or to stop smoking in publicly owned buildings. The individual must change his or her behavior in order to comply with the law.

Nurses' involvement in political activity can facilitate the development of partnership relationships between nurses and consumers in working toward shared goals, which are promoting health, self-reliance, and competence. This relationship is at the core of nurses' professional ideology, which focuses on community interest, not self-interest, to promote health. In health care nurses' political activity can promote consumer participation in health decision making. Nurses understand that appropriate changes of the health care system need the input and joint decision making from consumers. These decisions are too important to be left to professionals alone. Health, self-reliance, and competence are total community concerns and require a partnership in health. For example consumers can be strong lobbying groups that support health care that is responsive to their needs. By working together, nurses, other professionals, and consumers can form coalitions aimed at similar goals.

An important and common role for nurses is **patient advocacy.** Nurses do this regularly when they interpret patient concerns to the physician and physician concerns to the patient and family. A natural outgrowth of this role is policy advocacy. As indicated earlier, nurses can translate scholarly work in the field of nursing to the media, to consumers, and to policy makers, such as legislators and administrators.

SOCIETY

Milio[18] differentiated between policies that reshape people's environments in health promoting ways from those that merely focus on personal health services for which people seek professional care for illness. Healthy public policies focus on primary prevention, alleviating environmental and social inequities, and promoting incentives or opportunities for people to select healthy options. Referring to Figure 25-1, we are concerned with the combinations in which both the costs and benefits are distributed or in which the costs are concentrated and the benefits distributed. In our previous example of seat belt legislation, the law does not address the broader environment, which would alleviate individual actions. Laws that require automobile manufacturers to install air bags in new cars, so that all persons would be safer if they were involved in accidents, are an example of addressing the broader environment. However, these laws do not affect people who drive older cars. Other examples include legislation promoting clean air and clean water. The benefits for these health policies are widely shared, but in most cases, such as the safe handling of toxic waste, the costs are borne by a few industries that produce the hazardous materials. The consumers who purchase the goods produced by those industries also pay for the benefits as costs are passed on to the purchaser. Certainly the greatest benefits to health of the population are when the benefits are shared by many.

Nurses are politically responsive citizens through visible involvement in the election process. One in 44 registered women voters is a registered nurse, and increasingly nurses are reviewing candidates' records carefully. Nurses are providing financial and other resources to candidates' campaigns and supporting elected officials on issues. More and more nurses are represented in the political process as an organized professional group. Through their involvements in PACS, nurses financially support candidates who share their concerns. Nurses need to continue to have positive relationships with powerful decision makers after they are elected. Nurses need to bring a strong, informed, constant, public voice to policies affecting health.

For example, after health promoting policies are authorized, appropriations are allocated to implement them. Without adequate levels of resources, these policies cannot be implemented. Nurses need to realize that this two-part process can have significant ramifications for policies and continue to participate in political activities to ensure an appropriate level of funding for the resources needed. An ongoing, informed, organized professional presence is essential at the national and state level in order to have the nursing voice heard by the right people at the right time. Although the Government Relations Office of the American Nurses' Association exists in order to coordinate and direct nursing's voice, it is dependent upon all professional nurses to help decide what that voice says.

With nurses' skills in interpersonal relations, the media can be used, eg, television, newspapers, radio, to advocate for health promoting policies. Through nurses' networks policy makers can be influenced to vote for policies that maximize health rather than focus primarily on personal health services. Leaders in nursing history, such as Lillian Wald and Margaret Sanger, were inspired to advocate health-promoting policies for the poor. Lillian Wald's advocacy efforts helped form the United States Children's Bureau, and Margaret Sanger helped form the birth control movement.

In essence, the political process provides nurses with opportunities to help solve problems facing nursing, consumers, and society today. By forming networks and coalitions, contributing to PACS, communicating with legislators, lobbying and providing expert testimony nurses will not only increase their political clout but also practice the ideology of nursing, which extends beyond the provision of individual care to patients. It is in the broad health policy arena that nurses can have the greatest influence on decisions that impact on the nurse, on the consumer, and on society.

Future Considerations

Future considerations will be addressed in relation to nursing education, nursing practice opportunities for political involvement, nursing research, and the role of vision in our future.

NURSING EDUCATION

How often have students and faculty alike said that baccalaureate education in nursing is jammed full and cannot incorporate additional content or learning experiences? Frequently liberal arts courses are dropped from the nursing curricula. The rationale often given for this decision is that student nurses need more time in nursing courses so that they will be better practicing nurses. However, the discussion in this chapter indicates that in order to practice good nursing, nurses also need to be astute about policy decisions that will affect their practice and the health of consumers and society at large. Nurses need political knowledge and skill in order to participate in the policy process. Political socialization occurs at the high school and college levels, yet nurses have very little academic background in these areas to help them with this socialization process.[19] Nurse educators need to reconsider course requirements and include political science and economics courses as part of the liberal arts requirements for the baccalaureate degree in nursing. It is through this academic socialization that nurses can gain the background needed for political involvement during college and after graduation.

NURSING PRACTICE

As members of a practice profession, nurses are in the front line of working on health concerns of people. They observe and address barriers to achieving health. By noting their observations over time and taking collective action, they are able to discern solutions that are not possible on an individual case basis. Nurses can take their unified voice of concern to make positive changes within and across health care settings.

An excellent example of nurses' collective action stemming from their practice in a number of health care settings was rewarding professionally and economically for seven Atlanta nurses. About five years ago these nurses were dissatisfied with their conditions of hospital work and formed a new venture, called Around The Clock (ATC) Nursing Services, Inc. They each contributed $25 to start ATC, a temporary nursing agency that provides nurses for short-staffed hospitals. After a three-year slow start, the company is growing at a rate of 300 percent each year. These nurses are well aware of the ongoing hospital nursing shortage that results from a variety of factors, including more job options outside hospitals for nurses and more lucrative job options for men and women outside of nursing. These nurses provided practice opportunities for nurses who wanted flexible working options not possible while employed as hospital staff. Yet by working through a temporary nursing agency, hospitals could find the nursing coverage they needed. In 1987 ATC administrators projected billings of $12 million—certainly a success story! Although these nurses initially found they lacked business experience, and because of this overlooked a number of important financial details, they saw a need in their practice and were able to utilize their collective action to gain business and political savvy and succeed.

OPPORTUNITIES FOR POLITICAL INVOLVEMENT

There are many opportunities for political involvement in the practice of nursing. The excellent skills nurses developed in the health care setting can be directly applied in the health policy arena. Skills in interpersonal relations can be put to good use in the political arena. Nurses have learned how to communicate with diverse groups of people of different ethnic and cultural backgrounds, and with persons of all ages and from various socioeconomic levels and different educational preparation. Nurses develop skill in dealing well with crises: they are accustomed to organizing workloads to do more with less and cope with the unplanned and unexpected. Their preparation in nursing prepares them well for involvement in political activities.

You may ask, but how do I get involved? One of the easiest ways to get involved is to work on a grassroots political campaign. Nurses can capitalize on their interpersonal skills and gain the strategic insights required for other levels of political involvement. However, nurses will need to choose the campaign carefully by checking on the issues and the groups that are supporting the candidate. In addition, nurses should try to work with a well organized campaign in order to learn how an ethical, effective campaign is run. Whether or not the candidate wins or loses, nurses who are involved will be better prepared to participate again.

Another opportunity for political involvement is to learn how to influence and persuade elected officials through planned meetings and providing testimony. As indicated previously, nurses have developed a variety of communication skills and need to select the most effective. For example, focused communication is more effective than reflective listening when talking with a busy legislator. In addition, nurses' clinical expertise can be useful because it provides authoritative arguments and concrete examples with human interest. In both situations nurses also can consider the teaching opportunities that could broaden the scope of influence. For example, nurses work with patients, family members, or groups in the community who are concerned with any number of health issues. These situations are natural forums for nurses to help people address their broader social concerns in productive ways, through participating in the policy process. Nurses can help educate the public in how to present information and personal experiences related to health issues that concern them.

Nurses are beginning to work with the media in seeking support for issues relevant to the profession and the population as a whole. For the average person the major sources are television, newspaper, radio, and magazines. Nurses need to watch, read, and use the media for collecting and disseminating information. Information presented as facts, figures, rationale, and concrete examples can be used to influence policy makers about issues.

For most nurses it is difficult to be interviewed, yet a few practical tips can make the experience effective.[15] If possible, nurses should establish relationships with reporters prior to being interviewed. In any case, they need to treat the reporter with respect. Before the interview they should prepare and practice, to be certain of what they are willing and not willing to discuss. They need to learn to speak in 30-second bites. They need to state their conclusion or most important information first; statements can be expanded if time allows. The preparation of a one-page sheet of facts is helpful. A key point to remember is to be identified with the interest of the public and convey a professional image by dress, mannerisms, and language. Remember, nothing is off the record and whatever is said can be quoted.

There are other ways nurses can provide information to the public, for example, becoming involved as a health reporter. One nurse concerned with minority health issues was recently asked to serve as the health reporter for a weekly televised program focusing on minority health issues in Indianapolis, Indiana. She has been able to present a wide range of factors influencing the health of blacks and the health services available to the population.

Another area that nurses can become more involved in is fund raising. Fund raising is an essential political activity, but most nurses would rather do anything than ask people for money. However, well-planned fund raising works.[15] Some suggestions for fund raising include first preparing a master plan that delineates who will be in charge, what will be done, and when. Once the director is selected, future plans need to include people and their activities, lists and record keeping, events and when they will occur, mailings and when they will be sent, face-to-face solicitation for large donors, solicitation to previous contributors, and a system for thank you notes. All funds collected in fund raising should go to a designated person, such as a treasurer. Many nonprofit organizations have developed sophisticated fund raising efforts so nurses can find opportunities to be involved in various stages of fund raising. Not only is it an opportunity to learn from these experiences, but also to find satisfaction in soliciting and receiving contributions for a worthy cause.

NURSING RESEARCH

Nurses are in key positions to participate in nursing research. Opportunities in research are numerous, ranging from being a subject of research, to generating practice problems for research, to assisting in data collection, to being the principal investigator of a research project. One may ask: what does all of this have to do with future involvements in political activities? Our response is that there can be a direct relationship between research and health policy. Altman[20] cited numerous examples where research findings have influenced public policy. The clearest example is related to the efforts of health services research to develop "clearly defined and statistically accurate case-mix adjustment mechanisms,"[20] which laid the foundation for the Medicare prospective payment system based on diagnostic related groups (DRGs).

Nursing research is not always utilized in practice and the relationship between nursing research and policy is even more complex, yet one of the key issues in participating in the policy process is information.[21] Nursing research is a mechanism by which policy information can be generated. Certain types of research have potential for achieving this knowledge. For example, research on cost-effective strategies of nursing interventions is needed. Also needed is conceptual and theory-based research that is tested repeatedly in order to generate information that is reliable. However, it is realized that policy decisions are made within time constraints and policy makers need to act within these constraints, whether or not enough information is available. The use and analyses of existing data can help overcome some of these obstacles.[22]

It is no longer sufficient to just produce such information; nurses also must become actively involved in promoting the results of nursing research. This will bring them into the advocacy and action phases of the policy process. Nurses need to secure a high profile for nursing research by presenting testimony in order to educate and alert legislators and the general public to the results of nursing efforts aimed at improving health and the health care system. Policy makers do not necessarily review research reports, but they do listen to experts. Nurses need to translate research-based knowledge into expert advice.

ROLE OF VISION

Last and foremost, nurses need to create and project a clear vision in policy making. Hayes indicates "that policy making is more than a series of i cremental responses to interest group demands."[7] We have indicated in this chapter that nurses' professional orientation is to community interest rather than self-interest. Hayes[7] indicates that both vision and interest are potent factors in the formation of policy. Nurses are uniquely situated in diverse health care positions and can clearly see what people need. They have the capability to articulate a new vision in health policy and as such "can make things happen." Since nursing is a practice profession, nurses can imagine the exciting future potentialities without forgetting the often mundane present necessities.

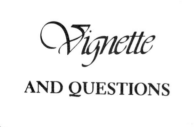

Vignette

AND QUESTIONS

The example that has been selected is a real life situation that could occur in any city or state, perhaps one in which you will find yourself at some point in your career. The situation that is unfolding is a cooperative venture in which nurses are taking a particular approach to reduce infant mortality in a large midwestern city.

First, nurses became aware that their city has the highest black infant mortality of any large city in the United States. This shocking piece of data set off a flurry of activity to collect additional related information. Comparative data for states and large cities was obtained from the Children's Defense Fund, which publishes an annual *Maternal and Child Health Data Book: The*

Health of America's Children.[23] The nurses learned that not only was the infant mortality rate high for blacks in the city, but the entire state did not compare favorably with the United States as a whole. For example, their state was not expected to meet the surgeon general's 1990 objective for infant mortality, whereas 37 other states would. More recent data about key maternal and child health indicators was obtained from the state and county health departments. That data indicated that although slight improvements were noted for blacks, the white infant mortality rate had increased. The nurses knew from their clinical knowledge base that black and teenage mothers are more likely to give birth to low-birthweight infants and that those infants are 20 times more likely to die in the first year of life. They also knew that the neonatal mortality rate is related to maternal health status and the provision of prenatal care; whereas postneonatal mortality is a sensitive indicator of the infant's basic environment. Therefore, the nurses obtained and analyzed additional information, including the proportion of low-birthweight infants by race and age of mother, the proportion of mothers who receive early prenatal care by race and age of mother, and the neonatal and postneonatal mortality rates. Two other states that had the same proportion of births to black and teenage mothers were used for comparison. The nurses found that, in the comparison states, the infant mortality rate and neonatal mortality rate were lower and a higher proportion of all mothers received early prenatal care, especially black mothers. The nurses also learned that eligibility criteria for Medicaid were less stringent, thus poor mothers in the comparison states had less financial barriers to early prenatal care.

The nurses joined hands with other organized health groups in the city and the state including the Healthy Mothers/Healthy Babies Coalition, the state nurses' association, the state public health association, the state health department, local health departments, and community and migrant health centers. Nurses from all those groups, in conjunction with nonhealth related community organizations, mobilized a door-to-door outreach effort to locate expectant mothers in selected communities and refer them for prenatal care. Care was taken to incorporate the extra outreach efforts into existing community groups and to provide continual follow-up for the referrals that were made. Prior to the outreach, plans were made to increase the capacities of the health department and community health centers in order to provide more prenatal care to low-income mothers.

Having knowledge and clinical expertise and working with other organizations was essential and perhaps sufficient for short-term solutions. However, the problem of access to prenatal care for poor mothers is not a short-term issue. Too many mothers have too few resources and clinics cannot provide an unlimited amount of uncompensated care. The nurses were able to draw on the results of studies that were done by others such as: the Institute of Medicine report, *Preventing Low Birthweight,*[24] the American Nurses' Association consensus conference report, *Access to Prenatal Care*,[25] and the Southern Governors Conference report, *For the Children of Tomorrow*.[26] These studies all pointed out that the lack of ability to afford care is central to any patient, provider, and system barriers to early prenatal care. The studies also demonstrated the cost-effectiveness of prenatal care. For example, each additional $1 spent on prenatal care to high-risk mothers is expected to save $3.38 in medical care costs for low-birthweight infants.[24] The savings mount up; $10 million of prenatal care can save nearly $34 million in low-birthweight infant care, a net cost savings of $24 million.

The nurses used this information to develop the broad-based consensus that is needed among health professionals and the general public regarding the definition of the problem and the proposed solutions. For example, the current infant mortality rate, especially for inner city blacks, needs to be viewed as a problem that can be solved and should be solved. There needs to be consensus that cost is a major deterrent to prenatal care as opposed to inadequate, unacceptable resources or the belief that mothers do not value prenatal care. Consensus can be built through listening to different opinions; collecting information that supports or refutes opinions; broadening outlooks through contacts with outside experts, literature, and conferences; and stating the problem and proposed solution in acceptable language.

To make significant changes, it will be important to have the support of some powerful people. These can be professionals, elected representatives, administrators, and community leaders. The media also can be a potent force for change. Good causes and good ideas are not enough; they need to be accepted and championed by key individuals. At the very least, key individuals need to not oppose the idea.

1. How is the infant mortality rate calculated? What is the infant mortality rate in your state or city? How does it rank with other cities and states? How can you find out?

2. Suppose you are convinced that access to prenatal care should be increased by expanding the Medicaid eligibility to include all pregnant women under 100 percent of poverty.

   a. Make a list of the categories of persons you would want to contact.
   b. Prepare a 30-second statement for each of the following: the general public through a television or radio public service announcement, a reporter from the local newspaper, a legislator who will likely be opposed to the idea, a legislator who you know supports you, the state maternal child health director, who is a pediatrician.

c. Make a list of information related to infant mortality that could be used for a one-page handout to be distributed as a fact sheet.

3. If you were going to form a coalition to reduce infant mortality in your state, which groups or individuals would you want to include?

INFORMATION SOURCES

Bagwell M, Clements S: A *Political Handbook for Health Professionals*. Boston, MA, Little, Brown, 1985

Dunn W: *Public Policy Analysis: An Introduction*. Englewood Cliffs, NJ, Prentice-Hall, 1981

Hayes C: *Making Policies for Children*. Washington, DC, National Academy Press, 1982

Lewin M (ed): *From Research into Policy-Improving the Link for Health Services*. Washington, DC, American Enterprise Institute for Public Policy Research, 1986

Lindblom C: *The Policy-making Process*, 2d ed. Englewood Cliffs, NJ, Prentice-Hall, 1980

Mason DJ, Talbott SW: *Political Action Handbook for Nurses*. Menlo Park, CA, Addison-Wesley, 1985

Solomon SB, Roe SC (eds): *Integrating Public Policy into the Curriculum*. New York, NY, National League for Nursing, 1986

REFERENCES

1. Rossi PH, Wright JD, Wright SR: The theory and practice of applied social research. Evaluation Quart 2:171, 1978

2. Dye T: *Who's Running America? The Reagan Years*, 3d ed. Englewood Cliffs, NJ, Prentice-Hall, 1983

3. Dahl R: *Pluralist Democracy in the United States: Conflict and Consent*. Chicago, Rand McNally, 1967

4. Schlotzman K, Tierney J: *Organized Interest Groups and American Democracy*. New York, Harper & Row, 1986

5. Isaacs J, Tames S: *Long-Term Care: In Search of National Policy.* Washington, DC, National Health Council, Inc, 1986

6. Dahl R: *Dilemmas of Pluralist Democracy: Autonomy vs Control.* New Haven, CT, Yale University Press, 1982

7. Hayes C: *Making Policies for Children.* Washington, DC, National Academy Press, 1982

8. Barber B: Some problems in the sociology of the professions. Daedalus, p15, 1963

9. Diers D: Policy and politics. In Mason DJ, Talbott SW (eds): *Political Action Handbook for Nurses.* Menlo Park, CA, Addison-Wesley, Health Sciences Division, 1985

10. American Nurses' Association: *Guidelines for Implementing the Code for Nurses.* Kansas City, MO, American Nurses' Association, 1980

11. American Nurses' Association: *1985 Report of N-CAP to the House of Delegates.* Kansas City, MO, American Nurses' Association, 1985

12. American Nurses' Association: *Nursing: A Social Policy Statement.* Kansas City, MO, American Nurses' Association, 1980

13. Fagin CM: Nursing as an alternative to high-cost care. Amer J Nurs 1:56, 1982

14. Walker D: The cost of nursing care in hospitals. In Aiken L (ed): *Nursing in the 80's: Crises, Opportunities, Challenges.* Philadelphia, Lippincott, 1982

15. Bagwell M, Clements S: *A Political Handbook for Health Professionals.* Boston, Little, Brown, 1985

16. Mason DJ, Talbott SW: *Political Action Handbook for Nurses.* Menlo Park, CA, Addison-Wesley, Health Sciences Division, 1985

17. Ferguson VD: Two perspectives on power. In Mason DJ, Talbott SW (eds): *Political Action Handbook for Nurses.* Menlo Park, CA, Addison-Wesley, Health Sciences Division, 1985

18. Milio N: *Promoting Health Through Public Policy.* Ottawa, Canada, Canadian Public Health Association, 1986

19. Torney-Purta J: Political socialization and policy: The United States in a cross national context. In Stevenson H, Siegel A (eds): *Child Development Research and Social Policy,* Vol 1. Chicago, University of Chicago Press, 1984

20. Altman SH: *Health Services Research: Do We Matter?* Paper presented at the Second Annual Meeting of the Association for Health Services Research and the Foundation for Health Services Research, Chicago, IL, June, 1985

21. Mitsunaga BK: The use of knowledge and health policy planning: Forms and functions of the relationships. West Coun Higher Educ 14:1, 1981

22. Bradham DD: Health policy formulation and analysis. Nurs Economics 3:167, 1985

23. Hughes D, Johnson K, Rosenbaum S, Simons J, Butler E: *The Health of America's Children: Maternal and Child Health Data Book*. Washington, DC, Children's Defense Fund, 1987

24. Institute of Medicine: *Preventing Low Birthweight*. Washington, DC, National Academy Press, 1985

25. Curry M: *Access to Prenatal Care*. Kansas City, MO, American Nurses' Association, 1987

26. Grad R: *For the Children of Tomorrow*. Washington, DC, Southern Governors' Association, 1985

Index

Health Promotion and Disease Prevention
    Branch, 258
Health trends, 433–434
Heart transplants, artificial, 164–166
HEW-Rush-Medicus Methodology, 147
HHA (home health aides), 397
Hierarchy, basis of, 11
High level issue, 459
Hill-Burton Act, 289, 356
Hippocrates, Oath of, 177
History, American, cycles of, 280
HMOs. *See* Health Maintenance
    Organizations
Holloran System, 139
Home health aides (HHA), 397
Home health care, 359–360, 379–398
    defined, 384
    factors influencing utilization of, 382–383
    marketplace demand in, 389–390
    models of, 383–386
    reimbursement sources for, 386–388
Horizontal integration, 357
Hospices, 360
Hospital advertising, 363–364
Hospital payment, 336–340
Hospitals, 281, 356–358
Hospital training schools, 282–283

I

ICD-9-CM (International Classification of
    Diseases—Ninth Revision—Clinical
    Modification), 335
ICFs (intermediate care facilities), 358
ICON (Integrated Competencies of Nurses)
    model, 22
Illness care. *See* Health care
Implementation, program, 440–441
Imprisonment, false, 184
Incrementalism, 292
Independent nursing care, 99–100
Independent prepayment plans, 408–409
Indigents, 314
Indirect nursing care time, 121
Individual Practice Association (IPA), 361
Inequalities in health care delivery, 309–328
Infections, nosocomial, 341

Infliction of mental distress, 184–185
Informed consent, absence of, 183
Institute of Nursing, National, 255–257
Institutional certification, 42
Institutionally housed agencies, 386
Institutional Review Board (IRB), 163, 164
Insurance, health, 363
    private, 387–388, 407–409
    self-insurance, 409
Integrated Competencies of Nurses (ICON)
    model, 22
Intellectual technique, 5, 8–9
Intensity of nursing care, concept, 120
Intentional torts, 183–185
Interdependent nursing care, 100
Interest groups, 437, 455–456
Intermediate care facilities (ICFs), 358
International Classification of Diseases
    —Ninth Revision—Clinical Modification
    (ICD-9-CM), 335
Interviews, 468
Intrapreneurs, 57
Invasion of privacy, 184
In vitro fertilization, 161–163
IPA (Individual Practice Association), 361
IRB (Institutional Review Board), 163, 164

J

Joint Commission on Accreditation of
    Hospitals (JCAH), 119, 147–148
Joint faculty/practice position, 74
Joint practice, 89
Journals, scientific, in nursing, 249
Jurisdiction, 182

K

Knowledge specialization, 5, 9

L

Law suits, 426
Legal actions, 180
Legislative process, national, 444–445